Essentials of Clinical MR

Thieme

Essentials of Clinical MR

Val M. Runge, MD
John Sealy Distinguished Chair in Radiology
Professor and Chair of Radiology
University of Texas Medical Branch
Galveston, Texas

John N. Morelli, MD
Department of Radiology
Texas A&M University Health Sciences Center
Scott and White Memorial Hospital
Temple, Texas

Thieme
New York • Stuttgart

Thieme Medical Publishers, Inc.
333 Seventh Ave.
New York, NY 10001

Executive Editor: Timothy Hiscock
Managing Editor: J. Owen Zurhellen
Editorial Assistants: Tess Timoshin and Elizabeth D'Ambrosio
Editorial Director, Clinical Reference: Michael Wachinger
International Production Director: Andreas Schabert
Vice President, International Marketing and Sales: Cornelia Schulze
Chief Financial Officer: James W. Mitos
President: Brian D. Scanlan
Compositor: Thomson Press
Printer: Sheridan Press

Library of Congress Cataloging-in-Publication Data

Runge, Val M.
Essentials of clinical MR / Val M. Runge, John N. Morelli.
p. ; cm.
Includes index.
Summary: "The objective of this book is to serve as a practical educational resource for clinical magnetic resonance imaging. The bulk of the text is organized along anatomic lines and discusses disease entities commonly encountered in clinical practice. The focus is illustrating and describing the MR appearances of the most commonly imaged disease entities, covering briefly in each area important points relative to imaging techniques then discussing in depth, the clinical MR interpretation. The breadth of clinical MRI is explored. For each subtopic within an anatomic region, clinical cases serve as the backbone for discussion, the most common pathologies affecting each anatomic region being illustrated. The final chapters discuss specifically contrast media and contrast enhanced MRA, two topics worthy of further description due to their present clinical importance. When relevant to diagnosis or essential for understanding, MR physics is discussed, however the reader is referred separately to Runge et al, The Physics of Clinical MR Taught Through Images 2nd Edition (New York: Thieme; 2009) for further elaboration. It is the goal that upon completing this text, the reader will have an appreciation for the complexity, utility, and versatility of MR in clinical imaging and will possess the knowledge essential for interpretation of basic clinical MR examinations"—Provided by publisher.
ISBN 978-1-60406-406-3
1. Magnetic resonance imaging. I. Morelli, John N. II. Title.
[DNLM: 1. Magnetic Resonance Imaging—methods. WN 185]
RC78.7.N83R863 2011
616.07'548–dc22

2010037829

Printed in the United States

978-1-60406-406-3

To my two daughters, Valerie and Sadie, with all my love.

– *VMR*

To my mother, Cecilia, and my sister, Kate.

– *JNM*

Contents

Foreword .... **xiii**

Preface .... **xv**

Contributors .... **xvii**

List of Abbreviations .... **xix**

Section I: Brain

1: Supratentorial Brain Neoplasms 2

2: Infratentorial Brain Neoplasms 4

3: Metastatic Brain Disease 6

4: Meningiomas 8

5: Internal Auditory Canal Neoplasms 10

6: Sellar/Parasellar Neoplasms 12

7: Diploic Space Lesions 14

8: Intraparenchymal Hemorrhage 16

9: Extraaxial and Subarachnoid Hemorrhage 18

10: Arteriovenous Malformations 20

11: Other Vascular Malformations 22

12: Aneurysms 24

13: Ischemia and Infarction I 26

14: Ischemia and Infarction II 29

15: Periventricular Leukomalacia 32
16: Diffuse Axonal Injury 33
17: Neurodegenerative Disorders 34
18: Multiple Sclerosis 36
19: Parenchymal Infections 38
20: Sinus Disease 40
21: Meningitis 42
22: Immunocompromise 44
23: Posterior Fossa Congenital Malformations 46
24: Arachnoid Cysts 48
25: Other Congenital Malformations 50
26: Inherited White Matter Disease 52
27: Neurofibromatosis and von Hippel-Lindau Syndrome 54
28: Tuberous Sclerosis and Sturge-Weber Syndrome 56

Section II: Cervical Spine

29: Congenital Abnormalities 58
30: Trauma 60
31: Disk Herniations 62
32: Degenerative Disease 64
33: Rheumatoid and Postoperative Changes 67
34: Other Inflammatory/Infectious Diseases 69
35: Metastatic Disease 72
36: Primary Neoplasms 74

Section III: Thoracic Spine

37: Disk Herniations 77
38: Canal Compromise 80
39: Primary Neoplasms 82
40: Vascular Abnormalities 84

Section IV: Lumbar Spine

41: Congenital Abnormalities 86
42: Common Incidental Findings 88
43: Compression Fractures 90
44: Disk Herniations 92
45: Postoperative Lumbar Spine 94
46: Degenerative Disk Disease I 96
47: Degenerative Disk Disease II 98
48: Infections 100
49: Metastatic Disease 102
50: Disorders of Marrow 104
51: Primary Neoplasms 106
52: Leptomeningeal Carcinomatosis 110

Section V: Head and Neck

53: Common Incidental Findings 113
54: Neoplasia I 116
55: Neoplasia II 118
56: Infections 120

Section VI: Heart and Chest

57: Cardiomyopathy 122
58: Ischemic Heart Disease 124
59: Valvular Heart Disease 126
60: Congenital Heart Disease 128
61: Thoracic Vasculature 130
62: Thoracic Neoplasia 132

Section VII: Breast

63: Breast Neoplasia 134
64: Breast Implants 136

Section VIII: Abdomen and Pelvis

65: Benign Hepatic Masses 138
66: Malignant Hepatic Masses 140
67: Diffuse Hepatic Pathology 142
68: Biliary Disease 144
69: Adrenal Disease 146
70: Renal Masses 148
71: Pancreatic Disease 150
72: Pediatric Abdominal Disease 152
73: Urinary Bladder and Male Pelvis 154
74: Benign Lesions of the Female Pelvis 157
75: Uterine and Cervical Cancer 160
76: Ovarian Pathology 162

Section IX: Musculoskeletal System

77: Meniscal Tears I 164
78: Meniscal Tears II 166
79: Cruciate Ligaments 168
80: Collateral Ligaments, Knee 170
81: Osteochondral Lesions, Knee 172
82: Rotator Cuff Tears 174
83: Glenohumeral Instability I 176
84: Glenohumeral Instability II, Labrum 178
85: Avascular Necrosis of the Hip 180
86: Insufficiency Fractures, Acetabular Labrum 182
87: Carpal Tunnel Disease and Wrist Fractures 184
88: Triangular Fibrocartilage Complex Tears 186
89: Carpal Fractures and Other Causes of Wrist Pain 188
90: Temporomandibular Joint Disease 190
91: Elbow Injuries 192

92: Tendinous Injuries of the Ankle and Foot 194
93: Ligamentous Injuries of the Ankle 196
94: Other Ankle and Foot Disorders 198
95: Musculoskeletal Neoplasms 200
96: Diseases of Marrow 202

Section X: MR Contrast Agents

97: Overview of MR Contrast Agents 204
98: Adverse Reactions 206

Section XI: Magnetic Resonance Angiography

99: MRA Principles and Carotid MRA 208
100: Peripheral MRA 212
101: Renal Artery MRA 216
102: Other MRA Applications 218
Index 221

Foreword

There are many ways to learn about magnetic resonance imaging—reading large textbooks, small subspecialized textbooks (e.g., on neuro or knees), journal articles (e.g., AJNR, radiology, JMRI, investigative radiology), and point-of-service information (e.g., StatDx); taking courses; and attending meetings. This book, *Essentials of Clinical MR*, has managed to compress the essential aspects of the field into a mere 200 pages or so—a tenth the size of multivolume textbooks like *Magnetic Resonance Imaging* by Stark and Bradley or *Clinical Magnetic Resonance Imaging* by Edelman, Hesselink, Zlatkin, and Crues. Val Runge, John Morelli, and their contributors have accomplished this compression by focusing on the practical clinical aspects of MR image interpretation with minimal physics, jokes, or references. In addition to being concise and pithy, the book is quite topical, featuring sections on newer MR contrast agents and MR angiography, with discussions of nephrogenic systemic fibrosis and contrast-free MRA. Where additional physics explanation is desired, the reader is referred to another of Dr. Runge's excellent works, the second edition of *The Physics of Clinical MR Taught Through Images* (Thieme, 2009).

Dr. Runge has been an MRI researcher and clinician for almost 30 years. He is one of the few people I know who could undertake what might be considered the "Cliffs Notes" or "Classics Illustrated" of MRI. This book has the most PPPPs (pearls per printed page) of any book I have read in years. I highly recommend it for physicians and technologists who desire to grasp the essentials of magnetic resonance imaging in a short period of time. By the same token, I recommend this book to radiology residents and to nonradiologists wanting a quick discussion of the utility of MRI and the MR findings in a particular disease state.

William G. Bradley, Jr., MD, PhD, FACR
Professor and Chairman, Department of Radiology
University of California, San Diego
San Diego, California

Preface

The objective of this book is to serve as a practical educational resource for clinical magnetic resonance imaging. The bulk of the text is organized along anatomic lines and discusses disease entities commonly encountered in clinical practice. The focus is illustrating and describing the MR appearances of the most commonly imaged disease entities, covering briefly in each area important points relative to imaging techniques then discussing in depth the clinical MR interpretation. The breadth of clinical MRI is explored.

For each subtopic within an anatomic region, clinical cases serve as the backbone for discussion with the most common pathologies affecting each anatomic region being illustrated. The final chapters discuss specifically contrast media and contrast-enhanced MRA, two topics worthy of further description due to their present clinical importance. When relevant to diagnosis or essential for understanding, MR physics is discussed; however, the reader is referred separately to Runge et al, *The Physics of Clinical MR Taught Through Images* (Thieme, 2009) for further elaboration. It is the goal that upon completing this text, the reader will have an appreciation for the complexity, utility, and versatility of MR in clinical imaging and will possess the knowledge essential for interpretation of basic clinical MR examinations.

Val M. Runge, MD
John N. Morelli, MD

Note about Figures

The white lines between figures (for example, between **Figures 5.1A** and **5.1B**) reflect the fact that images are taken from different patients. If two figures are otherwise contiguous, they are from the same patient.

Contributors

Fei Ai, MD
Department of Radiology
Tongji Hospital
Tongji Medical College
Huazhong University of Science and Technology
Wuhan, China

Ulrike Attenberger, MD
Department of Clinical Radiology and Nuclear Medicine
University Medical Center Mannheim
Medical Faculty Mannheim, Heidelberg University
Mannheim, Germany

John A. Carrino, MD, MPH
Associate Professor of Radiology and Orthopaedic Surgery
Johns Hopkins University School of Medicine
Section Chief, Musculoskeletal Radiology
Russell H. Morgan Department of Radiology and Radiological Science
Baltimore, Maryland

Peter Fries, MD
Clinic of Diagnostic and Interventional Radiology
Saarland University Hospital
Homburg, Germany

Xiaoming Li MD, PhD
Professor of Radiology
Vice Chair, Department of Radiology
Tongji Hospital
Tongji Medical College
Huazhong University of Science and Technology
Wuhan, China

Debra L. Monticciolo, MD, FACR
Professor of Radiology
Texas A&M University Health Science Center
Vice Chair for Research
Chief, Section of Breast Imaging
Department of Radiology
Scott & White Memorial Hospital
Temple, Texas

John N. Morelli, MD
Texas A&M University Health Sciences Center
Department of Radiology
Scott and White Memorial Hospital
Temple, Texas

Val M. Runge, MD
John Sealy Distinguished Chair in Radiology
Professor and Chair
Department of Radiology
The University of Texas Medical Branch
Galveston, Texas

Günther Schneider, MD, PhD
Clinic of Diagnostic and Interventional Radiology
Saarland University Hospital
Homburg, Germany

Spencer T. Sincleair, MD
Assistant Professor of Radiology
Texas A&M University Health Science Center
Department of Radiology
Scott & White Memorial Hospital
Director, Division of Diagnostic Imaging
Chief, Section of Diagnostic Radiology
Temple, Texas

Lan Vu, PhD
Texas A&M University Health Sciences Center
Scott and White Memorial Hospital
Temple, Texas

David M. Watkins, MD
Assistant Professor of Radiology
Texas A&M University Health Science Center
Department of Radiology
Scott & White Memorial Hospital
Temple, Texas

Wei Zhang, MD
Department of Radiology
Tongji Hospital
Tongji Medical College
Huazhong University of Science and Technology
Wuhan, China

List of Abbreviations

2D	two-dimensional
3D	three-dimensional
AC	acromioclavicular
ACA	anterior cerebral artery
ACL	anterior cruciate ligament
ACTH	adrenocorticotrophic hormone
ADC	apparent diffusion coefficient
ADEM	acute disseminated encephalomyelitis
AICA	anterior inferior cerebellar artery
AP	anteroposterior
ASA	anterior spinal artery
ASD	atrial septal defect
ATP	adenosine triphosphate
AVF	arteriovenous fistula
AVM	arteriovenous malformation
AVN	avascular necrosis
BBB	blood-brain barrier
CIDP	chronic inflammatory demyelinating polyneuropathy
CN	cranial nerve
CNS	central nervous system
CPA	cerebellopontine angle
CSF	cerebrospinal fluid
CT	computed tomography
CTM	continuous table movement
DAI	diffuse axonal injury
DCIS	ductal carcinoma in situ
DISI	dorsal intercalated segment instability
DAI	diffuse axonal injury
DPVS	dilated perivascular space
DSA	digital subtraction angiography
DTI	diffusion tensor imaging
DWI	diffusion weighted imaging
ECG	electrocardiogram

EG	eosinophilic granuloma
FASI	foci of abnormal signal intensity
FLAIR	fluid-attenuated inversion recovery
FMD	fibromuscular dysplasia
FNH	focal nodular hyperplasia
FACI	foci of abnormal signal intensity
FOV	field of view
FS	fat suppression
FSE	fast spin echo
GBM	glioblastoma multiforme
GFR	glomerular filtration rate
GI	gastrointestinal
GRE	gradient echo
HAGL	humeral avulsion of glenohumeral ligament
HASTE	half-fourier acquisition single-shot turbo spin echo
HCC	hepatocellular carcinoma
HIV	human immunodeficiency virus
HSV	herpes simplex virus
IAC	internal auditory canal
ICA	internal carotid artery
IR	inversion recovery
IV	intravenous
JPA	juvenile pilocytic astrocytoma
LCL	lateral collateral ligament
MCA	middle cerebral artery
MCL	medial collateral ligament
MIP	maximum intensity projection
MR	magnetic resonance
MRA	magnetic resonance angiography
MRCP	magnetic resonance cholangiopancreatography
MRI	magnetic resonance imaging
MRS	magnetic resonance spectroscopy
MRV	magnetic resonance venography
MS	multiple sclerosis
NAA	N-acetyl-aspartate
NF	neurofibromatosis
NSF	nephrogenic systemic fibrosis
PC	phase contrast
PCA	posterior cerebral artery
PCL	posterior cruciate ligament
PC-MRA	phase-contrast magnetic resonance angiography
PDWI	proton density weighted image
PICA	posterior inferior cerebellar artery
PLL	posterior longitudinal ligament
PML	progressive multifocal leukoencephalopathy
PNET	primitive neuroectodermal tumor
PVL	periventricular leukomalacia
RF	radiofrequency
SAH	subarachnoid hemorrhage

SCA	superior cerebellar artery
SDH	subdural hematomas
SE	spin echo
SI	signal intensity
SLAP	superior labrum anterior posterior
SNR	signal-to-noise ratio
SPIO	superparamagnetic iron oxide
SSFP	steady-state free precession
STIR	short Tau inversion recovery
SWI	susceptibility weighted imaging
T1WI	T1-weighted image
T2WI	T2-weighted image
T	tesla
TE	echo time
TFC	triangular fibrocartilage
TMJ	temporomandibular joint
TOF	time-of-flight
TR	repetition time
TREAT	time-resolved echo-shared angiographic technique
TRICKS	time-resolved imaging of contrast kinetics
TWIST	time-resolved angiography with interleaved stochastic trajectories
VHL	von Hippel-Lindau
VIBE	volumetric interpolated breath-hold examination
VISI	volar intercalated segment instability
VSD	ventricular septal defect
WHO	World Health Organization

Essentials of Clinical MR

1 Supratentorial Brain Neoplasms

Astrocytomas are the most common primary intraaxial tumor, arising predominantly supratentorially in adults and infratentorially in children. The World Health Organization's (WHO) criteria divide astrocytomas into four grades: grade 1 is circumscribed astrocytoma (usually pilocytic astrocytomas); grade 2 is low-grade astrocytoma; grade 3 is anaplastic astrocytoma; and grade 4 is glioblastoma multiforme (GBM). The magnetic resonance imaging (MRI) appearance of grade I astrocytomas is typified by increased signal intensity (SI) on T2-weighted images (T2WIs) and decreased signal intensity on T1WI, reflecting increased extracellular fluid due to abnormal capillary walls. These lesions typically do enhance. Unlike other astrocytomas, the prognosis for grade 1 lesions is usually favorable, and they are often cured by resection alone. Juvenile pilocytic astrocytomas (JPAs), the most common grade 1 lesion, will be discussed in Chapter 2. Grade 2 astrocytomas demonstrate a relatively homogeneous appearance with well-defined borders on MRI (**Fig. 1.1A,B**)—an appearance that may belie an infiltrative pathology and poor prognosis. These tumors may grow large enough to exhibit significant mass effect, such as midline shift (mild left-to-right in the instance of **Figs. 1.1A,B**), but they generally lack the degree of edema (**Fig. 1.1A**) seen in higher-grade counterparts. Their lack of enhancement also helps distinguish them from a GBM. MR perfusion scans may help distinguish borderline cases, with higher-grade tumors demonstrating elevated cerebral blood volume. Grade 2 tumors may arise from multiple cell lines. The mass in **Figs. 1.1A,B**, for example, is an oligoastrocytoma. Oligodendrogliomas are uncommon, slow-growing tumors. Their distinctive feature is calcification, which is not well visualized on MRI. Oligodendrogliomas cannot be differentiated from astrocytomas on MRI, and to further complicate matters, hybrids of the two occur. The presence of calvarial erosion (with peripherally located lesions, due to slow growth) favors an oligodendroglioma.

GBM (**Figs. 1.1C,D**) is the most common astrocytoma, comprising roughly half of solitary brain lesions (the other half being metastases). Overall 2-year survival for GBMs is 10 to 15%. Most GBMs involve the frontal and temporal lobes and arise from a lower-grade lesion; however, GBMs may be newly found in patients in whom prior MRIs were negative. They frequently involve the meninges and subarachnoid space, although they tend to not metastasize outside the CNS. GBMs have the most characteristic MRI appearance of the astrocytomas. A heterogeneous central lesion associated with prominent mass effect and margin irregularity is typical (**Figs. 1.1C,D**). Areas of necrosis, correlating with high SI on T2WI (**Fig. 1.1C**) and low SI on T1WI (**Fig. 1.1D**), occur where the GBM has outgrown its blood supply. Vascular flow voids are also commonly seen. Calcification is less common than in lower-grade astrocytomas but may be seen in GBMs arising secondarily to these. Peripherally the tumor may be surrounded by areas of high SI on T2WI (**Fig. 1.1C**) and low SI on T1WI (**Fig. 1.1B**), correlating with vasogenic edema. All GBMs enhance, with an irregular, thick rim (**Fig. 1.1D**, *arrow*) being the most characteristic pattern. Areas of enhancement in GBMs reflect the locations of maximal blood–brain barrier (BBB) disruption and help demarcate, possibly along with areas of maximal cerebral blood volume on perfusion studies, optimal sites for stereotactic biopsy. Histologically, GBMs extend beyond the area delineated by abnormal contrast enhancement, and even beyond areas of high SI on T2WI. Characteristically, GBMs spread via white matter tracts, and can cross the corpus callosum to the opposite hemisphere (i.e., to produce a "butterfly glioma").

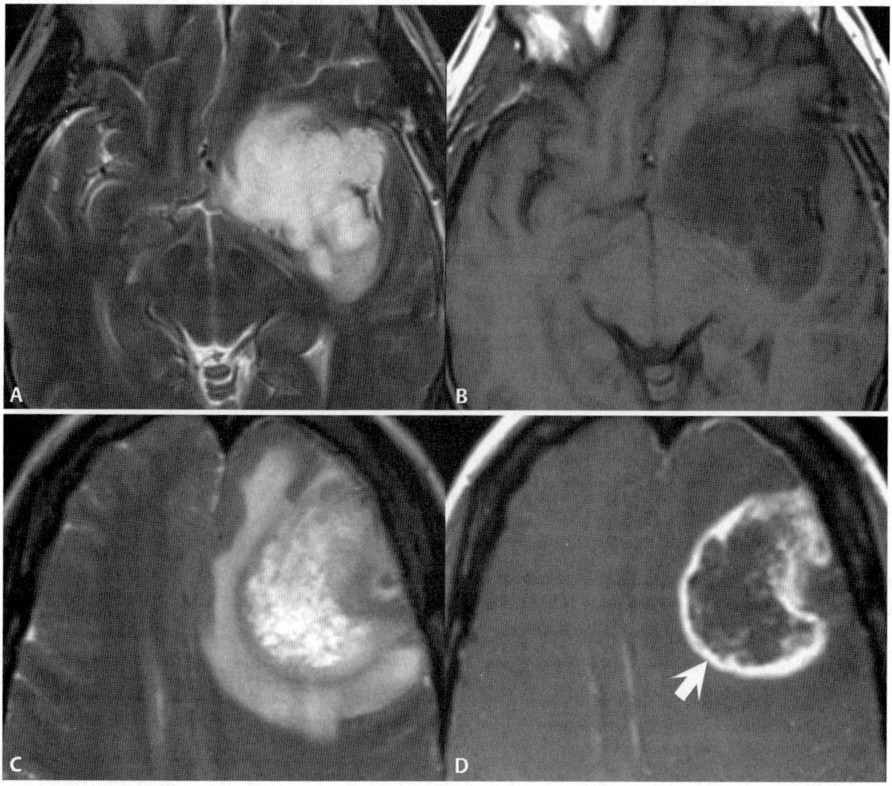

Fig. 1.1 (A–D)

Along with lymphoma and metastases, GBMs are one of the few neoplastic lesions that involve the callosum. Grade 3 lesions, or anaplastic astrocytomas, may arise from lower-grade astrocytomas and about half progress to GBM. Anaplastic astrocytomas demonstrate less distinctive imaging characteristics than GBMs: margins are not as irregular, there is less mass effect, enhancement is variable, and the SI heterogeneity is less. Unlike GBMs, not all anaplastic astrocytomas enhance. The presence of necrosis strongly implies the lesion is a GBM.

Differential considerations for a GBM include metastases and lymphoma. The presence of a second tumor focus favors the diagnosis of metastases, although multicentric GBMs do rarely occur. The incidence of CNS lymphomas has risen with the increase in the population of HIV (human immunodeficiency virus) and transplant patients. CNS lymphomas are primarily white matter tumors, frequently involving the basal ganglia, thalamus, corpus callosum, and periventricular areas. They are typically of homogeneous low SI on T2WI, unlike GBMs. Restricted diffusion may be present in CNS lymphomas, due to the dense cellularity of the tumor. Enhancement tends to be uniform, though it may be tempered by steroid treatments. Necrotic tumors (more common in HIV patients) may demonstrate ring-enhancement, mimicking toxoplasmosis. Periventricular location and lack of mass effect favor lymphoma.

2 Infratentorial Brain Neoplasms

Medulloblastoma, primarily a pediatric tumor, is the most common infratentorial neoplasm; 75% originate in the cerebellar vermis (**Figs. 2.1A,B**). Though medulloblastomas were once thought to be a type of primitive neuroectodermal tumor (PNET), studies have shown their molecular profile to be distinct. Medulloblastomas are highly malignant, commonly spreading via the cerebrospinal fluid (CSF). Thus, lumbar puncture and contrast-enhanced MRI of the entire neural axis are essential with a medulloblastoma. Metastasis outside the CNS is rare, most commonly involving the bone marrow. Treatment consists of some combination of resection, craniospinal radiotherapy, and chemotherapy. Like most brain tumors, medulloblastomas have low SI on T1WI (*white arrow*, **Fig. 2.1A**). On T2WI, their appearance varies from isointense to mildly hyperintense relative to brain parenchyma. Medulloblastomas show restricted diffusion, a point of distinction from astrocytomas. Intense, heterogeneous contrast enhancement (**Fig. 2.1B**, *black arrow*) is typical, although some lesions demonstrate only patchy enhancement. Medulloblastomas tend to extend into the 4th ventricle, leading to obstructive hydrocephalus, reflected in part by ventricular enlargement in **Fig. 2.1A**. The increase in ventricular pressure leads to compensation by transventricular absorption, with a thin uniform band of abnormal high SI present on T2WI in the periventricular white matter (**Fig. 2.1C**, *white arrow*)—a phenomenon known as transependymal CSF resorption. Spectroscopy reveals a marked elevation in the ratio of choline to *N*-acetyl-aspartate (NAA)—a finding typical of malignant tumors—and taurine. Medulloblastomas tend to be more aggressive in adults, with these lesions often demonstrating calcifications, cystic change, and location within the cerebellar hemispheres. Medulloblastomas may be difficult to distinguish from an ependymoma on MRI. Ependymomas tend to enlarge the 4th ventricle, but maintain its shape, whereas medulloblastomas tend to distort the appearance of the 4th ventricle (**Fig. 2.1A**).

Cerebellar astrocytomas closely follow medulloblastomas in incidence; they are the second most common posterior fossa neoplasm. A midline, vermian mass exhibiting restricted diffusion favors medulloblastoma; a hemispheric cerebellar mass favors astrocytoma. JPAs are WHO grade 1 astrocytomas and comprise the majority of cerebellar astrocytomas. These tumors carry a good prognosis (90% survival after 10 years) and high rate of surgical cure. They are associated with neurofibromatosis type 1 (NF1). JPA tends to be a round, cystic lesion (**Figs. 2.1D,E**) with a solid component (or nodule). The tumor in **Figs. 2.1D,E** is dominated by a cystic component, which characteristically appears similar to CSF on T1WI and T2WI, but can be differentiated from such on FLAIR scans. Lack of high SI intensity on T2WI argues against JPA. Because of elevated protein content, the cystic components will appear bright on FLAIR images. Unlike medulloblastomas, both the cystic and solid components of a JPA typically demonstrate increased apparent diffusion coefficient (ADC) values, due to increased water mobility. Though the nidus of the tumor in **Figs. 2.1D,E** is clearly seen on T2WI, this may not always be the case. Thus, every cystic cerebellar lesion warrants further evaluation with contrast administration to distinguish a JPA from a purely benign fluid collection. The tumor nidus will invariably enhance, and the cyst rim may as well (**Fig. 2.1E**). Though benign, JPAs can be associated with substantial edema (**Fig. 2.1D**, *asterisk*) Non-JPA cerebellar astrocytomas, including fibrillary astrocytomas, tend to be

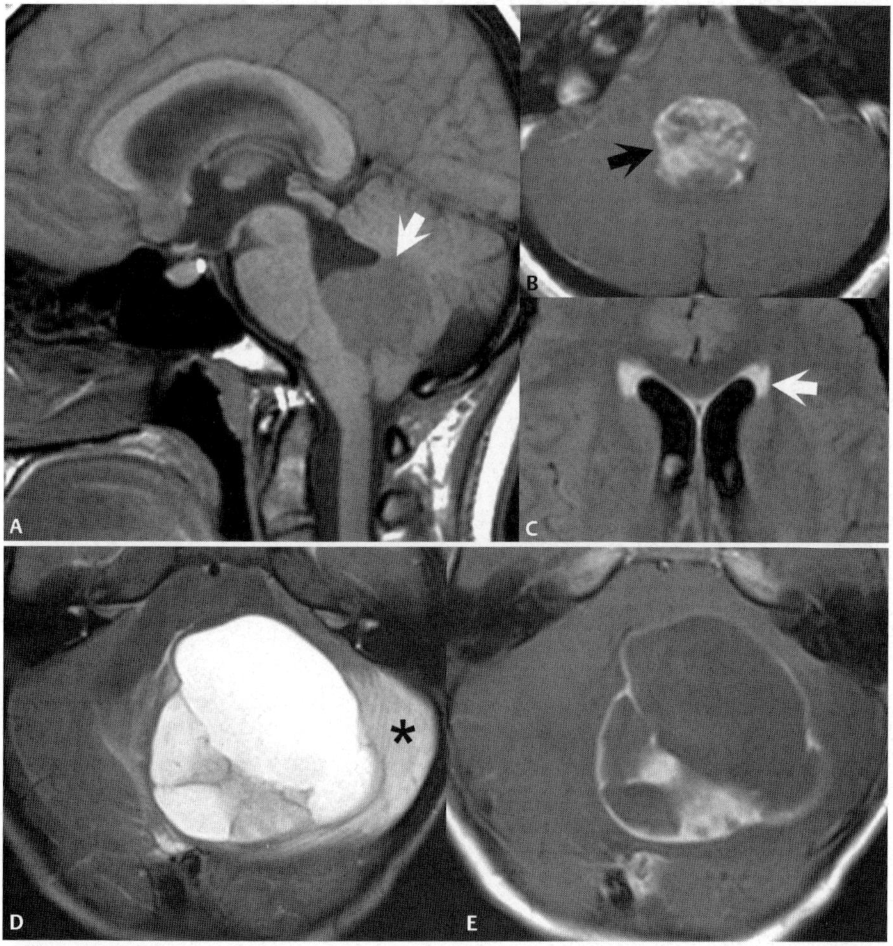

Fig. 2.1 (A–E)

solid, pathologically more infiltrative, and thus associated with a poorer prognosis. The latter lesions often fail to enhance, thus further distinguishing them from JPA.

Other brainstem and posterior fossa tumors include hemangioblastoma, choroid plexus papilloma, and brainstem glioma. Hemangioblastomas are benign vascular neoplasms of the young, which occur both sporadically and in von Hippel-Lindau (VHL) disease. An enhancing mural nodule with a nonenhancing cystic component, which may be confused with the cysts of JPA, is characteristic. Hemangioblastomas tend to be smaller and affect an older (>15 years of age) population than JPA. Choroid plexus papillomas are strongly enhancing, lobulated intraventricular lesions, with the most common locations being the lateral and 4th ventricles. Brainstem or pontine gliomas are usually grade 2 astrocytomas of the diffusely infiltrating or fibrillary type. These carry a worse prognosis (<1–2% 5-year survival) than JPA and show high SI on T2WI and FLAIR. They are less likely to enhance than other astrocytomas.

3 Metastatic Brain Disease

Metastases comprise about half of all intracranial tumors. Lung cancer followed by breast cancer then melanoma are the most common tumors to metastasize to the brain. Metastatic lesions are confirmed by the presence of multiple intracranial masses (**Figs. 3.1A,B,C,D**), although this differential also includes less common entities such as multifocal primary brain tumors and abscesses. Solitary brain metastases—seen frequently in breast, uterine, and gastrointestinal (GI) cancer—comprise about half of all brain metastases and pose a diagnostic challenge. Other imaging features suggestive of metastatic brain cancer include well-defined lesions (although pathologically metastases are less well defined than they appear on imaging) and a location at the gray–white matter junction (**Figs. 3.1A,B,C,D**). The predilection for this region likely

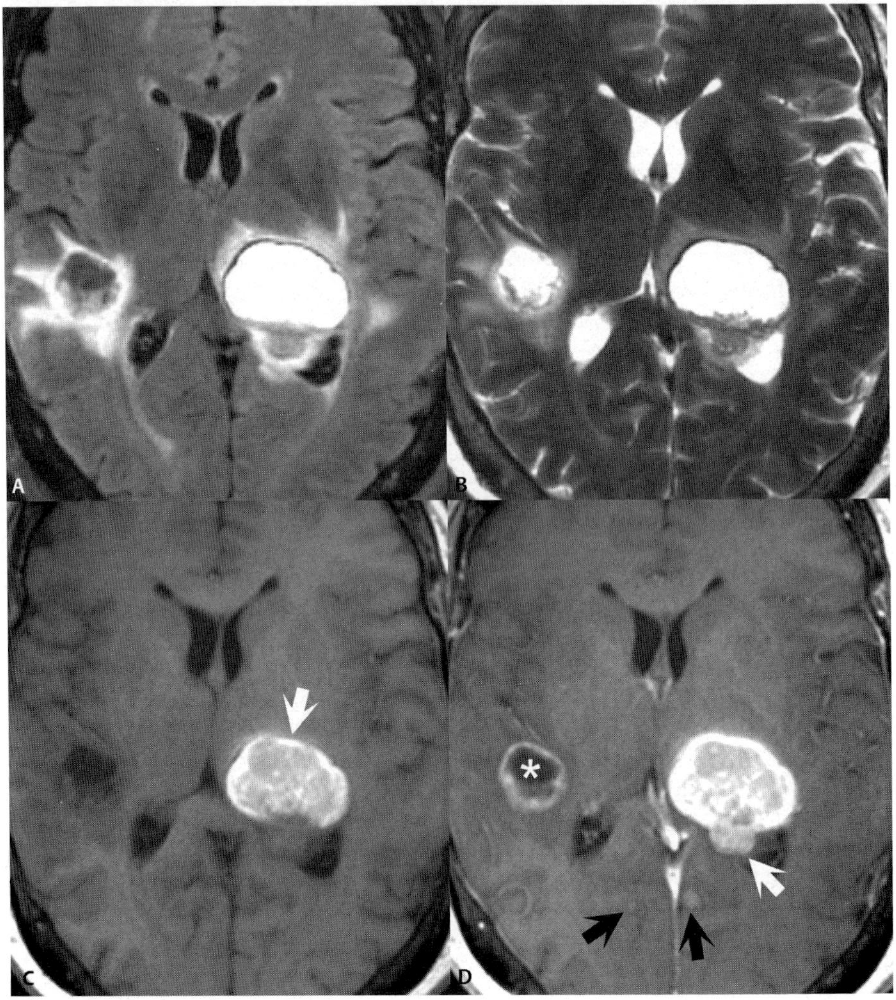

Fig. 3.1 (A–D)

relates to the inability of hematogenously spreading tumors to move freely through the smaller vascular structures found there. This hematogenous spread may form the basis for the preponderance of metastatic cancer found in the supratentorial region, reflecting the dominance of the carotid over the vertebrobasilar system.

Of unenhanced scan sequences, T2WIs (and in particular fluid attenuated inversion recovery [FLAIR] T2WI, **Fig. 3.1A**) are preferred for the visualization of metastatic cancer due to the high SI of the associated edema. Vasogenic edema from metastatic lesions tends to follow white matter tracts without crossing the corpus callosum (in distinction to a glioblastoma) and tends to be disproportionately large/prominent in extent when compared with the size of the tumor foci. Unfortunately, metastatic lesions at the cortical gray–white matter junction (and in other locations) may lack sufficient edema to be visualized using T2WI alone. This is illustrated in **Fig. 3.1D** by the two small occipital lesions (*black arrows*), which are visualized postcontrast, but are inconspicuous on FLAIR and T2WI (**Figs. 3.1A,B**). The demonstration of solitary versus multiple lesions dictates surgical versus nonsurgical (chemotherapy and/or radiation) management. Contrast administration is mandated for ease of diagnosis and improved lesion detection (the latter essential for therapy planning). If only a solitary lesion is apparent on first review, a careful search of the enhanced scans for a second metastatic lesion must be performed. Contrast-enhanced MRI detects far more lesions than enhanced CT, with the latter modality no longer employed for diagnosis. It should be noted, irrespective of the sensitivity of MRI for lesion detection, that some lesions can be difficult to visualize even on postcontrast T1WI. There are many ways to improve lesion detectability on MRI. These include thin section imaging and the use of high-field (3 Tesla [T]) MRI. Due both to the higher available signal-to-noise ratio (SNR) and the improved sensitivity to intravenous (IV) contrast enhancement, preferential use of 3 T in screening for intracranial metastatic disease is suggested. Triple-dose (0.3 mmol/kg) contrast administration further improves the number of visualized metastases (by $\approx$ 30%). Cost has led to high-dose brain MRI not being widely used in the United States.

Contrast administration also aids in distinguishing benign hemorrhagic disease (which may appear similar to the lesion denoted by the *white arrow* in **Fig. 3.1C**) from hemorrhagic metastases by more clearly demonstrating the enhancing tumor focus (**Fig. 3.1D**, *white arrow*). On nonenhanced studies, hemorrhagic metastases—most common in melanoma, renal cell carcinoma, and choriocarcinoma—demonstrate signal on T1WIs and T2WIs more heterogeneous and delayed in evolution than the expected signal changes of hemorrhage (see Chapter 8). Hemorrhagic metastases also lack the uniform, hypointense hemosiderin-rim seen in the later stages of benign hemorrhage. Metastases may appear as solid or ring-enhancing lesions. Ring-enhancing metastatic lesions (**Fig. 3.1D**, *asterisk*) may be distinguished, to some extent, from those of more benign entities (e.g., abscess) by the thickness and irregularity of the enhancing wall. A cystic appearance is also common for metastatic lesions (**Fig. 3.1D**, *asterisk*). These tend to be of CSF-like intensity on T2WI and T1WI (**Figs. 3.1B,C**), but differentiated from CSF on FLAIR scans (**Fig. 3.1A**) due to the presence of protein. Finally, certain metastatic tumors demonstrate signal characteristics on MRI that provide hints to their origin. For example, (nonhemorrhagic) melanotic melanoma is characteristically high SI on T1WI due to the paramagnetic effects of melanin, whereas mucinous adenocarcinoma of the colon is suggested by hypointensity on T2WI. Leptomeningeal metastatic disease, a less common finding, presents on imaging as abnormal enhancement of the leptomeninges, often focal and somewhat nodular. Bacterial, viral, or tuberculous meningitis, as well as sarcoidosis can mimic leptomeningeal metastases on postcontrast MRI.

4 Meningiomas

After glioblastomas, meningiomas are the second most common primary brain tumor, and the most common extraaxial tumor. They occur most commonly in females with risk factors including ionizing radiation, head trauma, and likely high exposure to estrogen and progesterone. Meningiomas are most commonly located over the cerebral convexity adjoining the mid or anterior one third of the superior sagittal sinus, but may occur, in decreasing order of frequency: along the lateral convexity, the sphenoid ridge, olfactory groove, suprasellar parasellar region, and in the posterior fossa.

Meningiomas may be relatively difficult to visualize on nonenhanced MRI as they tend to be relatively isointense to brain on T1WI, T2WI, and FLAIR (**Fig. 4.1A**). The presence of surrounding edema, demonstrating increased SI on T2WI and decreased SI on T1WI, may aid in lesion recognition on unenhanced scans. Approximately half of meningiomas, however, do not demonstrate significant associated edema (**Fig. 4.1A**). Thus, contrast administration (as in **Fig. 4.1B**) greatly aids in the detection of these lesions. Due to their lack of a BBB, meningiomas demonstrate prominent (and typically homogeneous) enhancement—a finding useful for lesion identification, characterization, and distinguishing surrounding edema (**Fig. 4.1C**, *asterisk*) from the tumor itself (**Fig. 4.1D**). The dura adjacent to a meningioma often enhances as well (**Fig. 4.1D**), with the presence of a "dural tail" characteristic, although this is occasionally seen with other lesion types. Meningiomas may appear mottled on T2WI secondary to cystic changes or areas of dense calcification. Though MRI does not demonstrate calcifications well, when extremely dense (like cortical bone) these are visualized as areas of low SI on both T1 and T2WI. These findings can be more obvious on gradient echo (GRE) T2WI and on imaging at a higher field (3 T). In both instances such scans are more sensitive to magnetic susceptibility effects and thus the detection of calcium. Hypointensity on GRE T2WI, however, is not specific for calcification as products of hemorrhage can lead to similar findings. MRI is vastly superior to computed tomography (CT) in localizing meningiomas as extraaxial. A broad margin along the dura (**Figs. 4.1B,D**) and the presence of an enhancing dural tail

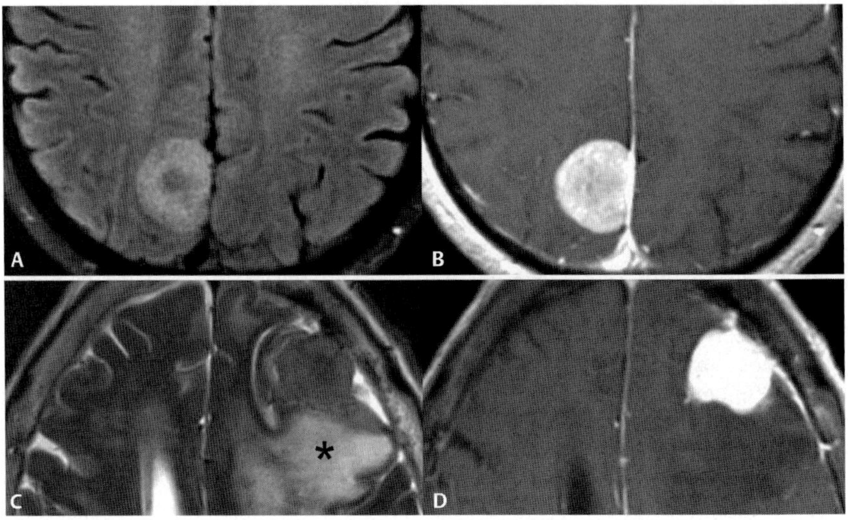

Fig. 4.1 (A–D)

(**Fig. 4.1D**) strongly support the diagnosis of meningioma. Even more specific is the so-called cleft sign (**Fig. 4.1C**) whereby CSF is visualized, usually best as a hyperintense cleft on T2WI, intervening between the tumor and brain parenchyma. As in **Fig. 4.1C**, an additional rim of hypointense parenchyma may separate the CSF cleft from surrounding parenchymal edema. Pial vasculature, appearing as hypointense flow voids, may similarly become trapped between the meningioma and adjacent brain parenchyma. Meningiomas within the cavernous sinus may demonstrate a similar phenomenon with the displacement of the dura, which manifests as a lateral hypointense line between the tumor and temporal lobes on postcontrast scans. Intraaxial tumors may grow outward to involve the dura, but only extraaxial tumors demonstrate interposed structures between the tumor and brain parenchyma. Another clue to the extraaxial location of these tumors is the bowing of adjacent white matter, due to compression of otherwise normal brain by the lesion. Meningiomas may also involve the vasculature or venous sinuses. Within the cavernous sinus, they are prone to displacement or encasement of the carotid artery: the latter finding may be confused for atherosclerosis on CT or digital subtraction angiography (DSA), but is easily visualized with MRI. A tumor displacing the carotid artery from its normal position is most likely a meningioma, as similarly located pituitary macroadenomas tend to encase it. Meningiomas may invade the venous sinuses as well, such invasion being demonstrated on enhanced T1WI (**Fig. 4.2**, *black arrow* showing transverse sinus invasion) but may also be seen, prior to contrast administration, on two-dimensional time-of-flight MR venography (2D TOF MRV). Postcontrast T1WI shows high SI venous sinuses abutted by the enhancing soft tissue of the meningioma. 2D TOF MRV depicts venous flow as high SI, which with an adjacent meningioma, demonstrates irregular contour or, if the obstruction is complete, absence of flow within the sinus.

Meningiomas are typically benign and slow-growing. Atypical (higher grade) and malignant meningiomas are less common and exhibit restricted diffusion, likely from a combination of necrosis, decreased cytoplasmic space (from an increased nuclear:cytoplasmic ratio), and decreased extracellular space (from tumor proliferation). En plaque meningiomas pose a therapeutic and diagnostic challenge. These tumors grow in a carpet-like fashion along the surface of the brain and frequently infiltrate through the dura and adjacent bone, thus rendering total resection impossible. Osseous invasion of meningiomas may be seen as bone thickening, and the tumors may also be visualized within the diploic space. Because en plaque lesions may simply appear as dural thickening, and are obscured due to beam hardening artifact from the adjacent skull, they are not seen on CT unless osseous invasion occurs. Even then, MRI comparatively easily makes the diagnosis because of the marked enhancement and extraaxial location of the lesion. When multiple or occurring in childhood, meningiomas (**Fig. 4.2**, *black arrow*) are often associated with NF2—an inherited condition for which presentation with bilateral vestibular schwannomas is pathognomonic (**Fig. 4.2**, *white arrows*).

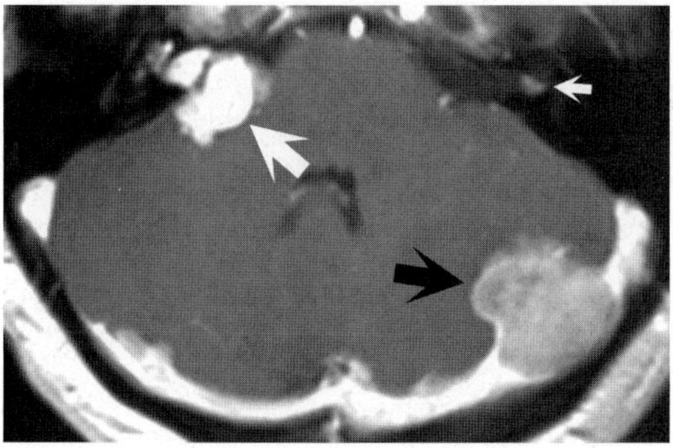

Fig. 4.2

5 Internal Auditory Canal Neoplasms

Schwannomas are the most common mass of the internal auditory canal (IAC) (**Figs. 5.1A,B**). They arise most frequently from the vestibular portion of cranial nerve (CN) VIII, although they may arise from CN VII as well. Risk factors include long-term exposure to loud noises, previous head or neck irradiation, and NF2. Bilateral vestibular schwannomas (10%) are pathognomonic for the latter. Symptoms are most frequently cochlear in nature—hearing loss and tinnitus—although vestibular nerve compression may result in an unsteady gate. MRI is vastly superior to CT and older invasive methods at diagnosing schwannomas as the lack of signal from adjacent bone allows CNs VII and VIII to be directly visualized. Most tumors are large enough to be well seen on precontrast scans with slice sections less than 3 mm. Schwannomas demonstrate moderate to low SI on T1WI and T2WI. SI on T2WI may, however, vary with tumor pathology: densely packed palisades of neural tissue (Antoni A areas) appear slightly hypointense; more loosely packed neural tissue (Antoni B areas) appears slightly hyperintense. About 10% of schwannomas are accompanied by an arachnoid cyst, the latter of high SI on T2WI. T2WI may also help predict recovery of auditory capacity postoperatively. Specifically, if there is a substantial amount of CSF between the schwannoma and the fundus of the auditory canal and if this, along with intralabyrinthine fluid, is of normal SI, then the likelihood of postsurgical hearing preservation is higher (due to implications for the operative approach). T2WIs allow visualization of disease processes that can clinically mimic a schwannoma, such as multiple sclerosis, mastoiditis, and vascular brainstem compression. Many schwannomas extend from the IAC to the cerebellopontine angle (CPA) cistern; however, purely intracanicular lesions occur and may be mistaken on T2WI alone for several different entities, including 8th nerve enlargement and IAC ectasia. Contrast administration further narrows the differential and is essential for the detection of tumors less than 3 mm in diameter (*white arrow*, **Fig. 5.1B**).

Contrast is also useful for preoperative evaluation of schwannomas and may demonstrate extension of tumor that is not otherwise seen. Enhancement of schwannomas is most frequently homogeneous, but may be heterogeneous (*black arrow*, **Fig. 5.1A**). Enhancement surrounding CN VII can represent either a schwannoma or neuritis (usually with a linear pattern), although CN VIII rarely enhances if affected by the latter. Inflammatory (i.e., sarcoid) and neoplastic conditions, which demonstrate meningeal enhancement, may be confused with neural origin lesions in the IAC. In this case, the diagnosis rests on clinical correlation and followup MRI. Glomus tympanicum (*white arrows*, **Figs. 5.1C,D**), a type of paraganglioma, may also be confused for a schwannoma. This lesion presents with pulsatile tinnitus and is the most common neoplasm of the inferior part of the middle ear, often at the cochlear promontory or semicircular canals. The location of this enhancing lesion, along with the classic presence of intratumoral flow voids, helps distinguish it from a schwannoma. Translabyrinthine approaches to the resection of schwannomas may complicate the MRI evaluation of recurrence. This approach involves resection of the mastoid and packing with autologous graft containing fat which may be superimposed over CN VIII in axial scans. Coronal imaging should be examined to separate this high SI graft from recurrent tumor.

Differentiation on MRI of a CPA schwannoma from a meningioma, the latter being much less common, can be challenging. Nearly 80% of CPA schwannomas contain an

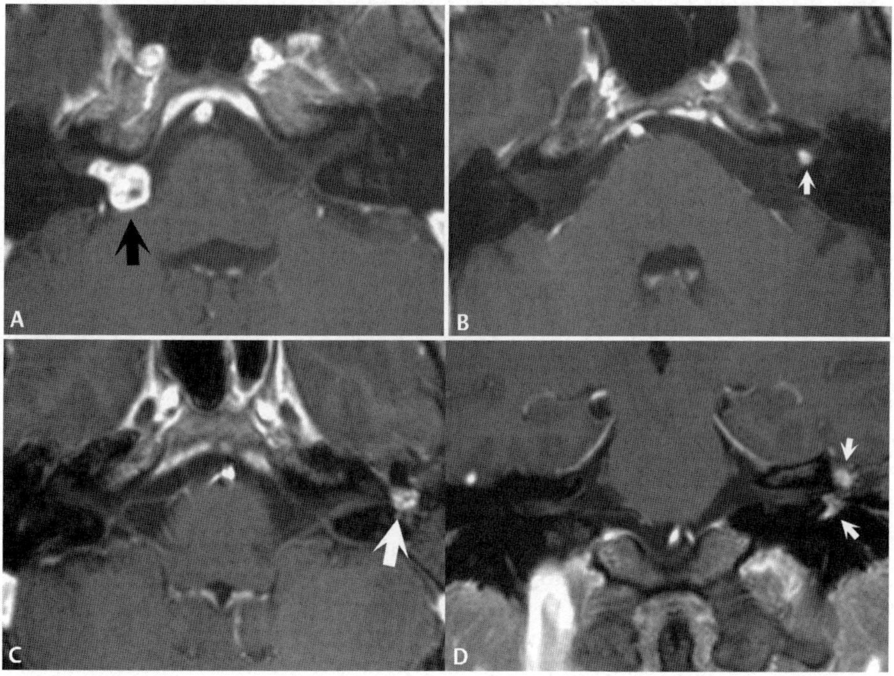

Fig. 5.1 (A–D)

intracanalicular component (**Fig. 5.1A**); however, meningiomas may extend into the IAC as well. The latter, however, do not enlarge the IAC. Though both may follow the contour of nerves, meningiomas frequently demonstrate a dural tail (see Chapter 4) and make an obtuse, rather than acute, angle with the petrous bone. Features favoring a schwannoma include areas of low SI on postcontrast T1WI (**Fig. 5.1A**) and high SI on T2WI correlating with cystic or necrotic changes as well as the presence of a concomitant arachnoid cyst. Schwannomas tend to enhance more heterogeneously and hemorrhage more frequently than meningiomas. Epidermoids (cholesteatomas) and dermoids are additional diagnostic considerations at both the CPA and IAC. Epidermoids result from incomplete cleavage of neural from cutaneous ectoderm, with inclusion of ectodermal elements at the time of neural groove closure. Dermoids contain additional dermal elements, such as skin appendages and sebaceous cysts. Both can occur at suprasellar or intraventricular locations as well as at the CPA. Dermoids are more frequently midline and due to the oil from intrinsic sebaceous glands, appear with high SI on T1WI. Both dermoids and epidermoids exhibit high SI on DWI. Epidermoids, however, have SI like that of CSF or an arachnoid cyst (low SI on T1WI and high SI on T2WI). Unlike the latter, epidermoids demonstrate slightly higher SI on FLAIR. Epidermoids, dermoids, and arachnoid cysts do not enhance, thus differentiating them from schwannomas and meningiomas.

6 Sellar/Parasellar Neoplasms

Pituitary adenomas are a frequent source of incidental findings, warranting serial MRI examinations. Three-fourths, however, are hormonally active and thus brought to early clinical attention. Microadenomas (<10 mm in diameter) appear as low to moderate SI focal lesions on T1WI, with variable SI on T2WI (**Fig. 6.1A**). This appearance, visualized against the moderate SI of the pituitary, render microadenomas often difficult to visualize without contrast. Early (<5 minutes) postcontrast MRI well demonstrates the minimally enhancing adenoma against the brightly enhancing pituitary gland (**Figs. 6.1B,C,** *white arrows*). On delayed postcontrast scans, the adenoma may be iso- to hyperintense to the gland. Contrast administration is essential preoperatively and when Cushing disease is suspected, as ACTH (adrenocorticotrophic hormone) secreting tumors tend to be the smallest of the microadenomas. MRI is not useful for distinguishing the various types of adenomas, although both prolactinomas—the most common functioning adenoma—and growth hormone-secreting adenomas tend to occur in the lateral aspects of the gland. 3 T MRI offers substantial advantages for imaging of pituitary microadenomas, making possible acquisition of images with a slice thickness of 2 mm.

Nonfunctioning pituitary adenomas are not as clinically obvious and thus comprise the majority of adenomas over 10 mm in diameter. Diagnostically, macroadenomas are rarely problematic even for CT. MRI is nevertheless markedly preferred for diagnosis given its superior ability to evaluate suprasellar extent, cavernous sinus invasion, and carotid artery encasement. Macroadenomas are low to intermediate SI on T2WI and T1WI (**Figs. 6.1D,E**). As lesions grow, their blood supply becomes more tenuous leading to

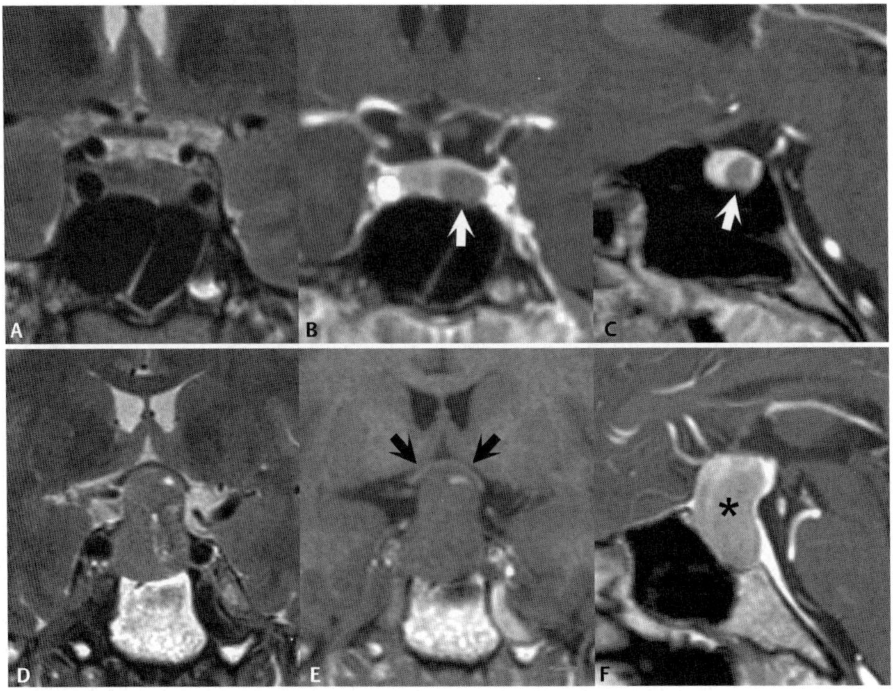

Fig. 6.1 (A–F)

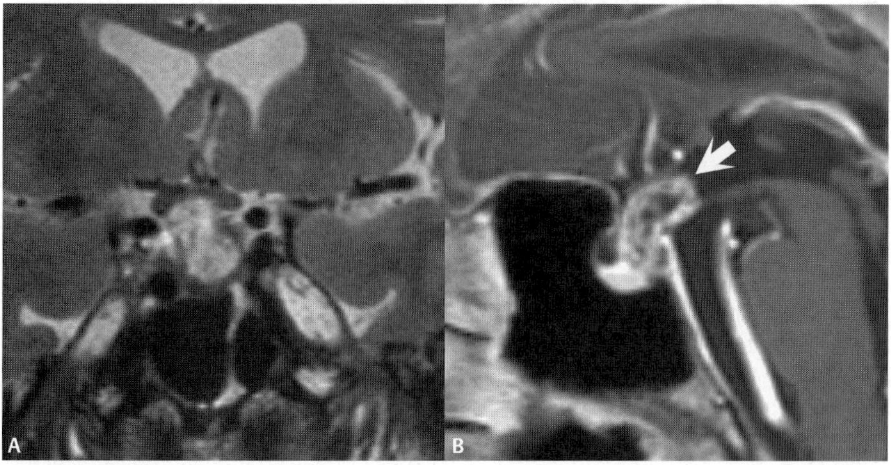

Fig. 6.2 (A,B)

necrosis and hemorrhage, which can manifest as areas of high SI depending upon the age of blood products. Chronic findings of hemorrhage (a rim of hypointensity on T2WI) will not be seen; the pituitary's lack of a BBB allows macrophages to successfully remove hemosiderin. Necrosis may lead to confusion in the differentiation of a pituitary adenoma from an inferiorly extending craniopharyngioma, but only adenomas enlarge the sella. Cystic changes also occur and are evident as low SI on T1WI and high SI on T2WI. As the tumor grows superiorly, splaying and compression of the optic chiasm (**Fig. 6.1E**, *black arrows*) is common. Inferior expansion is also common with enlargement of the sella into the sphenoid sinus. Macroadenomas thus commonly acquire a characteristic dumbbell-shaped appearance, with central compression/constriction by the diaphragma sellae (**Figs. 6.1D,E**). Macroadenomas tend to homogeneously enhance (**Fig. 6.1F**, *asterisk*), although this may be patchy in tumors with prominent necrosis. Enhancement helps define tumor extent, often underestimated in precontrast sequences especially with cavernous sinus involvement.

Craniopharyngiomas are histologically benign suprasellar tumors arising from the Rathke pouch. Unlike Rathke cleft cysts, these lesions typically enhance heterogeneously, calcify, and present with a concomitant (enhancing) soft tissue mass. Craniopharyngiomas are divided into adamantinoma and squamous-papillary subtypes with the former portending a worse prognosis and affecting a younger population. Adamantinomas demonstrate heterogeneous hyperintensity on T2WI (**Fig. 6.2A**) and enhance heterogeneously on T1WI (**Fig. 6.2B**). Cystic components are of high SI on T2WI and low SI on T1WI, although squamous and papillary types are more likely to be solid. In all types, high cholesterol content or methemoglobin from prior hemorrhage may result in foci of increased SI on T1WI. Contrast enhancement improves identification of lesion margins and differential diagnosis. Contrast administration can also assist in demonstrating compression of the pituitary, which enhances brightly (**Fig. 6.2B**, *arrow*), and well delineates craniopharyngiomas that are not large enough to obliterate the suprasellar cistern (the intensities from these two may not be distinguishable on T2WI). Adamantinomas may have calcified regions, which are not well seen on MRI; however, lesion location, contrast enhancement, and a dominant cystic component are usually sufficient for diagnosis.

7 Diploic Space Lesions

The diploic space is the marrow-containing area in the skull vault between the inner and outer layers of compact/dense bone. In adults, in whom yellow marrow has supplanted the red marrow of childhood (or in whom there is simply a greater proportion of yellow marrow), this space is visualized as increased SI on T1WI. The SI pattern of the diploic space may vary on T1WI, ranging from uniform high SI to patchy areas to only a small nidus of high SI. Regardless of the distribution of elevated SI, these areas should be symmetric; any asymmetry suggests pathology. Evaluation of the diploic space must be specifically included in the normal search pattern; otherwise subtle lesions will be missed. Metastases to the diploic space may be subtle (**Fig. 7.1A**) on nonenhanced MRI, but are usually readily evident with contrast administration (**Fig. 7.1B**). Any diploic space enhancement other than the arachnoid granulations and the occasional diploic venous channel is likely pathologic. The arachnoid granulations are best seen on coronal scans flanking the superior sagittal sinus along the midline convexity. These are hyperintense on T2WI. Diploic venous channels, which are of low SI on nonenhanced studies, are often seen to enhance in a recognizable linear pattern. Fat-saturated postcontrast images allow for optimal visualization of diploic space metastases, as there is no confusion between enhancing tumor and high SI fatty marrow. However, if these are not obtained, a simple comparison between pre- and postcontrast T1WI should suffice to distinguish normal marrow hyperintensity from metastatic enhancement.

Fibrous dysplasia is a classically painless, benign condition most commonly affecting females and patients under 30 years of age. Three forms are described: monostotic, polystotic, and fibrous dysplasia associated with McCune-Albright—a triad completed by café au lait spots and precocious puberty. Craniofacial fibrous dysplasia occurs in approximately half of polyostotic cases and a quarter of monostotic cases. Commonly involved bones include the frontal, temporal, sphenoid (**Figs. 7.1C,D,E**), maxillary, and ethmoid. Diffuse involvement of the jaw—cherubism—may also occur, leading to an "angelic" appearance, although these typically regress by adulthood. The pathologic findings of fibrous dysplasia involve the replacement of medullary bone with expansile fibroosseous tissue, which gives the bone an enlarged appearance (**Figs. 7.1D,E**). Fibrous dysplasia is most often an incidental finding on brain MRI. Lesions demonstrate low to intermediate SI, typically homogeneous, on T1WI (**Fig. 7.1C**, *asterisk*) and low SI on T2WI (**Fig. 7.1D**) secondary to fibrous and osseous tissue. These lesions enhance (**Fig. 7.1E**, *asterisk*), often with areas of more prominent enhancement that correspond to hyperintense parts of the lesion on T2WI (and lucent on CT). In distinction from enhancing metastatic lesions, fibrous dysplasia tends to follow the normal bone contour. Rapid lesion enlargement implies malignant transformation—most frequently to osteosarcoma.

Eosinophilic granuloma (EG) or Langerhans cell granulomatosis are the preferred terms for the clinical entity also known as histiocytosis X. Unifocal EG is found predominantly in male children and young adults, presenting with a solitary osteolytic lesion in the femur, skull, ribs, or pelvis. On brain MRI, the typical appearance is a solitary skull lesion (usually within the temporal bone), centered in the diploic space with destruction of adjacent bone. EG tends to demonstrate high SI on T2WI and low SI on T1WI. The lesion may also extend into the epidural or subgaleal space. EG enhances prominently, so again contrast administration is useful. Multifocal EG is a more aggressive childhood

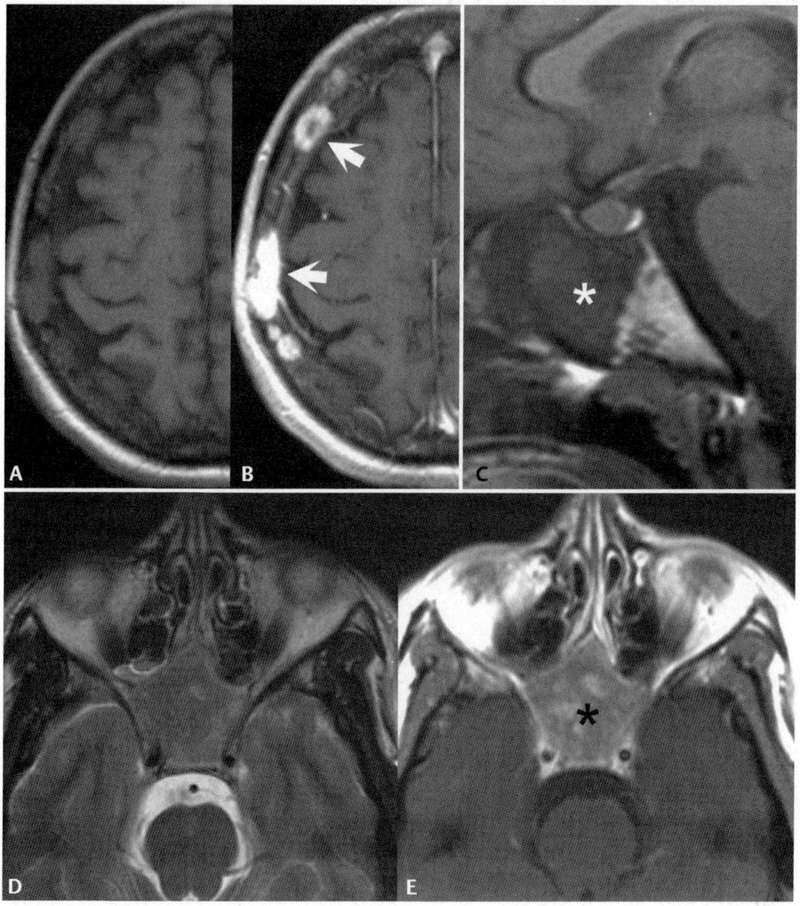

Fig. 7.1 (A–E)

disorder that is associated with Hand-Schüller-Christian syndrome—a triad of osseous EG, diabetes insipidus, and exophthalmos—in a quarter of patients. The imaging correlates of diabetes insipidus may be seen on brain MRI as pituitary stalk thickening or atrophy. Definitive diagnosis of EG is by biopsy of an osseous lesion. In terms of differential diagnosis, when a solitary lesion of the skull is encountered, a hemangioma should also be included.

8 Intraparenchymal Hemorrhage

Understanding the MRI appearance of hemorrhage requires a discussion of hemoglobin byproducts in the local proton environment. T1 and T2 are the times needed, following a radiofrequency (RF) pulse, for the higher energy level protons to longitudinally relax and to lose phase coherence, respectively. With free water protons, dipole-dipole interactions result in inefficient relaxation—a long T1 and T2. The degradation products of hemoglobin—which are all paramagnetic except oxyhemoglobin—affect T1 and T2 in various ways. When water protons closely approach a paramagnetic substance, proton-electron dipole-dipole interactions lead to efficient energy release, decreasing T1 (and less so T2). The T2 effects of paramagnetism are more complicated. When exposed to an external field, paramagnetic substances are induced to produce additional magnetic fields augmenting the external field locally. When these substances are intracellular, their distribution (across the tissue) is heterogeneous and thus so is the overall magnetic field. T2*WI (GRE T2WI) is sensitive to these fixed field heterogeneities (susceptibility), but spin echo (SE) and fast spin echo (FSE) T2WI are not. SE, however, is sensitive to spin diffusion effects arising from heterogeneous differences in field strengths. Specifically, stronger fields predominate in intact red blood cells (due to paramagnetic contents), resulting in differentials between intra- and extracellular proton spin frequencies. As water diffuses, these protons with differing spin frequencies interact, leading to more rapid dephasing (<T2).

Oxyhemoglobin is the main component of hyperacute (<2 hours) hemorrhage. It lacks paramagnetism, so hyperacute bleeds appear as fluid like SI on MRI—moderate high SI on T2WI (**Fig. 8.1A**, *asterisk*) and moderate to low SI on T1WI (**Fig. 8.1B**). Peripheral (more hypoxic) areas of hemorrhage may begin to undergo reduction to deoxyhemoglobin, resulting in a thin, low SI rim on T2WI. Acute hemorrhage (3–6 hours) is typified by the presence of intracellular deoxyhemoglobin throughout the hematoma. The protein structure of paramagnetic deoxyhemoglobin does not allow for close interaction with water protons, leaving T1 unchanged. However, the intracellular distribution of deoxyhemoglobin decreases T2, which is seen as low SI on T2WI (**Fig. 8.1C**, *asterisk*), by spin diffusion effects. As seen in **Fig. 8.1C**, extracellular water initially representing serum from the retracting clot (together with vasogenic edema) typically surrounds the area of hemorrhage resulting in a high SI border on T2WI. Continued clot resorption as illustrated in this case leads, long term, to the formation of a hemosiderin cleft (**Fig. 8.1D**). In early subacute hemorrhages (>2 days old) the iron of deoxyhemoglobin is oxidized intracellularly to form methemoglobin. Unlike deoxyhemoglobin, the structure of methemoglobin allows for the close approach of water protons, resulting in a reduction in T1 (high SI on T1WI) by proton-electron dipole-dipole interactions. By the late subacute stage, red blood cells have lysed, spilling methemoglobin and eliminating T2 effects from magnetic field heterogeneities. Because T2 relaxation effects are lost, late subacute hematomas appear as high SI on both T2 and T1WI (**Figs. 8.1E,F**). As clot transitions to the chronic stage (>1 month), a low SI rim may begin to develop (**Figs. 8.1E,F**) due to the presence of hemosiderin within infiltrating, phagocytic macrophages. Hemosiderin, a paramagnetic substance, is not water-soluble, and thus does not decrease T1, but its intracellular distribution decreases T2, resulting in a low SI on T1 and T2WI. Eventually, the remaining central methemoglobin is degraded and resorbed. If central fluid persists, the CSF-like SI of a chronic clot may be surrounded by a rim of low SI. If not, then only a low SI hemosiderin cleft may remain (**Fig. 8.1D**).

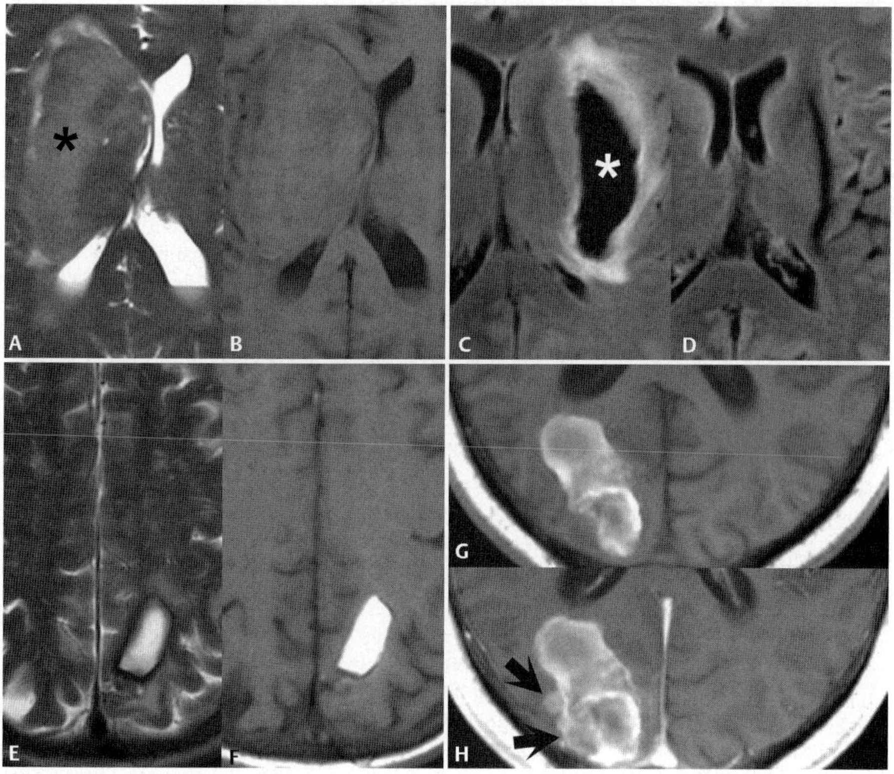

Fig. 8.1 (A–H)

The time course of the stages of blood product degradation described above may vary based on the local oxygen environment. For example, in hemorrhagic arterial infarcts, the formation of deoxyhemoglobin will be delayed compared with formation in a poorly oxygenated hemorrhagic venous infarction. Additional MRI sequences may be useful for the detection and evaluation of hemorrhage. GRE T2WI and high-field MRI are highly sensitive to susceptibility (T2*) effects and thus more easily detect acute, early subacute, and chronic hemorrhages. Diffusion is markedly restricted in hemorrhagic lesions until red blood cell lysis occurs in the late subacute phase. With conventional FSE, increasing the interecho interval (the time between the refocusing pulses) allows diffusing water molecules to encounter greater local magnetic heterogeneity, increasing dephasing and thus the loss of SI. Contrast administration may demonstrate a benign-appearing hemorrhage, as seen in the subacute phase in **Fig. 8.1G**, to be associated with an otherwise poorly visualized neoplastic lesion (**Fig. 8.1H**, *black arrows*). Other features suggestive of neoplasia include the delayed evolution of blood products, particularly in the deoxyhemoglobin stage (from hypoxia), heterogeneous SI, and a lack of the complete low SI rims seen in various stages of benign hemorrhage.

9 Extraaxial and Subarachnoid Hemorrhage

Subdural hematomas (SDH) are most frequently seen in the setting of trauma, particularly in older individuals, and result from injury to the veins bridging the subdural space. Because their signal characteristics may at many stages be isointense to parenchyma (**Fig. 9.1A**, T2WI) or the diploic space, they may be difficult to detect on MRI, depending in particular on the pulse sequence acquired. SDH typically exhibit a crescentic shape and do not cross dural attachments at the venous sinuses (**Fig. 9.1B**, *arrows*, T1WI). The evolution of SDH SI follows that of intraparenchymal hemorrhages (see Chapter 8). In a child, the presence of multiple SDH of various temporal stages (**Fig. 9.2A**, T2WI, **Fig. 9.2B** 1–4, T1WI) is pathognomonic of abuse. Unlike intraparenchymal bleeds, SDH (except in recurrent bleeds) do not demonstrate a hemosiderin phase: the lack of a dural BBB allows the macrophages that scavenge hemosiderin to return into the bloodstream. The appearance of chronic SDH, therefore, correlates with methemoglobin resorption which leads to a progressively lower SI on T1WI. The appearance of SDH may be confused for brain atrophy in these chronic or even subacute phases, and the presence of contrast enhancement (of the lining membrane) may help to confirm the presence of SDH. Chronic SDH may further degrade into a subdural hygroma, although this may also arise from a CSF leak (typically from an arachnoid membrane tear). Hygromas contain less methemoglobin than do chronic SDH, and thus appear isointense to CSF on T1WI and T2WI. Hygromas with greater protein concentrations may demonstrate higher SI on FLAIR scans, while areas of residual hemorrhage correlate with low SI on GRE T2WI. In distinction, arachnoid cysts are isointense to CSF on all sequences. Epidural hematomas are lens-shaped and are most commonly associated with fractures of the temporal bone. **Figure 9.3A** (*white arrow*), a T1WI, demonstrates an epidural hematoma with two distinct signal components, which crosses the tentorium. Although epidural hematomas may cross the falx or tentorium they do not cross the suture lines connecting the dura to the inner bone table. A band of low SI dura compressed against brain parenchyma also suggests an epidural location (**Fig. 9.3A**, *white arrow*).

Unlike the entities above, subarachnoid hemorrhages (SAHs) usually result from rupture of berry aneurysms or arteriovenous malformations rather than from trauma. Hyperacute and acute SAH are not well seen on most MRI sequences, as the high oxygen content of CSF prevents reduction of oxyhemoglobin to deoxyhemoglobin. The presence of CSF also tends to dilute the hemoglobin, decreasing the effect of its

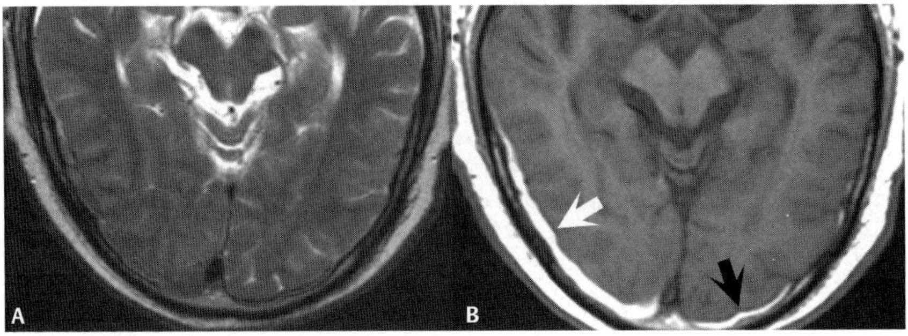

Fig. 9.1 (A,B)

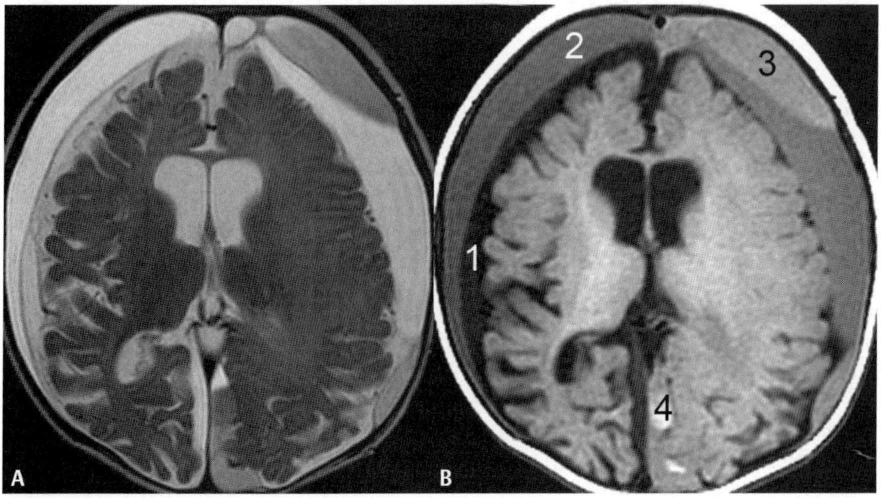

Fig. 9.2 (A,B)

byproducts on SI. The presence of additional protein within a hemorrhagic region, however, decreases T1, and results in hyperintensity to the normal low SI of CSF on FLAIR scans. Thus, FLAIR imaging is exquisitely sensitive to the detection of SAH (likely even more so than CT), and demonstrates SAH as areas of abnormally high SI either within the basal cisterns or cortical sulci (**Fig. 9.3B**, *arrows*). Leading differential considerations include meningitis and meningeal carcinomatosis, although oxygen administration at the time of MRI and pulsation artifacts, particularly in the basal cisterns, may have a similar appearance. GRE T2WI (and susceptibility weighted imaging [SWI]) identify the paramagnetic byproducts of hemorrhage, and may be of equal sensitivity to FLAIR. Chronic or recurrent hemorrhage, as seen in patients with vascular abnormalities, may result in superficial hemosiderosis, often seen as a thin rim of hypointensity lining the parenchymal surface on T2WI. Intraventricular hemorrhage, seen in trauma and preterm infants, is similar to SAH in its SI and delayed temporal evolution. FLAIR scans demonstrate hyperintensity against attenuated CSF, most often in the dependent portions (i.e., atria and occipital horns) of the lateral ventricle. Layering of blood products and CSF is commonly seen in interventricular hemorrhage.

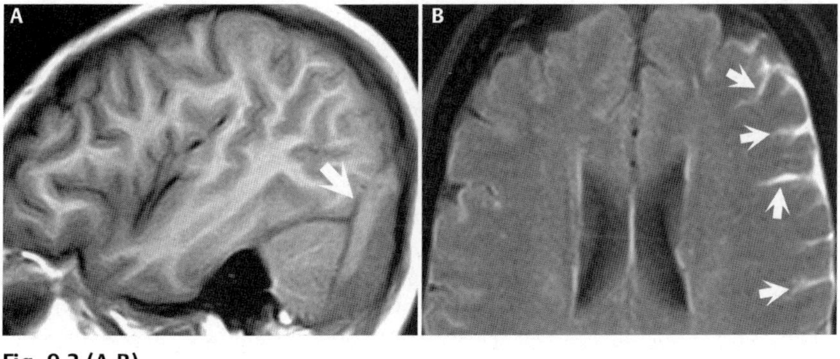

Fig. 9.3 (A,B)

10 Arteriovenous Malformations

Arteriovenous malformations (AVMs) are the most common cerebrovascular malformation, consisting of direct communication between the arterial and venous circulations without intervening capillaries. Their most serious complication is hemorrhage (4% annual rate) with a yearly mortality of 1%. Symptoms of AVMs include headache, seizures, and neurologic defects. These may be caused by mass effect or a steal phenomenon whereby blood flow is diverted from the surrounding parenchyma to an AVM, underperfusing the former. AVMs are associated with a variety of inherited conditions such as Sturge-Weber (port-wine stain, mental retardation, glaucoma, and seizures), Osler-Weber-Rendu (mucocutaneous telangiectasias and AVMs), and Wyburn-Mason (midbrain AVM, facial nevus in distribution of the trigeminal nerve, and retinal angioma ipsilateral to the facial nevus).

The most common major feeding vessel is the middle cerebral artery, and 80% of lesions are supratentorial. Classically, an AVM is visualized on MRI as a tangled nidus (**Fig. 10.1A,** *arrow*) of dilated vessels supplied by enlarged feeding arteries, with multiple enlarged, tortuous draining veins. AVM arterial supply is most frequently pial but may be dural, especially in infratentorial malformations. Feeding arteries are identified by location and dilatation. As shown in **Fig. 10.1B** where the anterior cerebral artery is feeding an AVM, TOF MRA may be useful in localizing the feeding artery. Aneurysms within feeding arteries occur in ~10% of patients and often regress after AVM treatment. Draining veins (**Fig. 10.1C,D** *black arrow*) appear even larger than feeding arteries—large enough to cause mass effect in some patients—and drain into deep or cortical veins. Because of rapid shunting, draining veins appear as serpentine flow voids on MRI. This differs from the intermediate or high SI typically seen with slow-flowing veins. Contrast administration demonstrates prominent enhancement of the nidus (**Fig. 10.1D**, *white arrow*) and slower flowing venous blood. Rapidly moving arterial blood may still not enhance. Pulsation artifacts, which often appear on nonenhanced images, may be more prominent with contrast administration. The parenchymal gliosis, edema, and ischemia resulting from steal may also be visualized on MRI, typically as increased SI on T2WI. With smaller, untreated lesions, the typical appearance is that of a nidus and associated large draining veins, without gliosis or edema, and little mass effect. MRI is also very sensitive for the detection of superficial siderosis, related to chronic SAH or parenchymal hemorrhage with an AVM. On nonenhanced FSE images, AVMs may be difficult to differentiate from hemorrhagic components (i.e., hemosiderin) or areas of calcification as the low SI of both of these may be confused for flow voids. These entities may be distinguished on GRE T2WI where flowing blood appears of high SI, in contrast to the low SI of dense calcification or hemosiderin. Of note, vessels on GRE T1WI also appear as high SI, an important fact to remember as such scans are often obtained for contrast-enhanced imaging at 3 T.

MRA is comparable to invasive angiography in assessing AVM nidus size and may also demonstrate feeding arteries (**Fig. 10.1B**) and allow visualization of associated aneurysms. Nidus size dictates course of therapy and inversely correlates with prognosis. MRA has several technical drawbacks that must be understood for proper image interpretation. Complex or tortuous arterial flow may appear as signal voids in feeding vessels and some draining veins may not be visualized due to spin saturation. Detection of AVM-associated thrombus on TOF MRA may also be difficult as methemoglobin clot is of high SI—indistinguishable from flow. Obtaining PC MRA avoids this

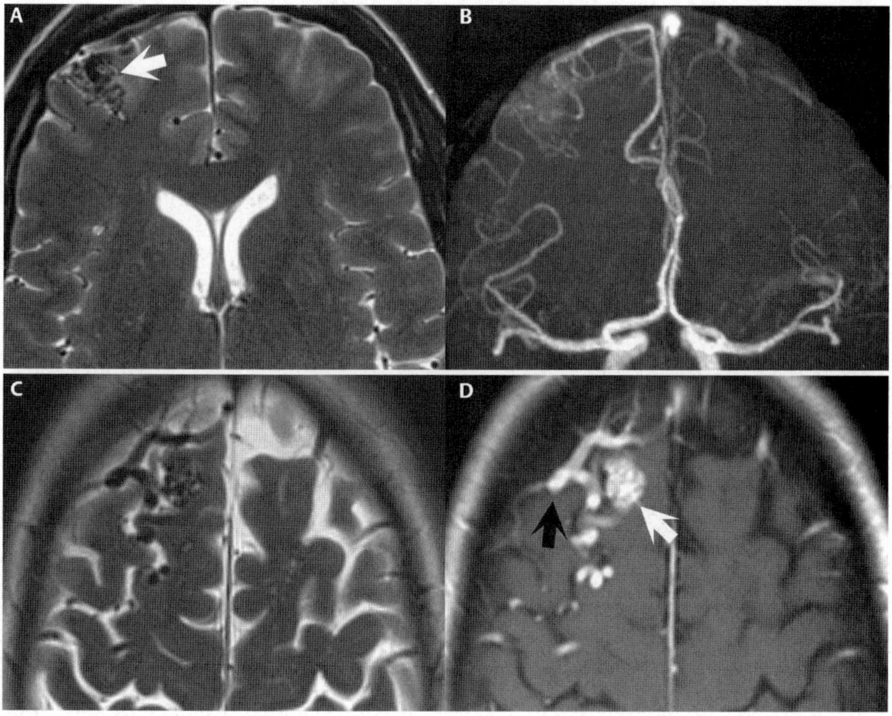

Fig. 10.1 (A–D)

latter problem, allowing differentiation of thrombus from flow. Catheter angiography, for now, remains the standard for preoperative evaluation of AVMs due to its more accurate detection of feeding and draining vessels. However, MRI and MRA are extremely useful, noninvasive preoperative adjuncts and are heavily relied upon for postoperative follow-up.

Dural-based AVMs, unlike the congenital variety above, are often secondary to trauma or inflammatory disease. These lesions may originate in areas of venous or sinus thrombosis where collateralization has occurred. Dural AVMs are usually fed by the external carotid artery and drain into the venous sinuses or cortical veins. Associated SAH or intraparenchymal hemorrhage is frequent. MRA is essential for detection of these lesions when they are adjacent to the inner skull table as both vascular flow and cortical bone appear as signal voids on conventional MRI. Although MRA is better for direct evaluation of dural vessels, clues to the diagnosis of a dural AVM on MRI include sinus thrombosis and dilated cortical veins.

The vein of Galen aneurysm is included in the spectrum of AVMs, and occurs when downstream venous obstruction results in increased flow through the vein due to an AV shunt. Hydrocephalus and increased intracranial pressure may result, as may heart failure in infants. MRI is useful in defining the anatomic extent of vein of Galen aneurysms and in evaluating blood flow patterns or thrombus within the aneurysm. Preoperative angiography remains essential because precise identification of the feeding arteries is necessary.

11 Other Vascular Malformations

Less common vascular malformations, such as cavernous angiomas (malformations), capillary telangiectasias, and venous angiomas, are more frequently angiographically occult than AVMs. MRI is thus the most sensitive imaging modality for their detection. Cavernous angiomas are the second most common type of vascular malformation after AVMs. They consist of a collection of sinusoidal vascular spaces with no intervening brain parenchyma. Cavernous angiomas are often asymptomatic but may present with hemorrhage or seizures. Supratentorial, subcortical lesions predominate, although lesions occur throughout the CNS and are multiple in up to one-third of cases. Cavernous angiomas are classically described as having a "popcorn-like" heterogeneity on T1WI, T2WI (**Figs. 11.1A,B**, *white arrows*), and FLAIR T2WI. Repeated hemorrhage leads to a characteristic thin, well-defined, low SI (on T2WIs), continuous rim of hemosiderin (**Figs. 11.1A,B**). Areas of hemosiderin deposition are best visualized on T2* weighted GRE T2WI (compare **Fig. 11.1B** vs **Fig. 11.1C**, same patient, FSE vs GRE T2WIs) because of the increased sensitivity of GRE to susceptibility effects. GRE T2WI are particularly advantageous over FSE T2WI for revealing additional lesions in patients with multiple cavernous angiomas. However, any type of lesion with a significant susceptibility effect may mimic a cavernous angioma on GRE. High-field (3 T) MRI similarly aids in the detection of hemosiderin. Due to their large vascular spaces, cavernous angiomas typically enhance, often heterogeneously (**Fig. 11.1D**). Cavernous angiomas, particularly one that has recently hemorrhaged, may appear similar to a hemorrhagic neoplasm. The latter is distinguished by its mass effect, the presence of concurrent edema, and the lack of a well-defined hypointense rim. Hemorrhagic cavernous

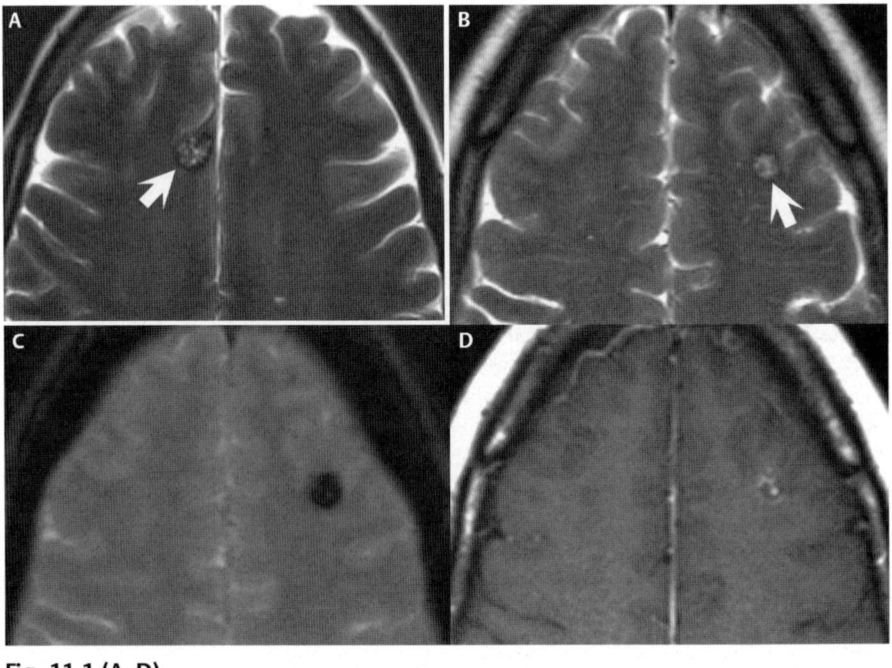

Fig. 11.1 (A–D)

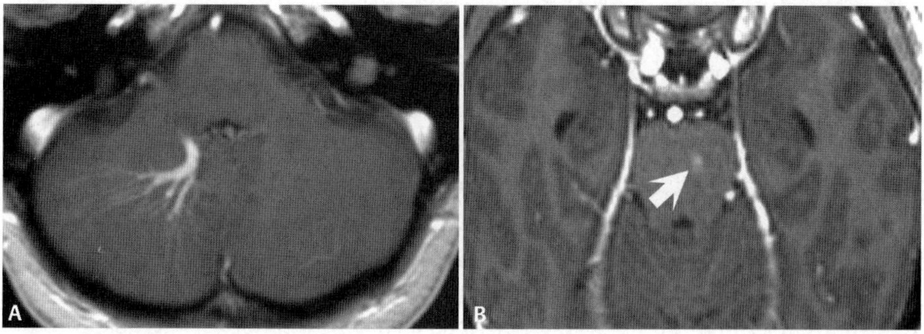

Fig. 11.2 (A,B)

angiomas are differentiated from a simple intraparenchymal hematoma principally by the orderly (temporal) changes in signal characteristics that occur in the latter.

Within the venous circulation, venous angiomas are the most common congenital malformation. They most frequently involve the frontal lobes and posterior fossa and are predominantly asymptomatic, nonsurgical lesions. Because venous angiomas are highly correlated with other cerebrovascular malformations, their identification in a clinically symptomatic patient warrants careful evaluation for the presence of additional vascular abnormalities. They are also part of the Sturge-Weber spectrum of disease (see Chapter 28). The accurate identification of a venous angioma is crucial because they are physiologically competent lesions. This means that if they are removed (in error), then ischemia to the area of brain previously drained by the angioma may occur. A venous angioma (**Fig. 11.2A**) consists of a group of dilated venous tributaries flowing into a larger draining vein in a radial pattern (classically described as caput medusae). On unenhanced MRI these tributaries are visualized as small, curvilinear areas of low SI arranged radially about a larger, solitary flow void—correlating with the draining vein. The flow void of the large draining vein may be the only obvious finding on conventional sequences, or the entire lesion may—due to slow flow—appear isointense to parenchyma, complicating its detection. Contrast-enhanced MRI avoids this problem, offering markedly improved visualization of venous angiomas. Venous angiomas typically enhance with contrast administration (**Fig. 11.2A**). Feeding tributaries are also more reliably visualized with IV contrast.

Capillary telangiectasias are almost uniformly asymptomatic. These lesions consist of dilated capillaries with intervening brain parenchyma. Capillary telangiectasias are predominantly solitary lesions <3 cm in diameter (**Fig. 11.2B**). Unlike cavernous angiomas, capillary telangiectasias most frequently demonstrate no significant abnormality on T1 and T2WI. However, capillary telangiectasias occasionally hemorrhage (mostly asymptomatically), in which case areas of hypointensity, correlating with blood products, may be visible on conventional MRI. GRE T2WI and high-field MRI may again better demonstrate these areas. The defining characteristic of a telangiectasia, however, is the presence of a small, lacy, nodular area of enhancement, in a lesion within the pons (**Fig. 11.2B**, *arrow*). Other differential considerations for an enhancing lesion, such as neoplasia or inflammatory conditions, rarely occur in the absence of signal abnormality on nonenhanced MRI.

12 Aneurysms

Aneurysms are the most common cause of SAH and a frequent cause of intraparenchymal hemorrhage, the imaging features of which were described in previous chapters. Non-ruptured aneurysms are usually asymptomatic, but may cause mass effect or produce emboli from areas of partial thrombosis. Risk factors include smoking and binge drinking, along with collagen vascular, connective tissue, and polycystic kidney diseases. Intracranial aneurysms frequently occur in the feeding arteries of AVMs, presumably from increased flow. Aneurysms are broadly classified into fusiform (spindle-shaped) and saccular (spherical) types. Fusiform aneurysms frequently occur secondary to arteriosclerosis and favor the basilar and intracranial carotid arteries. Saccular or berry aneurysms are far more common and result from a congenital defect in the tunica media. These aneurysms involve, in decreasing frequency, the anterior communicating (**Fig. 12.1A**, *white arrow*), posterior communicating (**Figs. 12.1B,C**, *white arrows*), and middle cerebral arteries (MCAs). MCA involvement frequently occurs at the bifurcation or trifurcation. Flow dynamics at arterial branch points render these favorable locations for aneurysm development.

MRI is the noninvasive screening test of choice for the detection and evaluation of intracranial aneurysms. TOF MRA is the specific sequence of choice, with maximum intensity projection (MIP; **Figs. 12.1A,B,F**) or volume rendering (**Fig. 12.1C**) used to create images for viewing. Although not commonly employed acutely, except in cases with a low clinical probability of hemorrhage or when angiography is contraindicated, MRI is also the preferred modality for monitoring previously treated aneurysms. Extreme care must be exercised to avoid imaging a patient with a ferromagnetic aneurysm clip (these were used in the distant past), as doing so may result in patient death. FSE sequences demonstrate areas of fast vascular flow as signal loss. This occurs when protons within blood do not remain within a selected slice long enough to acquire both the 90- and 180-degree pulses needed to produce a spin echo (SE). Saccular aneurysms are no exception, appearing as an enlarged flow void (**Fig. 12.1D**) corresponding with the focally dilated vasculature. Regions of slower-flowing blood within an aneurysm produce high or mixed SI rather than flow voids. The identification of one aneurysm on MRI warrants a careful search for additional lesions as aneurysms are multiple in up to one-fourth of cases. Pulsation artifacts, propagating in the phase-encoding direction, may be seen with patent aneurysms. Identification of this artifact, however, is not a reliable marker for aneurysms in the prepontine cistern as CSF pulsation artifact may simulate a basilar artery aneurysm in this region. Pulsation artifacts are more prominent following contrast administration. Both normal vasculature and patent aneurysms fill with contrast during the arterial phase and are thus high SI on T1WI. Giant aneurysms are defined as having a diameter >2.5 cm (**Figs. 12.1D,E,F).** Giant aneurysms frequently involve the internal carotid artery (ICA; as illustrated), MCA, and the tip of the basilar artery. A partially thrombosed giant aneurysm may appear similar to an intraparenchymal hematoma on MRI. The former demonstrates flow voids within any residual patent lumen, commonly surrounded by a high SI rim corresponding to extracellular methemoglobin. This is in distinction to the peripheral pattern of methemoglobin formation initially seen in an intraparenchymal hematoma. Different stages of organized clot within the thrombosed portion of an aneurysm manifest as layers of various mixed SI surrounding the high SI methemoglobin rim. The location of a parenchymal hemorrhage (and likewise SAH)

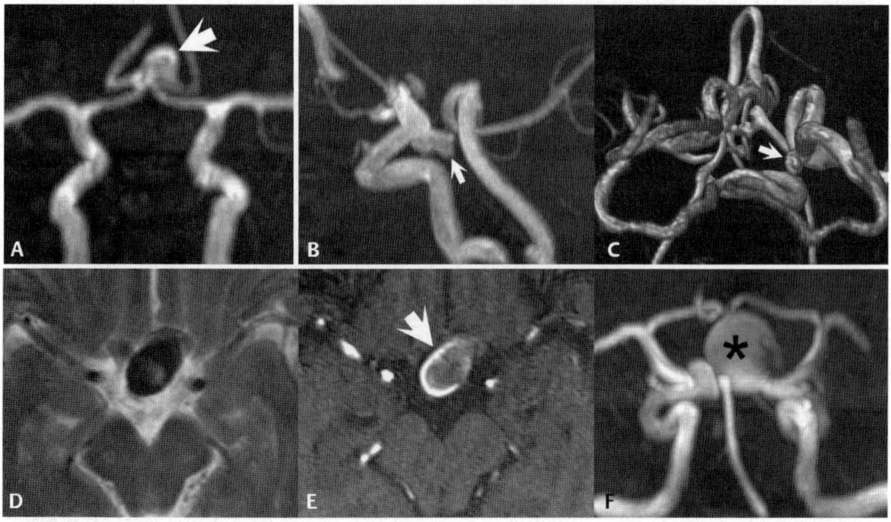

Fig. 12.1 (A–F)

may suggest the location of the culprit aneurysm. An intraparenchymal hematoma adjacent to the anterior interhemispheric fissure may be caused by a ruptured ACA aneurysm, while a hematoma adjacent to the sylvian fissure suggests a ruptured MCA.

TOF MRA depicts over 90% of aneurysms >3 mm in diameter. Aneurysms <3 mm in diameter typically do not rupture. Both the thin-section (source) images (**Fig. 12.1E**) and MIP images—rotated both right to left and tumbled—should be reviewed. MIP images oriented in sagittal (**Fig. 12.1B)** and coronal (**Figs. 12.1A,F**) planes are illustrated. Volume-rendering technique reconstructions may also aid in aneurysm visualization (**Fig. 12.1C**). Particularly in internal carotid lesions, the neck of an aneurysm may not be visualized. In this case, targeted reconstructions, shorter TEs, and a smaller voxel size may be helpful.

With TOF MRA, the SI of stationary tissue is suppressed. Rapidly flowing blood is identified due to its relatively high SI. In large aneurysms, however, the flow within may be sufficiently slow to be suppressed. Thus, as demonstrated in **Fig. 12.1E** (*white arrow*), large or giant aneurysms may demonstrate heterogeneous SI on TOF MRA, with a fast-flowing, relatively small stream of blood—appearing as high SI—flowing into a larger area of relatively stagnant blood—appearing as low SI. Because of this heterogeneous signal, MIP images (**Fig. 12.1F**, *asterisk*) may not fully visualize the aneurysm. Comparison of pre- and postcontrast images and the use of phase-contrast MRA (PC-MRA) are possible alternatives in this instance. These two approaches also allow better differentiation of intraaneurysmal clot than TOF MRA where the high SI clot (from methemoglobin) may not be distinguishable from the high SI of flowing blood.

13 Ischemia and Infarction I

Cerebrovascular disease is the most common neurologic disease encountered by the practicing radiologist. Diffusion-weighted MRI (DWI) demonstrates a high sensitivity for ischemia within 15 to 30 minutes of symptom onset. DWI exploits the differences in the diffusibility of intra- and extracellular water. The lack of availability of adenosine triphosphate (i.e., ATP) in ischemic tissue results in the failure of sodium–potassium exchange pumps. Pump failure results in increased intracellular sodium and thus water. This increase in intracellular water without an increase in overall tissue water is known as cytotoxic edema. Intracellular water is relatively restricted in its diffusion by the cell membrane and intracellular organelles, and this restriction is visualized as high SI on DWI scans. Although DWI is sensitive for the detection of cytotoxic edema, it is also a T2WI. An area of increased SI on DWI may represent either pure restriction of diffusion or additional components of increased SI from its T2-weighted component ("T2 shine through"). Thus an area of high SI on DWI must be correlated with an ADC map on which a true diffusion restriction appears as low SI. In the absence of DWI abnormality, ADC maps need not be examined. DWI detects brain ischemia much earlier than FLAIR or T2WI on which ischemia is visualized commonly after 6 hours and almost uniformly after 24 hours of symptom onset. These sequences detect the vasogenic edema present in later stages of brain ischemia. Vasogenic edema occurs when edematous cells lyse and vascular endothelium is destroyed, resulting in the release of water into the extracellular space. Increasing extracellular edema may lead to mass effect and compression of adjacent vessels, thus extending the original infarct. FLAIR images, in which CSF SI is suppressed, are preferred over conventional T2WI for the visualization of vasogenic edema, particularly in periventricular and sulcal locations.

Strokes may be characterized by timeframe as hyperacute, acute, subacute, and chronic. Hyperacute strokes are defined as being <6 hours after symptom onset. Although these may not be commonly seen clinically due to delays in patient presentation, the detection of hyperacute strokes is essential as IV thrombolytic intervention is often utilized within 3 hours of ischemic insult. As demonstrated in **Fig. 13.1A**, a hyperacute stroke is not accompanied by SI changes on T2WI or FLAIR (illustrated) scans. DWI, however, clearly demonstrates a hyperacute stroke as an area of high SI (**Fig. 13.1B**, *arrow*), which is confirmed as a true diffusion restriction by a corresponding region of decreased SI on an ADC map (**Fig. 13.1C**). An acute stroke is defined as being from 6 to 24 hours from symptom onset. These are typically well-seen on DWI, FLAIR, and T2WI (**Fig. 13.1D**) as areas of increased SI. Because a multitude of other entities may appear similar on T2WI and FLAIR, DWI may be useful to distinguish the restricted diffusion typical of stroke (**Fig. 13.1E**, *asterisk*) from neoplasia or other entities in which the diffusibility of water often remains unchanged. The appearance of subacute (24 hours to 6 weeks) stroke is dominated by vasogenic edema, which correlates with high SI on T2WI and low SI on T1WI. SI on DWI begins to decline in the first week following stroke and typically normalizes by week 2. ADC values likewise normalize within the first week and increase thereafter, owing to increased water diffusibility allowed for by the destruction of neurons. Resorption of extracellular edema typifies the chronic phase of stroke (after 6 weeks). Gliotic changes are prominent, correlating with increased SI on FLAIR (**Fig. 13.1F**, *white arrows*) and T2WI (**Fig. 13.1G**) and decreased SI on T1WI. Encephalomalacia results from the replacement of atrophic brain parenchyma with free water. These areas are distinguished from gliosis by their isointensity with CSF on

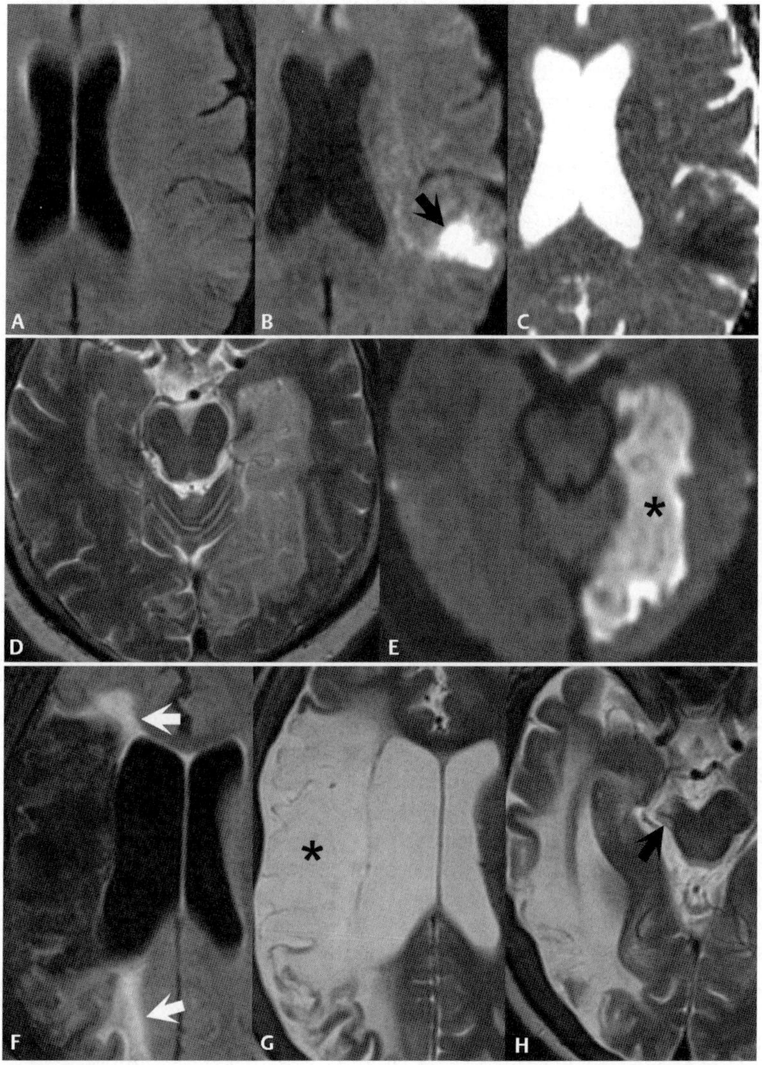

Fig. 13.1 (A–H)

all pulse sequences (**Figs. 13.1F,G**, *asterisk*). **Figure 13.1G** also demonstrates widened cortical sulci and ex vacuo ventricular dilatation, which provide further MRI evidence of parenchymal atrophy. Wallerian (anterograde) degeneration of the myelinated axons distal to the site of ischemic injury may be appreciated on MRI as asymmetry of the cerebral peduncles (**Fig. 13.1H**, *black arrow*) resulting from the loss of axonal mass ipsilateral to the infarct. The peduncles may also demonstrate gliotic changes (**Fig. 13.1H**, *black arrows*) correlating with increased SI on T2WI.

The distribution of supratentorial strokes corresponds with the vascular supplies of the ACA, MCA, and PCA. The MCA supplies the majority of the lateral surface of the cerebrum, the insula, and the anterior and lateral parts of the temporal lobes. It is the most commonly infarcted vascular territory. MCA infarctions most commonly involve either the anterior or posterior (**Figs. 13.1A,B,C**) portion of the MCA distribution but may involve the entire territory of the artery (**Figs. 13.1F,G,H**). The MCA is divided into named segments (M1–M4). The M1 segment is proximal to the bi- or trifurcation of the artery; the M2 segment extends from this location to the origin of the MCA's cortical branches. The M3 segment consists of the portion of the artery within the sylvian fissure, and M4 refers to those branches emerging from the fissure and extending onto the surface of the hemisphere. The PCA is the second most common vascular distribution involved in ischemic stroke and supplies the occipital lobe along with the medial parietal and temporal lobes. The posterior communicating artery divides the PCA into proximal (P1) and distal (P2) segments. **Figures 13.1D and 13.1E** demonstrate an infarction involving the entire distribution of the PCA including its medial temporal component. Infarcts of the distribution of the ACA account for less than 3% of cases. This is due in part to the access of the ACA to the circulation of its contralateral counterpart via the anterior communicating artery. The ACA supplies the anterior two-thirds of the medial cerebral surface, the corpus callosum, and 1 cm of superomedial brain over the convexity. ACA infarctions involving the callosum may be confused with lymphoma on MRI with the latter also demonstrating restricted diffusion due to its dense cellularity. Clinical correlation and the progression of the lesion's appearance over time may aid in diagnosis. Thrombosis of the distal portion of the internal carotid artery may, in individuals without effective cervical collateral vasculature or an incomplete circle of Willis, result in infarction of both the ACA and MCA territories.

Although contrast administration is not routinely used in the evaluation of stroke, often ischemic lesions are visualized on enhanced studies. Enhancement of the meninges adjacent to a large territorial infarct is rare but may be seen in infarcts 2 to 6 days old. The vessels supplying an infarct may enhance in strokes of 1 to 3 days of age. Vascular enhancement persists as long as the infarcted area remains without perfusion and dissipates with the establishment of collateral flow. With collateral flow, endothelial damage and loss of the BBB lead to parenchymal enhancement within the infarct in either an early intense or progressive pattern. Early intense enhancement occurs within 2 to 3 days and may predominate in cases of incomplete ischemia whereby contrast material is still delivered to ischemic tissues even at early stages of infarction. Progressive enhancement is first seen at 1 week and develops in a gyriform (if cortical) or uniform (if noncortical) pattern. Because of the time required for contrast to infiltrate the parenchymal space, scans obtained 5 to 10 minutes postinjection best demonstrate parenchymal enhancement. Disruption of the BBB and thus parenchymal enhancement rarely persists beyond 8 weeks.

14 Ischemia and Infarction II

Lacunar infarcts are small deep parenchymal lesions involving the basal ganglia, internal capsule, thalamus, and brainstem. The vascular supply of these areas includes the anterior choroidal artery of the supraclinoid portion of the ICA, the lenticulostriate branches of the ACA and MCA, the thalamoperforating branches of the posterior cerebral arteries (PCA), and the paramedian branches of the basilar artery. These infarcts are associated with chronic hypertension and may present clinically with pure motor or sensory deficits. On MRI lacunar infarcts appear as focal slitlike or ovoid areas, progressing in appearance similarly to the infarcts described in Chapter 13. The lenticulostriate branches of the MCA originate prior to the artery's bi- or trifurcation (M1 segment) to supply the basal ganglia and the anterior limb of the internal capsule. Thus ischemic disease involving the MCA prior the branching of the lenticulostriate arteries may involve its hemispheric distribution along with deep gray and white matter structures. A similar phenomenon is seen with the thalamoperforating arteries of the PCA. **Figure 14.1A** demonstrates acute ischemia of the lentiform nucleus, which consists of the globus pallidus (medially) and the putamen (laterally), shown on a DWI scan. Note that the susceptibility effects of iron within the globus pallidus result in this structure's low SI on T2WI (such as DWI) at 3 T (**Fig. 14.1A**). **Figure 14.1B** demonstrates in the same patient an acute infarction of the head of the caudate as seen on DWI. The head of the caudate is supplied by the recurrent artery of Heubner, which arises from the ACA to also supply the anterior limb of the internal capsule and part of the putamen. The anterior choroidal artery, arising from the supraclinoid internal carotid, also supplies portions of the caudate, along with the posterior limb of the internal capsule and parts of the thalamus, globus pallidus, and cerebral peduncles. DWI is particularly useful in the evaluation of lacunar strokes, due to the tendency of chronic small vessel ischemia to obscure the appearance of high SI infarcts on FLAIR (**Fig. 14.1C**) and T2WI. Such lesions are clearly differentiated from chronic ischemic changes on DWI (**Fig. 14.1B**). Lesions of multiple sclerosis (see Chapter 18), Binswanger disease (a triad of hypertension, hydrocephalus, and dementia), and hypertensive encephalopathy are similarly easily distinguished from acute and early subacute lacunar infarcts.

The thalamoperforating arteries arise from the P1 segment of the PCA. These supply the medial ventral thalamus and the posterior limb of the internal capsule. An infarction of this region, as seen on DWI, is denoted by a *white arrow* in **Fig. 14.1D**. Dilated perivascular spaces (DPVSs) surrounding vessels coursing through the brain may also masquerade as lacunar infarcts on T2WI because of their high SI and location. DPVSs are seen in the basal ganglia, periatrial and supraventricular white matter, and at the midbrain junction of the substantia nigra and cerebral peduncle. Unlike lacunar infarcts, they are isointense to CSF on FLAIR and do not demonstrate restricted diffusion.

The vertebrobasilar arterial system supplies the posterior fossa. Of brainstem strokes, isolated infarctions of the midbrain are rarest. The midbrain derives its vascular supply from perforating arteries arising from the posterior communicating artery and the PCA. The PCA arises as a branch of the basilar artery, while the posterior communicating arteries connect the carotid and vertebrobasilar systems by linking the MCA and PCA. Pontine strokes are more common. The paramedian branches of the basilar artery supply the medial aspect of the pons—an infarction of which is demonstrated in **Fig. 14.1E** on DWI. The lateral pons is supplied by the anterior inferior cerebellar artery (AICA) caudally and the superior cerebellar artery (SCA) rostrally. Infarctions of the lateral medulla result in a constellation of symptoms known as

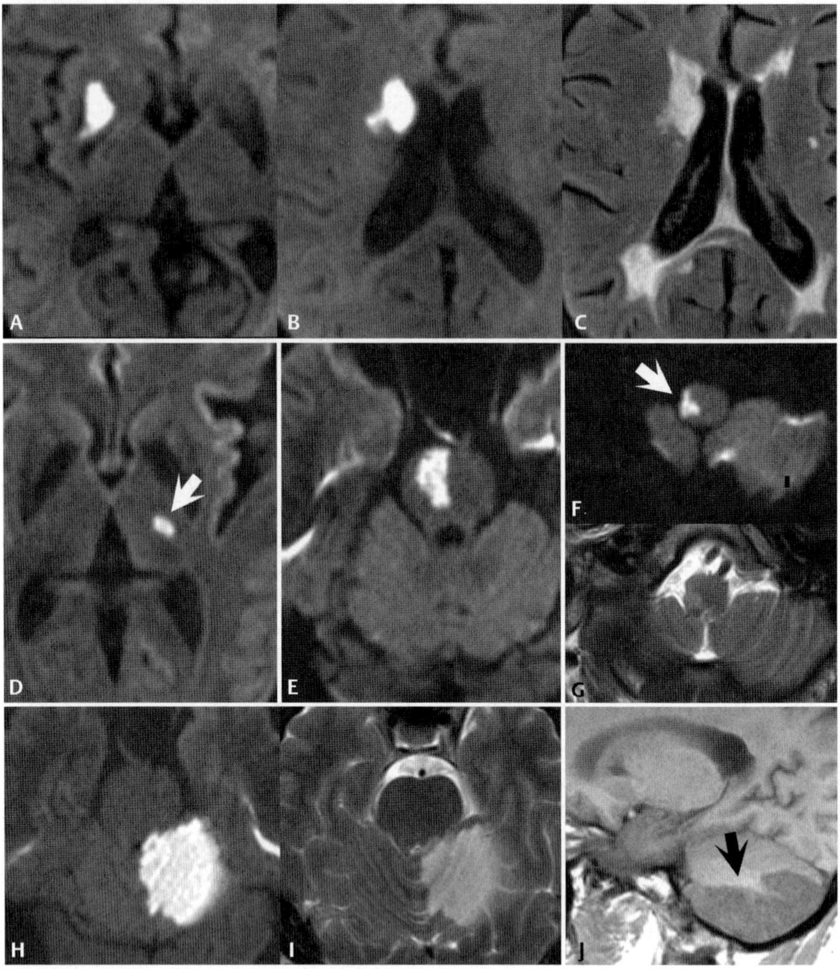

Fig. 14.1 (A–J)

Wallenberg syndrome. These strokes (as seen on DWI and T2WI in **Fig. 14.1F,** *white arrow* and **Fig. 14.1G**, respectively) are particularly devastating and result from interruption of blood supply to the posterior inferior cerebellar artery (PICA). Occlusions of the perforating branches of the basilar artery or vertebral arteries result in medial medullary infarcts. PICA, AICA, and the SCA supply the cerebellum. The SCA arises from the basilar artery just prior to its termination as the PCA. **Figures 14.1H** and **14.1I** demonstrate an infarct affecting the entirety of the SCA's distribution on diffusion and T2WI, respectively. **Figure 14.1J** demonstrates an infarct of the PICA territory, seen with low SI (*black arrow*) on this T1WI. PICA is the largest intracranial branch of the vertebral artery and supplies the posterior inferior portion of the cerebellum and the lateral medulla. Infarctions of PICA may also involve the cerebellar tonsils. AICA arises from the basilar artery just subsequent to its origin at the junction of the vertebral arteries and supplies the anterior inferior portion of the cerebellum and the lateral pons.

Distinct underlying etiologies of stroke may result in differing MRI appearances. In addition to the infarctions described above, thrombotic, embolic, hemodynamic, and venous (see Chapter 20) infarctions may occur. Arterial thrombotic infarctions are most common, usually resulting from atherosclerotic narrowing and eventual occlusion of vessel lumen. The extent of infarction is determined by the location and extent of obstruction (proximal lesions are less likely to develop infarctions), the availability of collateral circulation, and the integrity of the systemic circulation. Thrombotic infarctions tend to be sharply demarcated, wedge-shaped lesions confined to a single arterial distribution and extending to the cortical surface. The appearance of the cerebellar infarct in **Figs. 14.1H,I** typify that of a thrombotic infarction of the SCA. This appearance of a cerebellar infarction is uncommonly encountered in clinical practice, however, as cerebellar infarctions appear more frequently as multiple, chronic, punctate lesions. Differential considerations for an early thrombotic infarct on DWI include hyperacute hemorrhage, neoplasm, and abscess. None of these localize to an arterial territory, while the former undergoes a classic progression in MRI appearance as described in Chapter 8. Neoplastic lesions and abscesses are usually centered in white matter, whereas thrombotic infarctions involve gray matter as well. Cortically extending neoplasms also demonstrate edema projecting in a finger-like pattern with ill-defined margins and an associated centrally enhancing mass. If enhancing, thrombotic infarctions should do so in a wedge-shaped pattern. Embolic infarctions, the source of which is most frequently the heart, are often multiple and may simultaneously affect more than one arterial distribution. The presence of septic emboli is suggested by the concurrent presence of infarction and abscess. Occluding emboli tend to fragment and lyse between days 1 and 5, reestablishing normal circulation. Luxury perfusion or hyperemia following embolic lysis may lead to hemorrhagic conversion of the infarct due to a higher perfusion pressure. These hemorrhages usually appear petechial in nature and cortical in location, although a large hematoma may occasionally develop.

The MRI appearance of a hemorrhagic infarct varies with the stage of its blood products. When hemorrhagic stroke is suspected clinically, GRE T2WI should be obtained due to their high sensitivity for paramagnetic blood products and the important implications that the presence of hemorrhage has for the clinical management of stroke. Hemodynamic infarctions occur because of the failure of the heart to pump sufficient blood to oxygenate the brain. Watershed regions at the margins of major arterial distributions—areas with the lowest perfusion pressure—are most frequently involved in these infarctions. Watershed areas include the junctions of the distributions of the anterior, middle, and PCAs. The parieto-occipital watershed region—at the junction of all three of the aforementioned arteries—is especially susceptible to injury. Within the cerebellum, the major watershed area is at the junction of the SCA and the PICA territories.

15 Periventricular Leukomalacia

Periventricular leukomalacia (PVL) is the most common ischemic brain injury of prematurity, occurring in up to one-fourth of such infants. Sequelae include cerebral palsy and mental retardation. PVL results from watershed hypoperfusion, which progresses to infarction. Premature infants have collateral circulation between the meninges and cerebral arteries, which protect the cortex from such infarction. Thus, the periventricular white matter, often specifically that adjacent to the atrial trigone or frontal horn, is most frequently involved. This produces a pattern of ischemia similar to that of chronic small vessel disease of the elderly, but distinct from that of severe prenatal asphyxia, which involves the brainstem and deep cortical white matter. MRI is rarely used acutely in preterm infants suspected of PVL, but may easily detect mild to moderate disease missed on ultrasound. DWI, in particular, may be extremely sensitive for the acute detection of PVL. A follow-up MRI in symptomatic infants often confirms the diagnosis, demonstrating areas of increased SI on T2WI and FLAIR scans (**Fig. 15.1A**) correlating with gliosis. Care must be taken to distinguish pathologic edema from the normal high water content of white matter, particularly in the occipital-parietal periventricular white matter where terminal zones of myelination may persist for years. PVL may be further distinguished by the presence of ex vacuo dilatation resulting from white matter loss. **Figure 15.1B** demonstrates a common appearance of such dilatation, showing the markedly enlarged, somewhat irregular posterior aspects of the lateral ventricles encroaching abnormally closely to the cortical gyri and sulci. Marked callosal thinning may also be apparent on sagittal images. Chronically, the lesions of PVL may progress to cystic cavitation manifesting as high SI on T2WI.

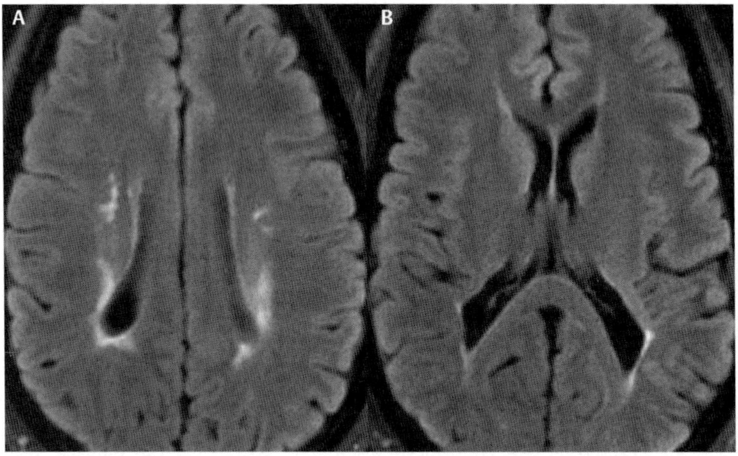

Fig. 15.1 (A,B)

16 Diffuse Axonal Injury

Diffuse axonal injury (DAI) is the most common parenchymal injury occurring in trauma, and results from acceleration–deceleration or rotational force injuries. In these injuries, force differentials in adjacent areas of brain result in axonal shearing. DAI is staged by lesion location. Stage 1 lesions have the best prognosis and occur in the lobar white matter, usually at the gray–white matter junction (**Figs. 16.1A,B**). Stage 2 lesions involve the corpus callosum (**Fig. 16.1C**, *black arrow*), most commonly in the splenium and posterior portions. This pattern is related to the relatively narrow anterior falx, which allows for transient hemispheric herniation in lieu of axonal shearing. Stage 3 DAI is the most severe and involves the brainstem (**Fig. 16.1D**, *black arrow*), most frequently the midbrain and superior pons. The appearance of DAI on conventional MRI is initially related to tissue swelling and edema. Thus, areas of axonal injury appear somewhat hypointense on T1WI and hyperintense on T2WI and FLAIR scans (**Figs. 16.1A,C**). Such lesions are classically described as ellipses with long axes paralleling the direction of axonal fibers. While T2WI are sensitive to DAI, the high SI of nearby CSF may make lesions that are near sulci or the ventricular system much less evident. Thus, FLAIR T2WI are the FSE sequence of choice for detection of DAI. The appearance of hemorrhagic DAI on MRI is variable, specifically depending upon the stage of blood products (see Chapter 8).

Because of their increased sensitivity to the susceptibility effect of paramagnetic substances, GRE T2WI (**Figs. 16.1B,D**) must be obtained when DAI is suspected. Such scans are used primarily to detect blood products, which are seen as areas of low SI (**Figs. 16.1B,D**), due to the presence of deoxyhemoglobin acutely. High sensitivity to hemosiderin also enables improved detection of chronic DAI with GRE: lesions remain hypointense for years with GRE after they have become unapparent on FSE MRI. DWI is less sensitive to DAI than the aforementioned sequences, but may detect mild shear injuries that are otherwise inapparent. DAI lesions demonstrate restricted diffusion within the first 2 to 3 weeks of injury. Diffusion tensor imaging may demonstrate decreased diffusion along white matter tracts (anisotropy) in the setting of DAI, correlating with axonal shearing.

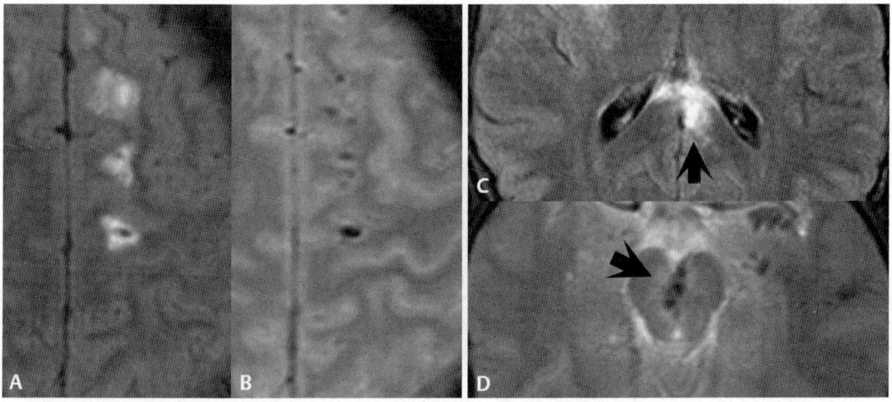

Fig. 16.1 (A–D)

17 Neurodegenerative Disorders

Age-related changes of the brain are commonly seen in clinical MRI. Findings include decreased SI in the basal ganglia from chronic iron deposition, atrophy, and foci of high SI on FLAIR and T2WI. These findings may be asymptomatic or pathologic. Diffuse atrophy is frequently visualized in Alzheimer disease as widening of the cortical sulci and dilatation of the ventricular system (ex vacuo hydrocephalus). The latter finding without corresponding sulcal widening, however, suggests a nonatrophic cause. In Alzheimer, atrophy of the hippocampal structures and temporal lobes may be especially prominent, as demonstrated in the sagittal T1WI and axial T2WI of **Figs. 17.1A,B**. Sulcal enlargement with diminution of the vermis and folia characterizes cerebellar atrophy as seen in **Figs. 17.2A,B**. Etiologies for cerebellar atrophy vary by age, with findings in a younger patient suggesting a primary cause like fragile-X syndrome, Friedreich, or spinocerebellar ataxia. Secondary atrophy may preferentially involve the vermis and pontocerebellar tracts and is seen in chronic phenytoin use (the etiology in **Fig. 17.2**) and alcoholism. Bilateral atrophy of the caudate nuclei (**Fig. 17.3A**, *black arrows*) is best visualized on thin-section, coronal T1WIs and is associated with Huntington chorea. The putamen, globus pallidus, and even cortex may demonstrate similar findings. Atrophy or enhancement (**Fig. 17.3B**, *white arrows*) of the mamillary bodies suggests Wernicke encephalopathy—another alcohol-related condition. In acute Wernicke encephalopathy, abnormal high SI on FLAIR images may be seen in the mamillary bodies, brainstem, and medial thalami.

Figure 17.4A demonstrates areas of white matter hyperintensity consistent with the appearance of chronic small vessel ischemic disease on FLAIR images. In **Fig. 17.4B** similar high SI white matter lesions are present, but the gray and white matter is readily differentiable and sulcal widening is absent suggesting a younger brain. In fact, white matter lesions such as displayed in these images are nonspecific and may reflect changes of small vessel ischemia (**Fig. 17.4A**, findings in an 80-year-old man), lupus (**Fig. 17.4B**, findings in a 30-year-old woman), multiple sclerosis (**Fig. 18.1D**), acute or subacute infarctions (**Figs. 14.1A,B,C**), or a variety of other conditions. Mild chronic small vessel white matter ischemic disease exhibits only a few, small, scattered hyperintense foci on FLAIR or T2WI, whereas severe disease is marked by lesion coalescence. Correlation with additional pulse sequences (on which small vessel ischemic disease is not typically apparent) may be diagnostically helpful. Lesions with restricted diffusion or contrast enhancement favor acute or subacute ischemia, although active multiple sclerosis (MS) plaques may also enhance. MS plaques involve certain locations characteristically, and some may appear as low SI on T1WI (see Chapter 18). Lupus and other vasculitides may involve gray and white matter (like MS) but tend to spare

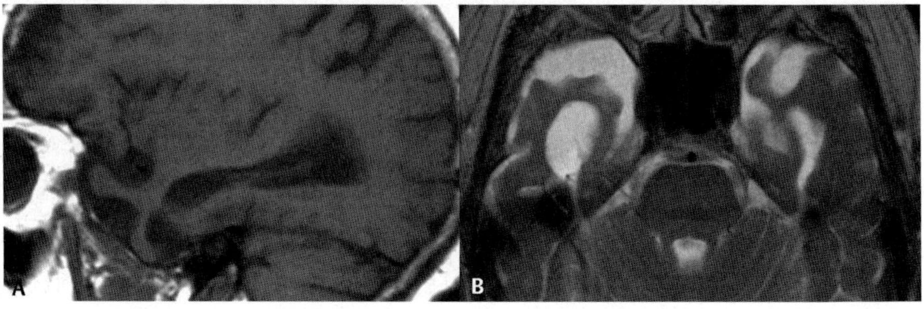

Fig. 17.1 (A,B)

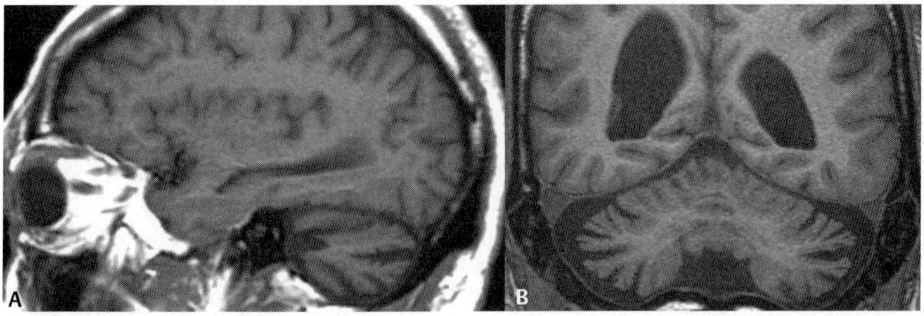

Fig. 17.2 (A,B)

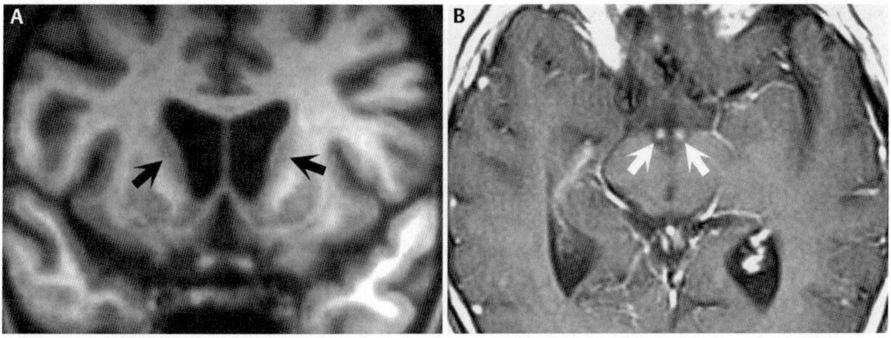

Fig. 17.3 (A,B)

periventricular tissue and may occur within a clear arterial distribution. Lesions may also be of low SI on GRE T2WI, correlating with hemorrhagic blood products. Secondary vasculitis is commonly caused by and may be seen concurrently with the MRI findings of meningitis (see Chapter 21). Reversible, occipital-dominant white matter lesions favor hypertensive encephalopathy. Additional differential considerations for the lesions in **Fig. 17.4** include sickle cell, migraine disorders, and Binswanger disease (a clinical triad of dementia, hypertension, and hydrocephalus).

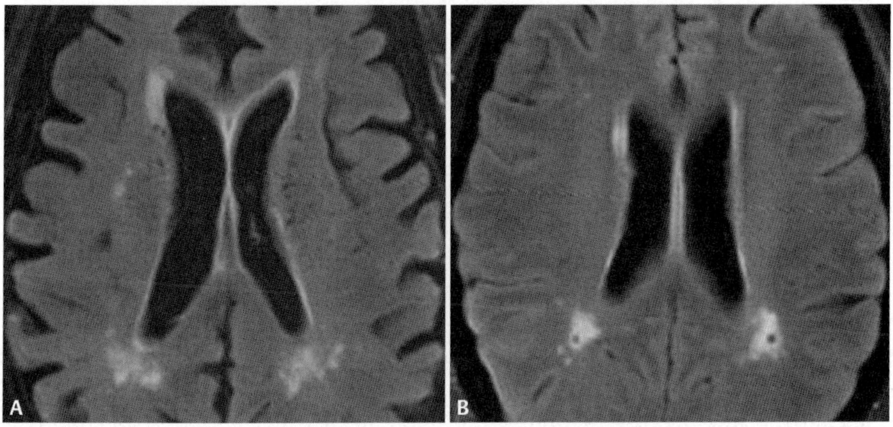

Fig. 17.4 (A,B)

18 Multiple Sclerosis

An international committee has developed specific MRI criteria for the diagnosis of MS, which include three of the following disseminated in time: (1) a gadolinium-enhancing brain or spinal cord lesion or a total of nine T2-hyperintense lesions, (2) one infratentorial or spinal cord lesion, (3) one juxtacortical lesion, and (4) three periventricular lesions. MRI is the most sensitive test for MS, although findings may be confused with those of small vessel ischemia. A younger, female patient favors MS, and given the high prevalence of small vessel disease, older patients must not be diagnosed with MS based solely on imaging. **Figure 18.1A** demonstrates the typical pattern of disease on FLAIR scans, with small focal areas of abnormal high SI—correlating pathologically with edema and gliosis—scattered throughout the periventricular white matter. Periventricular lesions are nonspecific for MS, as opposed to callosal lesions—best seen on sagittal FLAIR images as in **Fig. 18.1B** (*white arrow*). These are typically oval-shaped with a flat inferior border, line the ependymal surface, and are oriented perpendicular to the lateral ventricle. Such findings are sometimes overlooked on axial scans (**Fig. 18.1A,** *black arrow*), with the clue being that they are medial to the lateral ventricles. Other more specific areas for plaques include the centrum semiovale, the major and minor forceps, and the white matter surrounding the atrial trigones, temporal, and occipital horns of the lateral ventricles. In the posterior fossa, lesions of the colliculi, middle cerebellar peduncles, and pons are characteristic. Gray matter is less frequently involved. The contrast-enhanced T1WI in **Fig. 18.1C** displays a nonenhancing plaque with low SI (*black arrow*). Such "black hole" lesions represent areas of axon loss and signify a poor prognosis. Because small vessel ischemic disease is not well-seen on T1WI, the presence of these lesions favors MS. With contrast administration, plaques may enhance in a uniform, punctate, or ringed pattern (*white arrow*), often with progression to the latter over time. Enhancement signifies an active lesion and is thus seen in a minority of cases, persisting for less than a month when present. Triple-dose contrast improves detection of active lesions; steroid therapy decreases enhancement. The concurrent presence of enhancing and nonenhancing lesions is fairly unique to MS and may help rule out otherwise similar appearing conditions.

The progression of MS over time is marked by increasingly confluent lesions with a resultant loss their punctate appearance, rendering them even less distinct from lesions of small vessel ischemia. The FLAIR images of **Figs. 18.1D,E** display the progression of high SI (correlating with gliosis in chronic MS) periventricular lesions in scans performed on the same patient but 3 years apart. Lesion confluence lends the periventricular lesions a "lumpy bumpy" outer margin, distinct from the often smooth outer margins of small vessel ischemia. Ventricular prominence, widening of the sulci (seen progressively from **Figs. 18.1D,E**), and callosal thinning (from Wallerian degeneration) may also occur in chronic MS. The lesions in **Fig. 18.1E** hint at the fact that consolidated plaques may acquire a tumefactive appearance. In about half of cases, tumefactive lesions enhance in a thin, open-ringed pattern, although their lack of mass effect, diminishment with steroid therapy, and loss of enhancement over time aid in distinguishing them from neoplasia. Unlike abscesses and vasculitic lesions, ADC values in tumefactive MS are elevated, whereas vasculitic disease may be further differentiated by areas of low SI on GRE T2WI correlating with hemorrhage. Cord and optic nerve lesions comprise the remaining spectrum of MS. Optic neuritis is the most common initial manifestation with findings including abnormal high SI on T2WI within the

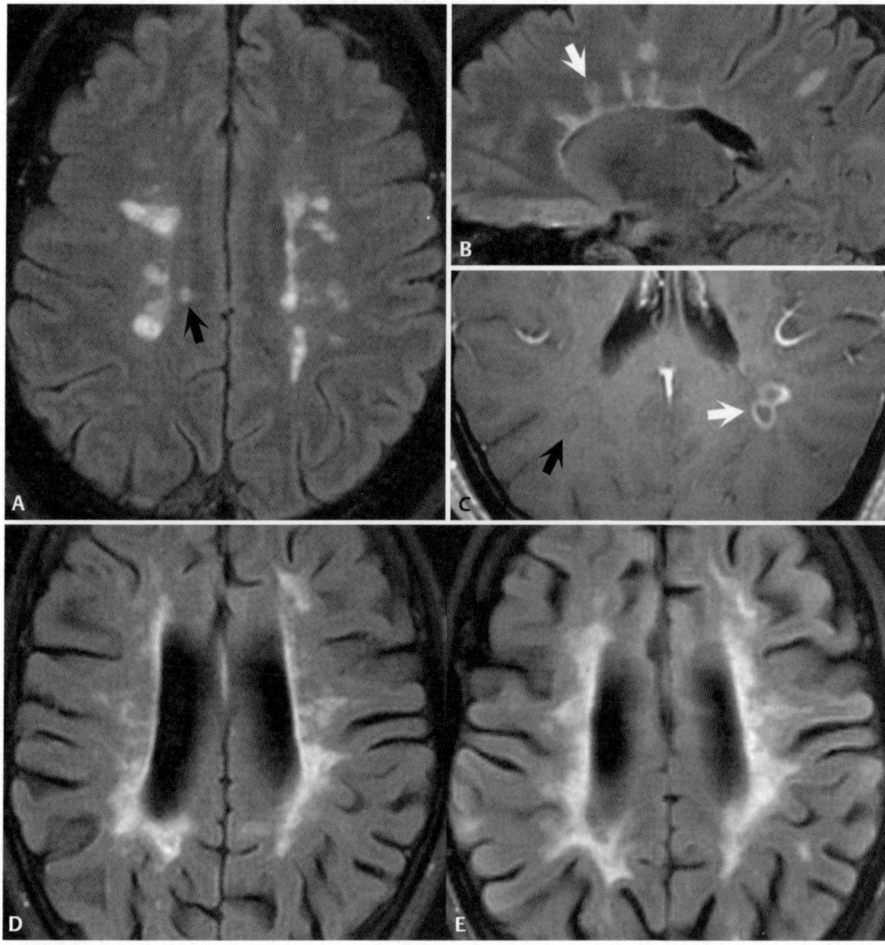

Fig. 18.1 (A–E)

optic nerve, best seen on images with fat suppression. Lesions of optic neuritis may also enhance.

Acute disseminated encephalomyelitis (ADEM) is an inflammatory, demyelinating disorder of white matter that may mimic MS on MRI. Unlike MS, it occurs predominantly in children (following viral infections and immunizations), and is associated with a monophasic course and near-complete clinical recovery. Multiple foci of demyelination may be seen on MRI, but are fewer in number than those of MS. Asymmetric involvement of the hemispheres along with the brainstem and cerebellum are frequent. With clinical improvement, MRI changes may completely resolve.

19 Parenchymal Infections

Pyogenic abscesses most frequently arise hematogenously, seeding the brain at the gray–white matter junction. They may also occur as sequelae of contiguously spreading sinus infections (see Chapter 20) or trauma. *Streptococcus* is the most common etiologic organism, followed by *staphylococcus* and *pneumococcus*. Abscesses favor the frontal and parietal lobes within the MCA distribution, and their early appearance is one of a diffuse cerebritis, consisting of infiltrating lymphocytes. This infiltrate enhances heterogeneously, and demonstrates high SI on T2WI with low to moderate SI on T1WI. Within the first week, a central necrotic area forms, an area subsequently enveloped by collagen in the second week. This collagen wall appears as a rim of low SI on T2WI and may be surrounded by a disproportionate amount of edema (**Fig. 19.1A**). The central area is necrotic and typically demonstrates restricted diffusion (**Fig. 19.1B**) due to its pustulant contents. Central ADC values rise with treatment, and any return in diffusion restriction foretells a recurrence in infection. Similar DWI findings may be seen, although are less common, in necrotic primary or metastatic cancers, which can also demonstrate ring-enhancement thus rendering differentiation from a pyogenic abscess difficult. In pyogenic abscesses, the enhancement (**Fig. 19.1C**) is distinguished by the completeness, uniformity, and lack of nodularity of the ring, although daughter abscesses may mimic nodularity. The distinction between an abscess and necrotic tumor is often clinical, although acetate and succinate peaks along with inverted branched chain amino acid peaks are fairly specific for abscess on MR spectroscopy (MRS). Ring-enhancement may persist for months after treatment and is a less reliable marker than ADC values for monitoring treatment response. Areas of ring-enhancement bordering a ventricle may be asymmetrically thin. Rupture into a ventricle with subsequent ependymitis can occur, although this is rare. This is seen as increased intraventricular SI on FLAIR scans along with ventricular margin enhancement on postcontrast T1WI.

Neurocysticercosis—a common cause of adult-onset seizures in the developing world—is caused by the pork tapeworm *Taenia solium*. Within the CNS, neurocysticercosis can involve the spinal cord, ventricles, brain parenchyma, and the subarachnoid space (**Figs. 19.1D,E**, *arrows*). Within these structures, the larvae progress through several stages. Larvae in the vesicular stage rarely enhance, and the cysts are typically seen as CSF-like SI. The colloidal vesicular phase is associated with larval death and degeneration, demonstrating a thick, enhancing capsule with surrounding edema on MRI. Fluid within the cyst, which appears as high SI on T2WI, is hyperintense to CSF on FLAIR and T1WI due to its high protein content. With particularly mucinous fluid, high SI is seen on all conventional sequences. Progression to the granular nodular stage is marked by diminished edema with continued enhancement, often in a rim pattern (**Fig. 19.1E**, *white arrow*). By this time, the cyst itself has shrunk into a nodule. The chronic lesions of neurocysticercosis are typified by an almost complete absence of edema and moderate SI on T2WI with areas of low SI representing dense calcifications (**Fig. 19.1D**, *black arrows*), which are best visualized on GRE T2WI.

Encephalitis involves the brain parenchyma more diffusely than the lesions above and is most frequently viral in origin. In adults, herpes simplex type 1 (HSV1) is a common culprit, presenting in a typical pattern initially affecting one of the temporal lobes. As seen in **Fig. 19.1F**, lesions may eventually extend to involve the bilateral temporal and inferior frontal lobes. Increased edema in these areas leads to high SI on

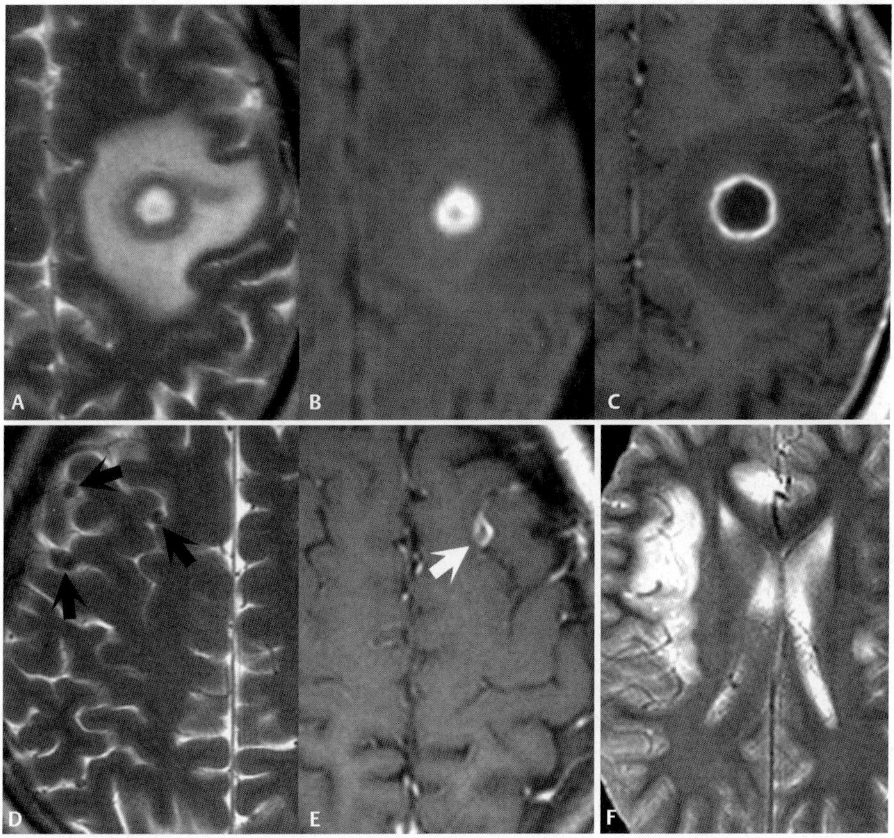

Fig. 19.1 (A–F)

FLAIR images and T2WI (**Fig. 19.1F**), although the presence of hemorrhage—a frequent finding—may interfere with the expected low SI appearance of edema on T1WI. Enhancement, particularly of the adjacent meninges, is frequently present in the acute phase of the disease. Diffusion is initially restricted in HSV encephalitis due to increased cellularity from lymphocytic infiltration, but may recover or even increase over baseline in later, more edematous lesions. Late in the disease, atrophy and parenchymal destruction may occur. Neonatal HSV infection, usually caused by HSV2, may include encephalitis as part of its usual spectrum of microphthalmia, microcephaly, mental retardation, and brain calcifications. MRI characteristics of the developing brain complicate the detection of neonatal encephalitis: the lack of myelinated white matter in the neonatal brain increases its normal SI on T2WI. Thus, the high SI edema of HSV encephalitis is not easily differentiated from normal brain parenchyma in neonates. Hemorrhagic lesions, calcification, and necrosis correlate with low SI on T2WI and make the presence of neonatal encephalitis on MRI more obvious. The loss of gray–white matter differentiation may provide an additional clue to the diagnosis of HSV neonatal encephalitis.

20 Sinus Disease

Incidental sinus disease is a common finding on MRI, with active sinusitis identified much less often. Most sinus infections are viral, but may result in the obstruction of outflow tracts predisposing the sinus to bacterial infection, frequently by *S. pneumonia*, *H. influenza*, or *M. catarrhalis*. MRI findings of retention cysts (with a CSF-like SI) and mucosal thickening are often seen in asymptomatic patients and are not specific for active sinusitis. True active disease is typified by the presence of both mucosal thickening and an air–fluid level, with sinusoidal fluid undergoing a characteristic evolution in appearance on MRI. Initially, the sinusoidal fluid appears as CSF-like SI replacing the normal low SI of the air-filled sinus. Eventually, as demonstrated in **Fig. 20.1A**, accumulation of protein decreases the SI of the fluid relative to that of CSF on T2WI. Higher protein content also hastens T1 relaxation, leading to a high SI on T1WI. Chronic desiccation of sinusoidal contents results in even higher protein concentrations, leading to low SI on T1 and T2WI that may be confused for the SI of a normal, patent sinus. In these cases, the characteristic peripheral enhancement of sinusitis may provide the only evidence of disease.

The major role of MRI in the evaluation of acute sinusitis is in delineating the spread of infection to surrounding structures. Such extension is demonstrated in **Fig. 20.1A** as an area of isointensity compressing the parenchyma adjacent to the frontal sinus on the right. This area is lined posteriorly by low SI dura and demonstrates restricted diffusion (**Fig. 20.1B**) consistent with the diagnosis of an epidural abscess. Contrast administration confirms the confinement of this abscess to the epidural space (**Fig. 20.1C**, *white arrow*), but also reveals more extensive enhancement of the dura, consistent with spreading meningitis (*black arrow*). **Figure 20.1C** also demonstrates an infected left frontal sinus showing the pattern of peripheral enhancement typical of sinusitis. Infections may also breach the meninges to involve brain parenchyma. **Figure 20.1D** demonstrates the high SI of acute sinusitis on a T2WI of the mastoid sinus, while the T2WI slightly superior to this plane reveals abnormal high SI in the posterior temporal lobe consistent with cerebritis (**Fig. 20.1E**, *white arrow*). As in **Fig. 20.1F**, cerebritis often enhances (*black arrow*) and is accompanied by peripheral edema, the latter appearing as low peripheral SI on this T1WI. Cerebritis may progress to an intracranial abscess, the classic appearance of which—a ring-enhancing lesion (*asterisk*) surrounded by copious edema—is shown on the contrast-enhanced T1WI in **Fig. 20.1G**.

The anatomic proximity of the mastoid sinus to the transverse venous sinus is evident in **Figs. 20.1D,E**. Proliferation of infection into venous sinuses may result in their thrombosis. Prior to the antibiotic era, this mechanism was the most frequent etiology of venous thrombosis, but today noninflammatory causes—pregnancy, oral contraceptives, trauma, dehydration, neoplasm, and L-asparaginase therapy—predominate. MRI findings of venous thrombosis progress in an orderly manner, beginning with the initial absence of a normal flow void seen on T1WI. At this early stage, the deoxyhemoglobin content of the thrombus results in a moderate SI on T1WI and low SI on T2WI. Venous collaterals may be seen bypassing the obstructed area. With reduction to methemoglobin, the clot appears as high SI on T1 and eventually T2WI. Upon vessel recanalization, flow voids are again visualized. Diagnostic pitfalls of venous thrombosis include slow flow in a patent vein masquerading as a high SI thrombus. True thrombus does not enhance and maintains a consistent SI in every plane and on scans performed

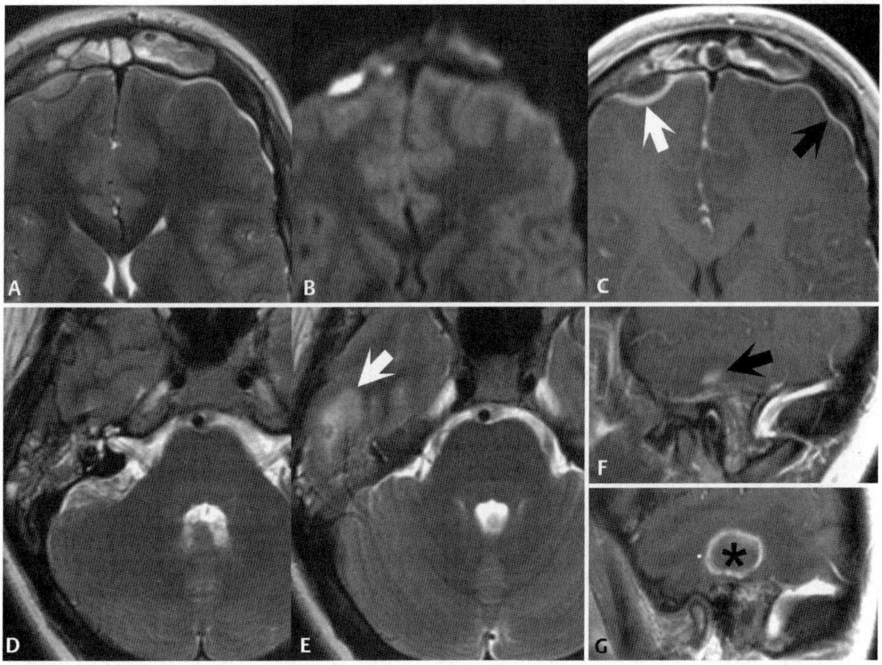

Fig. 20.1 (A–G)

at different times. MR venography (MRV) is not strictly necessary for the diagnosis and assessment of venous thrombosis, although commonly employed and often making diagnosis simpler. Ancillary findings include suggestions within the venous system of increased intracranial pressure, including visible emissary veins, prominent flow in the deep medullary veins, and hemorrhage. The thrombosed sinuses lack the hyperintensity seen on T2WI with normal venous flow and may demonstrate a frayed appearance if previously recanalized. Acute thrombus appears as a focus of intermediate SI, whereas subacute thrombus is less consistently visualized due to the confusion of the high SI of methemoglobin with that of venous flow. These may be better distinguished on pre- and post-contrast T1WI. Congenitally hypoplastic or asymmetric sinuses may also be confused with thrombosis, as may the signal voids of in-plane venous flow.

Venous thrombosis may result in parenchymal infarction. Venous infarctions tend to affect a younger age group than their arterial counterparts and do not follow the patterns of arterial distributions described in Chapters 13 and 14. Instead, they classically consist of multiple, bilateral, parasagittal, high-convexity lesions sparing the cortex, unilateral hemorrhagic temporal lobe infarctions, or bilateral lesions of the deep gray matter. Venous infarctions are also more frequently hemorrhagic than their arterial counterparts—a characteristic that may interfere with the classic temporal MRI changes in infarction (see Chapter 13). Acute hyperintensity on DWI may be more heterogeneous in venous infarctions. Venous infarctions are frequently accompanied on imaging by the signs described previously of venous thrombosis and of elevated intracranial pressure like hydrocephalus.

21 Meningitis

Clinically, meningitis presents as a combination of headache, nuchal rigidity, fever, and altered mental status. Infections of the meninges are most commonly of hematogenous origin, but may result from trauma, surgery, or the extension of local infections. Bacterial etiologies vary by age: neonates are affected most commonly by *Escherichia coli* and group B *Streptococcus*, older children by *Neisseria meningitidis*, *Streptococcus pneumoniae*, and type B *Haemophilus influenza*, and adults by *Streptococcus* and *N. meningitidis*. MRI and CT may be performed prior to lumbar puncture to rule out masses and assess for SAH. Nonenhanced MRI is relatively insensitive to the detection of meningitis, particularly aseptic (usually viral) forms, but due to the necessity of early antibiotic treatment, when present, these features must be recognized. An early MRI finding of meningitis is subarachnoid distension, most prominently seen as widening of the interhemispheric fissure and basilar cisterns. FLAIR is the most sensitive nonenhanced sequence, the higher protein content of the subarachnoid space manifesting as high SI compared to the normally low SI CSF. **Figure 21.1A** demonstrates posterior cortical sulci with normal low SI on FLAIR along with the high SI sulci (*black arrow*) that typify meningitis. Enhanced scans must be performed immediately after contrast administration, as delays result in the dilution of contrast agent within the CSF. The degree of enhancement is dose-dependent, and occurs in pachymeningeal—along the contours of the inner skull—and leptomeningeal patterns—extending to the sulci, fissures, and basilar cisterns. The degree of contrast enhancement does not correlate well with the extent of disease (in general underestimating the severity of involvement), as exemplified by **Fig. 21.1B** (*black arrow*) where mild leptomeningeal enhancement is seen in a patient who died of herniation secondary to meningitis the following day. Contrast-enhanced MRI is similar in sensitivity to FLAIR, but may be positive when the former is negative and vice-versa, as in **Fig. 21.1 C,** which displays a case of meningitis with clear sulcal enhancement (*black arrows*) in which FLAIR images were normal. Findings of meningitis on FLAIR and contrast-enhanced studies are nonspecific with differential considerations including SAH, meningeal carcinomatosis, and posttraumatic and postsurgical changes. The blood due to acute SAH is hyperdense on CT, and the enhancement of meningeal carcinomatosis on MRI tends to be thick and nodular, preferentially involving the pachymeninges, which lack a BBB. Trauma or surgery may result in indefinitely persisting dural enhancement, whereas leptomeningeal enhancement is more suggestive of acute disease. Bacterial and viral causes of meningitis are most common, although fungal, tubercular, and chemical etiologies are possible. In the appropriate clinical situation, neurosarcoidosis must be considered as a cause of noninfectious meningitis. This presents as a granulomatous leptomeningitis involving the skull base in a focal or diffuse pattern with possible extension along CNs. Parenchymal involvement results from the spread of disease via the Virchow-Robin spaces, presenting clinically as a mass lesion and with a SI pattern on MRI that may be similar to MS.

Complications of meningitis include empyema, hydrocephalus, and infarction. **Figure 21.1D** demonstrates a low SI subdural fluid collection on postcontrast T1WI extending along the interhemispheric fissure that could represent either a subdural effusion or empyema. The leptomeningeal enhancement flanking the lesion (*black arrow*) and the marked hyperintensity (restricted diffusion) on DWI (**Fig. 21.1E**) suggest the presence of meningitis complicated by a subdural empyema. Pediatric meningitides

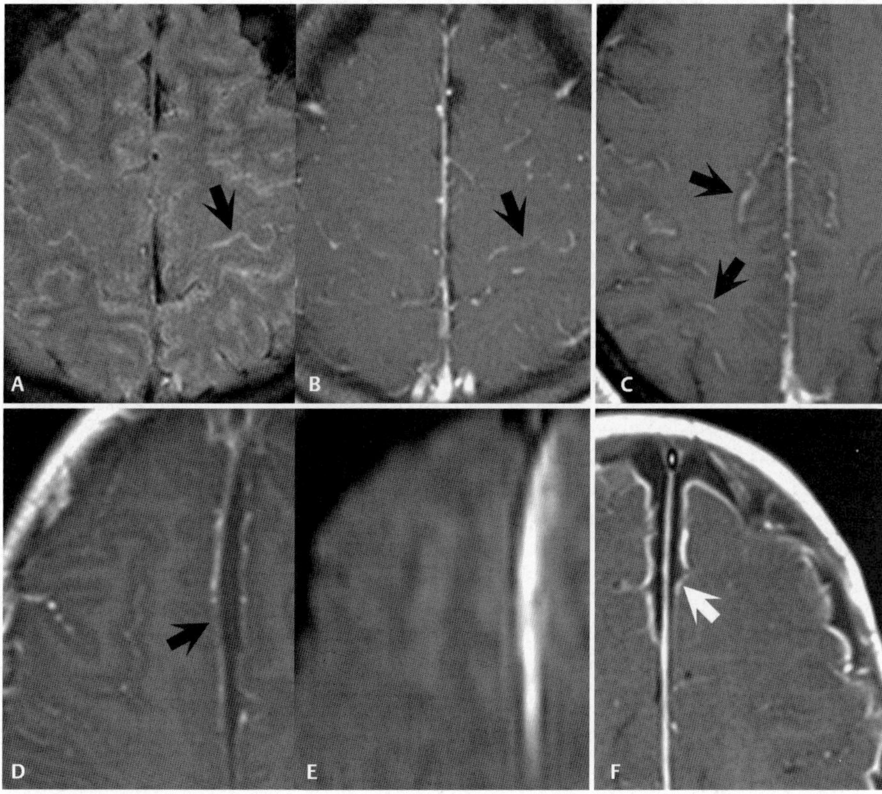

Fig. 21.1 (A–F)

caused by *S. pneumoniae*, on the other hand, produce sterile fluid collections. **Figure 21.1F** demonstrates such a subdural collection—extending laterally across cranial sutures of the attached dura, but not medially across the midline—with prominent associated leptomeningeal (*white arrow*), but not dural enhancement. This lesion lacked any restriction in diffusion, consistent with a sterile subdural fluid collection associated with *S. pneumoniae* meningitis.

Hydrocephalus may result from meningitis due to adhesions or loculations impairing CSF resorption at the arachnoid villi. MRI findings include dilated ventricles and transependymal resorption. The high SI of ependymitis on FLAIR and T2WI may mimic transependymal resorption, but the former usually enhances. The most common complication of adult meningitis is infarction, resulting from the inflammatory involvement of the pial vasculature, leading to thrombosis and subsequent infarction. The temporal changes of MRI SI in infarction have been previously described in Chapters 13 and 14. The disruption of the pia in infarction predisposes the parenchyma to cerebritis and subsequent abscess formation (see Chapters 19 and 20).

22 Immunocompromise

The availability and efficacy of highly active antiretroviral treatment has rendered the CNS manifestations of HIV—HIV encephalopathy, progressive multifocal leukoencephalopathy (PML), and toxoplasmosis—somewhat less common. The recognition of these entities on MRI is nevertheless important, HIV encephalopathy being the most frequent. The mechanism of this condition involves the direct viral infiltration of neurons, which correlates with diffuse hyperintensity of the cortical gray matter and subcortical white matter on T2WI. Eventually these changes may involve the periventricular white (**Figs. 22.1A,B**) and deep gray matter. Such lesions are typically isointense brain to parenchyma on T1WI (**Fig. 22.1.C**) and rarely enhance. With treatment, initial worsening of the lesions is seen on MRI, and although white matter disease usually resolves, central and peripheral cortical atrophy often persists. Such atrophy is in fact the most common MRI finding in HIV encephalopathy, demonstrated in **Fig. 22.1C** along with the loss of gray–white matter differentiation, another common finding. DWI and DTI (diffusion tensor imaging) changes may precede those of conventional MRI, and spectroscopic findings include a decrease in NAA (from neuronal loss), an increase in choline (from membrane turnover), and increased myoinositol (a marker for neuroglial activation).

PML is another CNS disease associated with immunocompromise and HIV. It is caused by the JC polyomavirus, which infiltrates and destroys oligodendrocytes while largely sparing the axons. The incidence of PML appears to be decreasing, although it is a rapidly progressive, fatal (10% 1-year survival) condition when present. Initial clinical findings include focal neurologic defects, in contrast to the diffuse encephalopathy seen in HIV encephalopathy. MRI findings mirror this relationship, PML being more asymmetric unifocal or multifocal pattern localized to the parietal or frontal lobes (**Fig. 22.1D**) as opposed to the diffuse, more symmetric pattern of HIV encephalopathy. PML may also occasionally involve the posterior fossa (**Fig. 21.1E**). The demyelinated lesions of PML appear as high SI on T2WI (**Figs. 22.1D,E**, *white arrow*) and low SI on T1WI. These lesions enhance more frequently than those of HIV encephalopathy. In PML, DWI may reveal central areas of increased diffusion, correlating with necrosis and reduced cellularity, and areas of restricted diffusion peripherally, correlating with ongoing tissue injury.

Toxoplasmosis is the most common intracranial opportunistic infection in HIV and is caused by an obligate intracellular protozoan transmitted through insufficiently cooked meat and cat feces. Clinical features in immunocompromised adults include fever, headache, seizures, mental status changes, and focal neurologic signs. MRI evidence of disease is commonly seen in the thalamus, basal ganglia, and gray–white matter junctions of the frontal and parietal lobes. **Figure 22.1F** demonstrates the characteristic appearance of toxoplasmosis on T2WI consisting of multiple hyperintense lesions with surrounding peripheral edema. A contrast-enhanced T1WI (**Fig. 22.1G**) reveals faint rim enhancement (*black arrows*)—indicative of active disease—surrounded by low SI edema. Alternatively, toxoplasmosis may present with multiple lesions <2 cm in diameter. Differential considerations for toxoplasmosis include necrotic metastases, pyogenic abscesses, and lymphoma. Unlike these, toxoplasmosis demonstrates increased central diffusion, likely from the decreased immune response within the lesion. Metastases and pyogenic abscesses may also be differentiated on the basis of clinical history, although CNS lymphoma, which frequently occurs in HIV

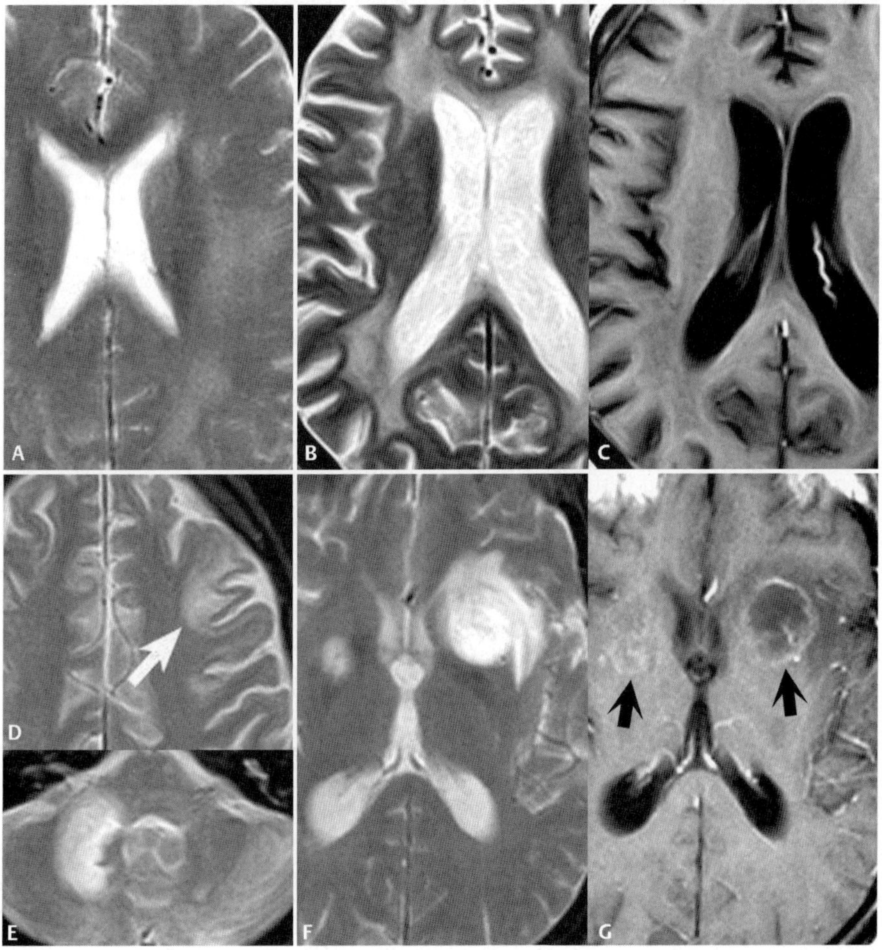

Fig. 22.1 (A–G)

patients, may prove more difficult. Lymphoma does, however, typically present with solitary lesions that are larger, less edematous, and enhance with a more irregular rim than those of toxoplasmosis. The inability to distinguish these two on imaging may necessitate empiric treatment for toxoplasmosis with MRI follow-up. Further workup may include MR perfusion or gallium nuclear medicine studies in which lymphoma and toxoplasmosis are hyper- and hypometabolic, respectively. Neonatal toxoplasmosis is associated with the triad of chorioretinitis, intracranial calcifications, and hydrocephalus.

23 Posterior Fossa Congenital Malformations

Chiari malformations are commonly encountered congenital abnormalities. Type 1 malformations are typically asymptomatic, although they may present with headaches, cerebellar signs, or lower CN symptoms. In addition to congenital etiologies, type 1 malformations may result from elevated intracranial pressure and conditions causing basilar invagination (e.g., Paget disease of bone). **Figure 23.1A** demonstrates the principle feature of a type 1 malformation—the herniation of wedge-shaped cerebellar tonsils (*black arrow*) below the foramen magnum. In this patient, the tonsils descend almost to the level of the posterior arch of C1. Herniation to the C1 level is seen in approximately two-thirds of patients; extension to the C3 level may occur in up to one-fourth of cases. Tonsils descending <5 mm below the foramen magnum are rarely of clinical significance. **Figure 23.1B** demonstrates another case of Chiari type 1 with the tonsils (*black arrow*) extending below the level of the posterior C1 arch. In this case, the malformation is associated with dilatation of the central canal of the cord, hydromyelia or (a more general term) syringohydromyelia (*asterisk*)—a longitudinally extending CSF-filled cavity commonly seen in this disorder. Hydromyelia demonstrates high SI on T2 and low SI on T1WI. Hydrocephalus is another frequent finding along with osseous abnormalities such as vertebral fusion, spina bifida occulta, and fusion of C1 to the occiput. The corpus callosum and quadrigeminal plate in **Fig. 23.1A,B** are normal, ruling out a Chiari type 2 malformation.

Type 2 malformations are almost uniformly associated with a myelomeningocele—the most severe variant of spina bifida in which both the spinal cord and intact meninges herniate at the lumbosacral midline. Detection of these defects at birth often leads to the diagnosis of Chiari type 2. In about half of cases, cervical or lumbar hydrosyringomyelia may also be present. As demonstrated in **Fig. 23.2 [1,2,3]**, type 2 malformations involve herniation below the foramen magnum of not only the cerebellar tonsils but also potentially the vermis, brainstem, and 4th ventricle. In severe cases, the medulla may kink, folding over itself at the cervicomedullary junction to rest posterior to the spinal cord. In **Fig. 23.2 [1]**, a portion of the cerebellum herniates through the foramen magnum, but only a smaller portion (the so-called "peg") protrudes through the C1 ring (**Fig. 23.2 [1]**). Compression of the vermis and the 4th ventricle may

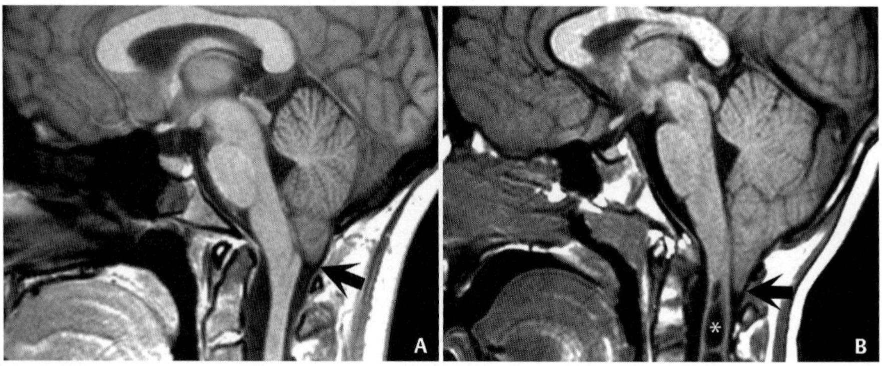

Fig. 23.1 (A,B)

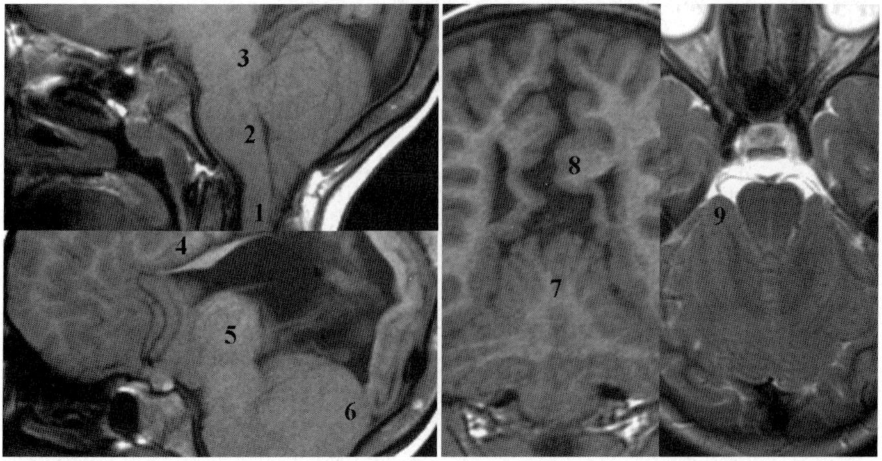

Fig. 23.2

occur—giving a slit-like appearance to the latter (**Fig. 23.2 [2]**). The midbrain colliculi of type 2 malformations (**Fig. 23.2 [3]**) are typically fused resulting in a beak-like appearance of the tectum. Complete or partial (**Fig. 23.2 [4]**) agenesis of the corpus callosum is seen in one-third of cases. The massa intermedia—bridging the 3rd ventricle and connecting the two lobes of the thalamus—is frequently enlarged in these patients (**Fig. 23.2 [5]**). The insertion of the tentorium may also be lower than normal (**Fig. 23.2 [6]**). As seen in **Fig. 23.2 [7]** the cerebellum may take on a towering appearance in coronal views with an exaggerated vertical orientation of the folia. Complete or partial absence of the falx (**Fig. 23.2 [8]**) may lead to an interdigitated appearance of the gyri. In addition, the gyri are often thin and numerous (stenogyria), not to be confused with polymicrogyria (in which the MRI appearance is grossly smooth), which is not associated with Chiari malformations. Anterior displacement of the cerebellar hemispheres relative to the pons may also occur in Chiari type 2 (**Fig. 23.2 [9]**). In extreme cases, the hemispheres may touch anterior to the pons, enveloping the brainstem. Hydrocephalus is also common with features including inferiorly pointing frontal horns of the lateral ventricles, large atria, and a prominent suprapineal recess of the 3rd ventricle. Chiari type 3 malformations share the features of Chiari type 2 but are also associated with a cervical-occipital encephalocele. These may herniate through osseous defects in the posterior vertebral elements or occipital skull.

A Dandy-Walker malformation is another congenital malformation of the posterior fossa, the differential considerations for which will be discussed in Chapter 24. In contrast to Chiari malformations, the 4th ventricle is enlarged in a Dandy-Walker malformation, communicating with a posterior cyst-like structure. This structure may expand the posterior fossa, elevating the tentorium and the torcular herophili (the confluence of superior, straight, and transverse sinuses). The partial or even complete absence of the cerebellar vermis is an important diagnostic clue. Associated embryonic dysgenesis of the foramens of Magendie and Luschka may alter CSF flow resulting in hydrocephalus—a frequent finding and important prognostic factor. A Dandy-Walker malformation may be associated with other intracranial defects—agenesis of the corpus callosum, cortical heterotopias, polymicrogyria, and brainstem lipomas. Extracranial abnormalities include craniofacial and cardiac septal malformations along with polydactyly.

24 Arachnoid Cysts

Arachnoid cysts are the most common congenital cystic brain entity, resulting from the failure to completely form an arachnoid villus or as sequelae of head trauma, leptomeningitis, or SAH. They form between the dura and arachnoid layers of the meninges or between the layers of the arachnoid. Along with berry aneurysms, they represent a frequent intracranial finding in polycystic kidney disease. Arachnoid cysts most commonly originate in the middle cranial fossa (**Figs. 24.1A,B**). Although typically much smaller than the lesion in **Figs. 24.1A,B**, arachnoid cysts are CSF-filled and thus characterized by isointensity to CSF on all MRI pulse sequences. This appearance includes high SI on T2WI (**Fig. 24.1A**), low SI on T1WI (**Fig. 24.1B**), and importantly low SI on FLAIR scans and DWI. Other characteristic locations include along the brain convexities and within the perimesencephalic cistern. Although typically asymptomatic, arachnoid cysts may become large enough to cause substantial mass effect on adjacent structures. **Figure 24.1C** demonstrates a large arachnoid cyst displacing the adjacent frontal lobe and also remodeling the inner table of the left frontal bone. Such erosions of the calvaria tend to be smooth. An expansile arachnoid cyst may grow large enough to obstruct the flow of CSF, resulting in ventricular dilatation, although this is quite rare.

Retrocerebellar arachnoid cysts (**Figs. 24.1D,E**) pose a particular diagnostic challenge due to the potential for confusion with the characteristic cyst of a Dandy-Walker malformation. Both entities may result in mass effect (note the displacement of the left cerebellar hemisphere in **Fig. 24.1D**) and elevation of the cerebellar tentorium (seen to some degree in **Fig. 24.1E**). However, whereas the 4th ventricle communicates with the retrocerebellar cyst in Dandy-Walker malformation and thus appears enlarged, an arachnoid cyst tends to compress the ventricle (**Fig. 24.1E**). Although the cerebellar vermis is often compressed (as seen partially in **Fig. 24.1E**), an otherwise intact vermis strongly favors the diagnosis of arachnoid cyst. Both an arachnoid cyst and the cyst in a Dandy-Walker malformation may be confused with a prominent cisterna magna (or cerebellomedullary cistern). This is a common benign, typically congenital, condition known as mega cisterna magna. Unlike the former other entities above, a mega cisterna magna characteristically does not exert mass effect. Along with the retrocerebellar space, infratentorial arachnoid cysts commonly involve the pontocerebellar and quadrigeminal plate cisterns.

Additional differential considerations for an arachnoid cyst include a subdural hygroma, an epidermoid cyst, a widened subarachnoid space from brain atrophy, and a choroidal fissure cyst. Subdural hygromas (see Chapter 9) result from a CSF leak through the meninges or resorption of blood products in a chronic subdural hematoma. Due to their location, these lesions are crescentic-shaped—an appearance not seen with arachnoid cysts. Subdural hygromas also do not erode bone, unlike arachnoid cysts and epidermoids. Epidermoids (see Chapter 5) are further distinguished from arachnoid cysts by a higher SI on T1WI, FLAIR, and PDWI along with restricted diffusion. Epidermoids also, in contrast to arachnoid cysts and hygromas, encase rather than compress vasculature and infiltrate rather than flatten the cortical sulci. A widened subarachnoid space secondary to atrophy will always appear isointense to CSF and will never demonstrate mass effect or erode bone. Choroidal fissure cysts represent a subtype of arachnoid cysts. They are benign collections of CSF, arising congenitally at the time of choroid plexus formation. The importance of choroidal fissure cysts and indeed their only distinction from arachnoid cysts lies in their location. The choroidal fissure is a CSF-filled space that runs between structures of the

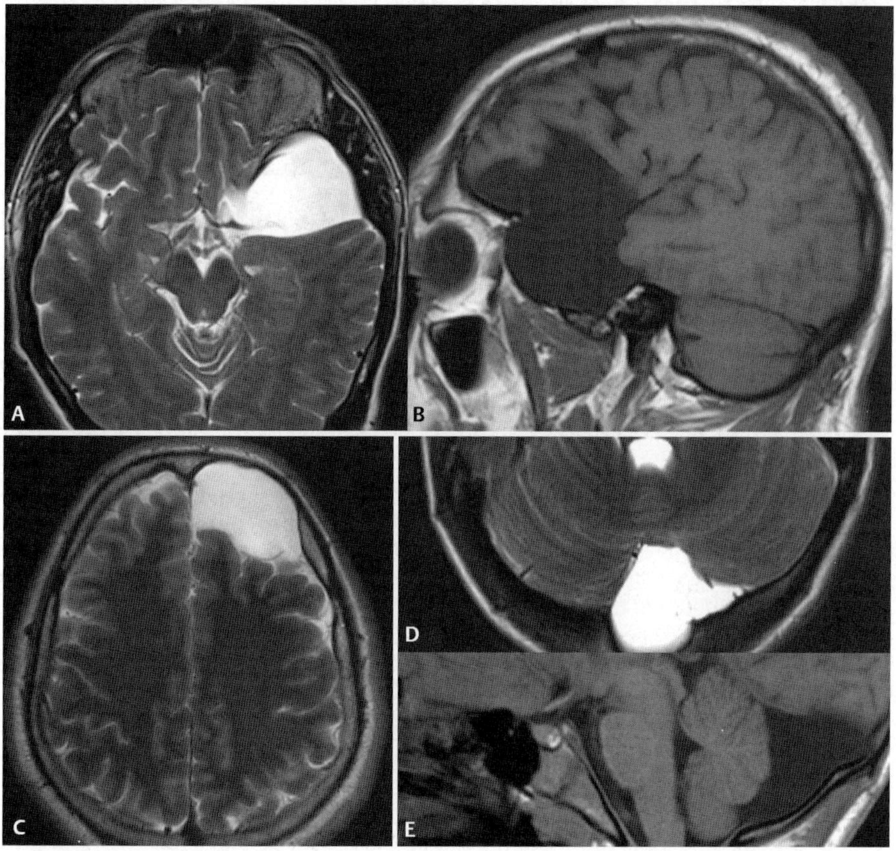

Fig. 24.1 (A–E)

diencephalon and the hippocampus—an area commonly evaluated for the presence of seizure foci. Choroidal fissure cysts, however, are almost always incidental findings, rarely producing seizures or mass effect within the temporal lobe. On sagittal MRI, these cysts are spindle-shaped and isointense to CSF on all sequences.

Additional benign entities warranting consideration include colloid cysts and intracranial lipomas. The most characteristic feature of colloid cysts is their location within the anterior portion of the 3rd ventricle, often obstructing the foramina of Monro and resulting in enlargement of the lateral ventricles. The spectrum of possible content—cholesterol, blood, and cellular products along with various metal ions—leads to variable signal intensity. Colloid cysts may rarely demonstrate peripheral enhancement. Intracranial lipomas are a benign congenital lesion occurring most frequently in the cisternal space. They are commonly midline, 80% being supratentorial, with the most common location being just superior (and along) the corpus callosum. The appearance of these lesions on MRI—increased SI on T1WI—reflects their fat composition. Chemical shift artifacts may be seen as a band of high or low SI at the margin between fat and adjacent fluid or brain.

25 Other Congenital Malformations

Malformations of the corpus callosum occur in complete or partial forms. Callosal formation proceeds from anterior to posterior, and thus in partial agenesis the anterior portion is typically preserved, as in **Fig. 25.1A** (although, in this instance, only a very small part of the corpus callosum is present). In this figure the cingulate gyri are aligned progressively radially in the posterior direction where the cingulate sulcus has not formed secondary to callosal absence. One gyrus extends to the cortical surface. In neonates, in whom the callosum is not readily visualized, radiating gyri may be diagnostic of agenesis. Mega cisterna magna (**Fig. 25.1A**), Chiari type 2, and Dandy-Walker malformations may be seen with agenesis. Parallel lateral ventricles (**Fig. 25.1B**) are characteristic, and on coronal images, the frontal horns may take a crescent shape from the white matter bundles (of Probst) lining their medial walls. Holoprosencephaly is also a congenital malformation and occurs in lobar, semilobar, and alobar forms. Alobar (the most severe) forms lack a third ventricle, falx, and interhemispheric fissure. Fused or absent thalami and a horseshoe-shaped monoventricle are common. **Figure 25.1C** demonstrates a case of semilobar holoprosencephaly in which the interhemispheric fissure is clearly absent anteriorly (although present posteriorly), and the thalami are mostly fused. The monoventricle divides into atrial but not anterior horns. Lobar holoprosencephaly is least severe and characterized by the absence of the septum pellucidum, a small amount of frontal lobe fusion, and nearly normal thalami, ventricles, and corpus callosum.

Lissencephaly refers to the gross MRI appearance of a "smooth brain" as seen in pachygyria and agyria. **Figure 25.1D** demonstrates the rudimentary gyral formation seen in the latter. A cell sparse area (*black arrows*)—consisting of mainly axons—may be seen as a region of high SI on T2WI between a thin, low SI cortex (representing successfully migrated neurons) and a deep layer of gray matter (where neuronal migration has been disrupted). In **Fig. 25.1E,** smooth, thickened gray matter (*white arrows*) lines the gyri in a focal case of pachygyria. The sulci in this case are shallow, but more prominent than in agyria. Polymicrogyria (in contrast to stenogyria where the gyri are grossly too thin and numerous) may appear grossly similar to pachygyria, but pathologically small gyri involve various cortical layers. Gray matter lobulation, known as cobblestoning (**Fig. 25.1F**, *black arrows*), is the characteristic MRI finding. Schizencephaly is a migration disorder resulting in a cleft traversing the hemisphere from the cortex to the ventricle. **Figure 25.1G** demonstrates an open lip schizencephaly with wide communication between the ventricle and subarachnoid space. The cleft's gray matter lining (*white arrows*) favors schizencephaly over porencephaly or other destructive lesions. Closed lip varieties consist of a double layer of cortex between the ventricle and the surface. In a separate patient, two areas of heterotopic gray matter are shown in **Fig. 25.1H** (*black arrows*) in their most common location—lining the ventricles. These lesions demonstrate isointensity to gray matter on all sequences, do not enhance, and are best identified with heavily T1WI where gray and white matter is better differentiated. Septooptic dysplasia (not illustrated) may result in blindness, seizures, hypothalamic–pituitary dysfunction, and growth retardation. The septum pellucidum is dysplastic or even completely absent, and there is optic nerve hypoplasia.

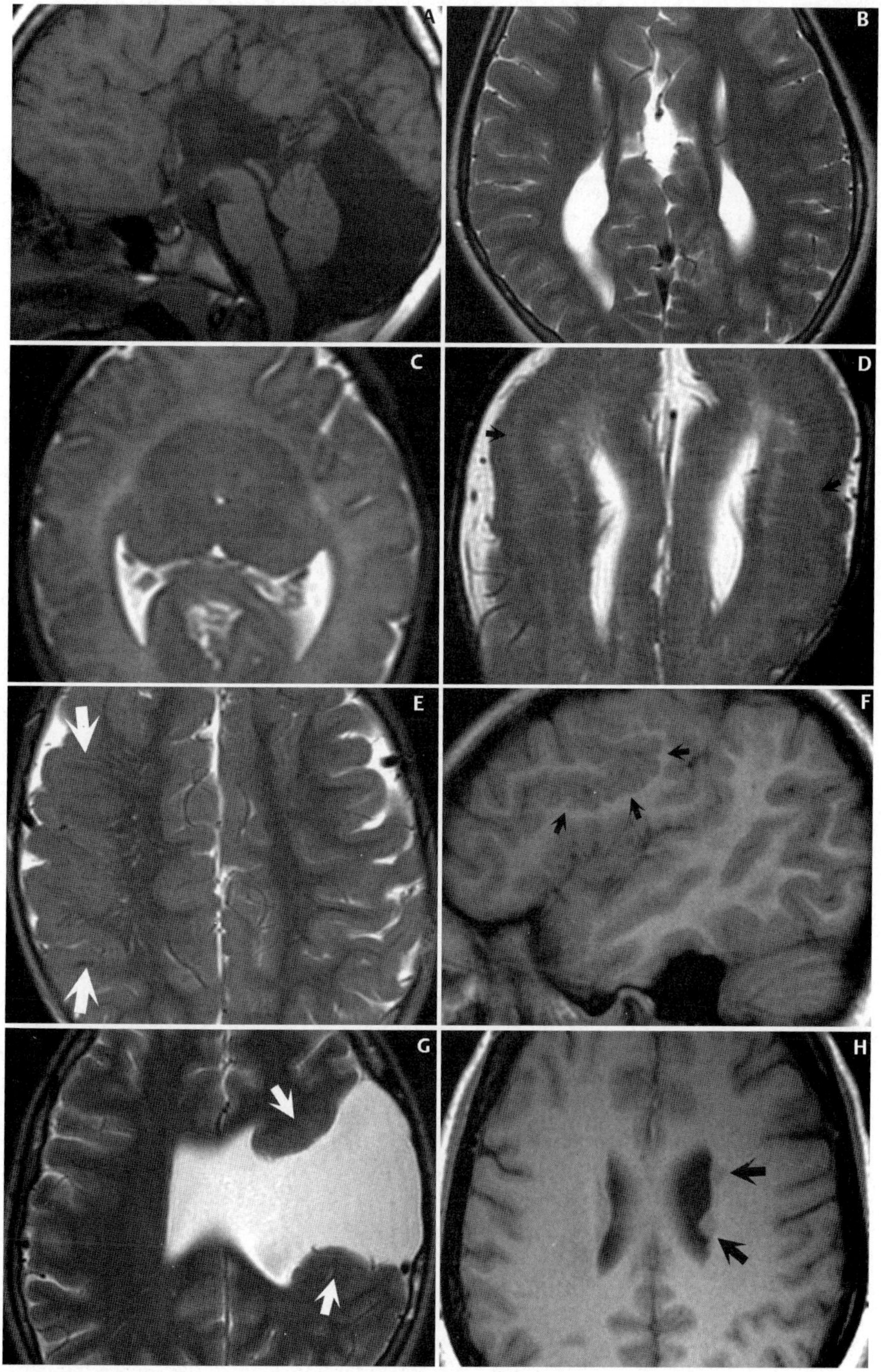

Fig. 25.1 (A–H)

26 Inherited White Matter Disease

Recognizing the progression of myelination in normal brain development is critical for detecting white matter diseases of childhood. The cholesterol content of myelin is responsible for the high SI appearance of white matter on T1WI. Thus, the MRI SI relationship between gray and white matter in neonates—in whom the latter is not yet myelinated—is reversed. Myelination begins in the occipital lobe, centrum semiovale, internal capsule, and corpus callosum and is best assessed with T1WI. Myelination progresses from central to peripheral, posterior to anterior, and from sensory to motor tracts. By one year of age, T1WI demonstrates close to the adult pattern of gray and white matter SI. As the water content of newly formed myelin progressively decreases, the SI of white matter on T2WI declines, with marked changes occurring between 1 and 2 years of age (at which time the appearance is close to that of the adult pattern). Terminal areas of myelination—the white matter of the parietal lobes surrounding the ventricular trigones—may demonstrate high SI on T2WI up until 10 years after birth.

The leukodystrophies are inherited dysmyelinating conditions characterized by the improper laying down or subsequent breakdown of myelin. Adrenoleukodystrophy is a congenital peroxisomal abnormality in very long-chain fatty acid metabolism presenting with adrenal insufficiency and rapid neurologic decline. Of the inherited leukodystrophies, its MRI appearance is the most characteristic. The T2WI of **Fig. 26.1A** demonstrates areas of high SI surrounding the atria of the lateral ventricles and extending across the slightly atrophic (due to disease involvement) splenium of the corpus callosum. Corresponding areas of low SI are seen on the sagittal T1WI of **Figs. 26.1B,C**. Involvement of the fornix and parietooccipital white matter is also common. Contrast enhancement may occur along the leading edge of these lesions correlating with active demyelination. MRI appearances of other leukodystrophies are less specific. The mucopolysaccharidoses—including Hurler, Hunter, and Sanfilippo syndromes—are inherited conditions resulting from defects in the lysosomal enzymes that degrade glycosaminoglycans. The T2WI of **Fig. 26.1D** demonstrates a case of Hunter syndrome (caused by a defect in iduronate sulfatase) with nonspecific patchy periventricular hyperintensities. Gray-white matter differentiation may also be poor; small cystic lesions, correlating with glycosaminoglycan-filled cells, are somewhat specific for the diagnosis of a mucopolysaccharidosis. Chronically, atrophic changes and ventriculomegaly (**Fig. 26.1D**) may be present.

The GM1 and GM2 (Tay-Sachs) gangliosidoses (lysosomal storage disorders) are leukodystrophies resulting from deficiencies in β-galactosidase and hexosaminidase, respectively. **Figure 26.1E** demonstrates a case of GM1 that highlights the importance of recognizing the progression in normal brain MRI appearances with age. In this T1WI there is diffuse hypointensity throughout the parenchymal white matter except within the posterior limb of the internal capsule. In a neonate, this appearance would be typical of a normally developing brain with early myelination in the internal capsule posteriorly. However, this child is 11 months of age. The T1WI should thus appear similar to that of an adult, and so—by age criteria—the white matter in **Fig. 26.1E** is diffusely abnormal. Findings on T2WI include areas of high SI corresponding in location with the abnormality seen on T1WI. These may predominate within the basal ganglia. Atrophic findings occur chronically. Metachromatic leukodystrophy is the most common lysosomal storage disease and results from the accumulation of ceramide sulfatide within Schwann cells secondary to a defective arylsulfatase A enzyme. Diffuse, symmetric high SI within the cerebellar and periventricular white

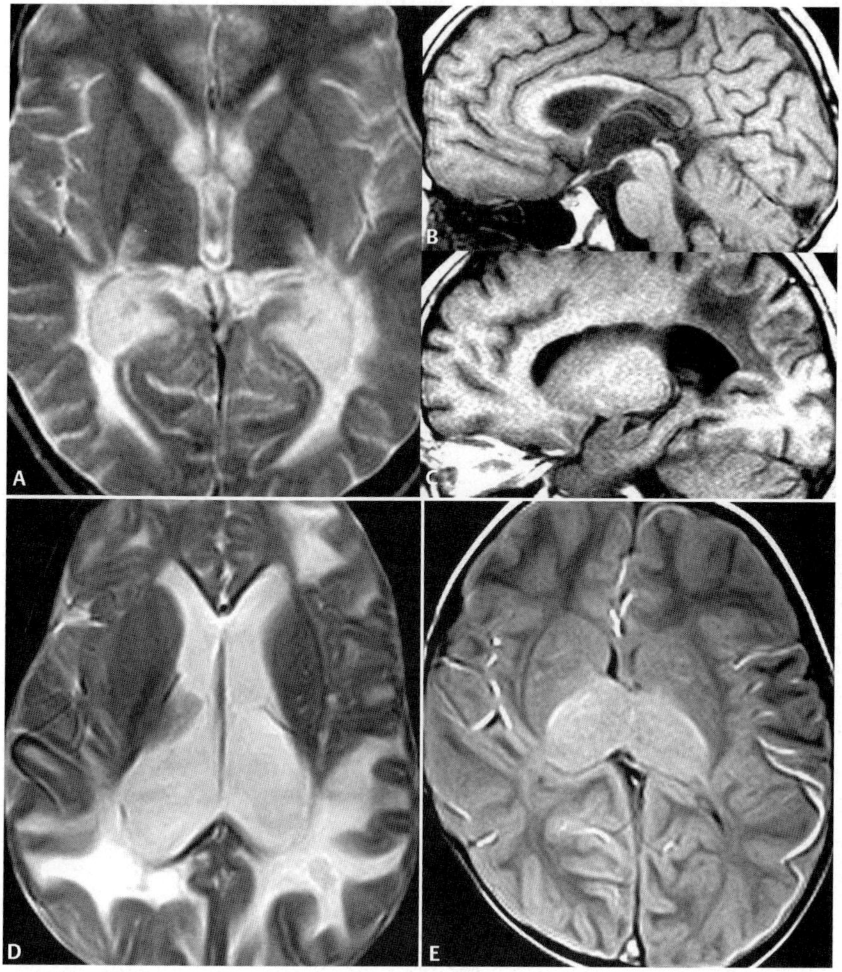

Fig. 26.1 (A–E)

matter on T2WI may be present with characteristic sparing of subcortical U-fibers and gray matter. Other early findings in leukodystrophies may be suggestive of an exact diagnosis, even though MRI findings in later-stage disease are typically indistinguishable. For example, deep gray matter involvement suggests a mitochondrial leukoencephalopathy; enhancing lesions are more typical of adrenoleukodystrophy, Krabbe, or Alexander disease. The latter along with Canavan disease characteristically presents with macrocephaly.

27 Neurofibromatosis and von Hippel-Lindau Syndrome

NF1 or von Recklinghausen disease is an autosomal dominant disorder with diagnostic criteria including two or more of the following: a first-degree relative with NF1, axillary freckling, distinctive bone lesions, an optic glioma, a plexiform neuroma, at least six café-au-lait spots, and more than one Lisch nodule or neurofibroma. Foci of abnormal signal intensity (FASI) are the most common NF1 findings on brain MRI. The FLAIR images in **Fig. 27.1A** demonstrate the typical high SI appearance of FASI within their characteristic location—the globus pallidus of the basal ganglia. Pallidal lesions, in particular, may also appear as high SI on T1WI—a characteristic relating to their possible pathologic identity as hamartomas or heterotopic Schwann cells. Less commonly, FASI may involve the pons (**Fig. 27.1B**) or cerebellum (**Fig. 27.1C**). Lesions often increase in prominence in middle childhood, fading by adolescence. Unlike a neoplasm, FASI do not demonstrate surrounding vasogenic edema or mass effect and will only rarely enhance. Optic gliomas—nearly always JPAs (WHO grade 1)—are the most common intracranial tumor of NF1. Bilateral lesions are nearly pathognomonic. NF1 gliomas appear most frequently as diffuse, isointense enlargements of the optic nerve, in distinction to the heterogeneous, cystic appearance of non-NF1 lesions. Enhancement (best seen on fat-suppressed images) is variable, but may aid in detection, along with the high SI on T2WI seen in some lesions. Differential considerations include perioptic meningiomas—characterized by a fusiform, tram-track appearance—along with sarcoidosis. Gliomas are rarely limited to the nerve itself. Involvement of the optic chiasm is frequent—particularly with non-NF1 gliomas—and often visible as diffuse chiasmal enlargement as in the T1WI of **Fig. 27.2A** (*white arrow*). Hypothalamic gliomas are also common (**Fig. 27.2A**, *black arrow*). Plexiform neuromas of the face and cranial nerves are less prevalent than optic gliomas, but are nearly pathognomonic for NF1. Lesions demonstrate low to moderate SI on T1 and high SI on T2WI. Heterogeneous enhancement is common. Additional common findings

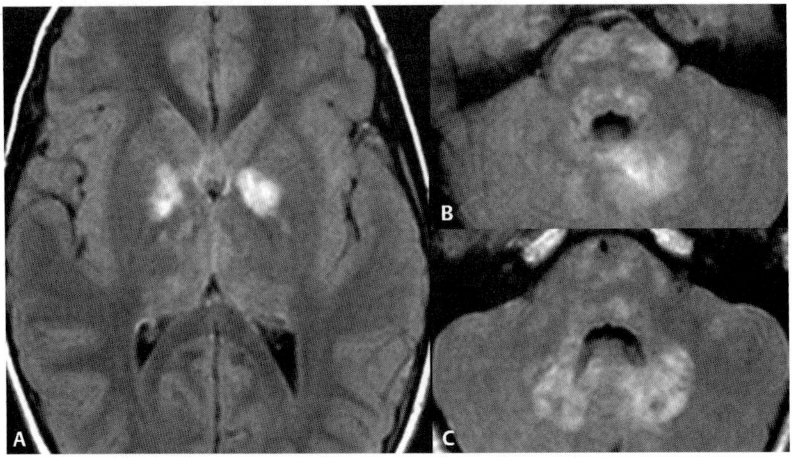

Fig. 27.1 (A–C)

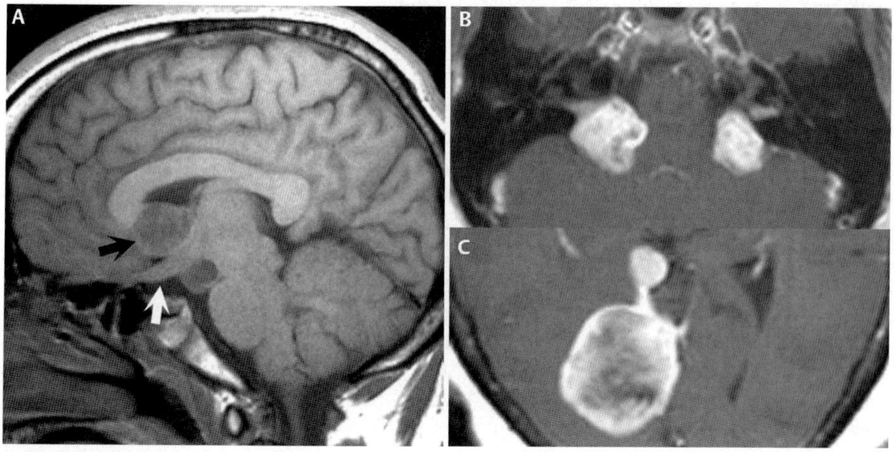

Fig. 27.2 (A–C)

include buphthalmos (enlargement of the globe) and sphenoid dysplasia (part of the NF1 diagnostic criteria).

NF2 is inherited in an autosomal dominant pattern with an incidence of about 1/10th that of NF1. No cutaneous neurofibromas or plexiform neuromas are present. Bilateral CPA masses (acoustic or facial schwannomas)—the enhancing lesions in **Fig. 27.2B**—are diagnostic and require no further pathologic confirmation. Other criteria for diagnosing NF2 include a first-degree relative with the condition plus either a unilateral CPA mass or two of the following: a glioma, schwannoma, neurofibroma, or juvenile capsular cataract. Compared with spontaneously occurring schwannomas, those of NF2 are more commonly bilateral, may occasionally arise from the cochlear portion of CN VIII, and tend to invade rather than compress nerves. They are otherwise similar in MRI appearance (see Chapter 5). The meningiomas of NF2 are also similar in appearance to their spontaneously occurring counterparts (see Chapter 4), except they occur in younger patients and are more frequently located intraventricularly or along the cranial nerves. **Figure 27.2C** demonstrates two bright, heterogeneously enhancing meningiomas similar in appearance to those previously illustrated in Chapter 4's **Fig. 4.1B**. The suggestion of intracranial NF2 warrants screening for spinal lesions (see Chapter 36) with contrast-enhanced MRI.

Von Hippel-Lindau (VHL) disease is an autosomal dominant condition consisting of pheochromocytomas; cysts and carcinomas of the kidney and pancreas; and hemangioblastomas of the posterior fossa, spinal cord, and retina. Multiple or spinal hemangioblastomas necessitate a full imaging workup of VHL. Hemangioblastomas are classically described as cystic masses with a solid, subpial, mural nodule. On MRI the cystic portions demonstrate high SI on T2 and low SI on T1WI. The SI of the mural nodule may be mixed due in part to low SI flow voids within or just peripheral to it. Enhancement of only the nodule without rim enhancement of the cyst is characteristic. 60% of all posterior fossa hemangioblastomas have this appearance, cystic with a "mural" nodule; 40% are solid. Cord hemangioblastomas are less prevalent, but more specific for VHL than cerebellar lesions.

28 Tuberous Sclerosis and Sturge-Weber Syndrome

Tuberous sclerosis is an autosomal dominant (and spontaneously occurring) condition defined by facial adenoma sebaceum, seizures, and mental retardation. Intracranial findings are hamartomatous lesions consisting of subependymal nodules and cortical tubers. **Figures 28.1A and 28.1B** demonstrate multiple subependymal nodules lining the walls of the lateral ventricles. Although these lesions are clearly seen in this instance as low SI on T2WI (**Fig. 28.1A**, *white arrows*) and high SI on T1WI (**Fig. 28.2B**), the SI of these nodules varies (in part due to calcification), potentially resulting in a more subtle appearance. GRE T2WI better detect this calcification, which is absent in heterotopic gray matter—a lesion that potentially could be confused with the subependymal nodules of tuberous sclerosis, but that does not enhance and is isointense to gray matter on all pulse sequences. The enhancement of subependymal nodules is variable, although its presence on MRI (unlike on CT) is not indicative of malignant transformation to a subependymal giant cell astrocytoma (WHO grade 1). Distinguishing between these two lesions may thus be difficult and require close MRI follow-up. Fortunately, giant cell astrocytomas are slow-growing lesions with the major morbidity being from ventricular outflow obstruction. The FLAIR image in **Fig. 28.1C** demonstrates a subtle heterogeneous area of high SI in the frontal horn of the left lateral ventricle that, because of its location

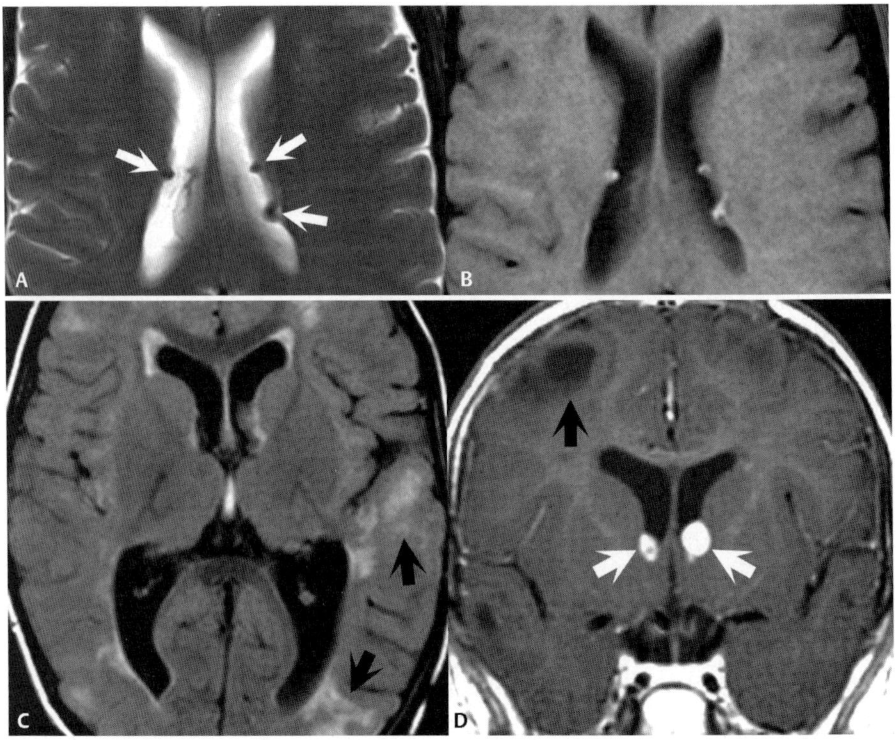

Fig. 28.1 (A–D)

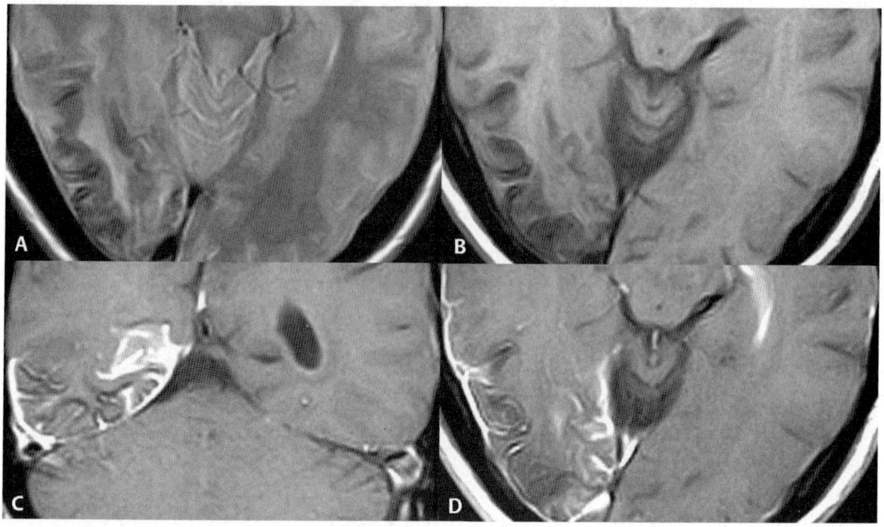

Fig. 28.2 (A–D)

and size, may represent a giant cell astrocytoma. Coronal imaging in **Fig. 28.1D** reveals the existence of bilateral lesions (*white arrows*), that enhance and are both in the characteristic location—near the foramina of Monro—for a subependymal giant cell astrocytoma. Cortical and subcortical tubers occur most frequently in the frontal, then parietal lobes and involve both gray and white matter. A "gyral core" pattern of tubers consists of an expanded gyrus surrounding a subcortical white matter hamartoma of high SI on FLAIR (**Fig. 28.1C**, black arrows) and T2WI with low SI on T1WI (**Fig. 28.1D**, *black arrow*). These lesions do not typically enhance. When two adjacent gyri are involved as above with sparing of the intervening cortex, a "sulcal island" pattern results. This is best seen on T2WI as two high SI subcortical lesions flanking a sulcal area of (normal) lower SI.

Sturge-Weber syndrome is defined by the presence of a facial port-wine stain, mental retardation, and seizures. The port-wine stain is a capillary angioma and ipsilateral to this lie the major intracranial pathologies of Sturge-Weber–cortical calcification, leptomeningeal angiomatosis, and parenchymal atrophy. **Figures 28.2A** and **28.2B** demonstrate a gyriform pattern of abnormal low SI on (**Fig. 28.2A**) T2WI and (**Fig. 28.2B**) T1WI that is most consistent with dense cortical calcifications. Contrast-enhanced coronal (**Fig. 28.2C**) and axial (**Fig. 28.2D**) images display mild focal parenchymal atrophy along with leptomeningeal enhancement typical of the pial-contained thin-walled venous structures of leptomeningeal angiomatosis. Evolution of the vascular abnormalities can be seen, thought to be due to further occlusion of draining veins. In neonates, transient hyperperfusion may lead to pseudo-early myelin maturation, which appears as decreased SI on T2WI. With subsequent ischemia and gliosis, increased SI on T2WI as well as enhancement may occur. An additional common finding is ipsilateral choroid plexus enlargement, together with prominent enhancement therein.

29 Congenital Abnormalities

Congenital posterior fossa abnormalities are frequently visualized on cervical spine MRI, often with accompanying neural axis and osseous findings. Sagittal images best evaluate the position of the cerebellar tonsils, which may normally lie as far as 5 mm below the foramen magnum. Extension of the tonsils below this level is seen in type 1 Chiari malformations, which are commonly asymptomatic. A symptomatic case—with the lack of space surrounding the medulla at the level of the foramen magnum leading to CSF obstruction—is demonstrated in **Fig. 29.1A**. Cerebellar herniation must be assessed with attention to tonsillar location relative to the anterior and posterior arches (*arrows*) of C1, as well as the foramen magnum. The tonsils frequently appear pointed in a type 1 malformation in contrast to their normal globular appearance. Clinical symptoms may also be due to the presence of hydromyelia, illustrated in addition in **Fig. 29.1A**. Hydromyelia occurs secondary to dilatation of the central canal of the spinal cord and thus appears on MRI as an area of CSF SI within an enlarged cord. Cord wall thinning (posteriorly in **Fig. 29.1A**) may occur in severe cases. Hydromyelia may occur at any location within the cord but favors the cervicothoracic junction when associated with Chiari malformations. With severe hydromyelia, the walls of the cord are markedly thinned and compressed against the adjacent dura. Intraspinal arachnoid cysts are a differential consideration but are quite rare. Hydromyelia involving the medulla is termed syringobulbia and is often symptomatic. The preservation of the 4th ventricle and the normal appearing midbrain colliculi help distinguish the Chiari 1 malformation of **Fig. 29.1A** from the type 2 malformation illustrated in **Fig. 29.1B**. In the latter, the ventricle is slit-like, and the tectum is fused resulting in a beak-like appearance. In addition, a cerebellar peg is present, the anteroposterior (AP) dimension of the pons is foreshortened, and the insertion of the tentorium is low—all typical features of type 2 Chiari. Associated osseous and spinal abnormalities include anomalies of the posterior arch of C1 and lumbar spinal dysraphism (commonly a myelomeningocele), the latter seen in nearly all patients. Additional cerebellar and brainstem findings as described in Chapter 23 may also be present along with hydromyelia.

The most significant osseous congenital abnormalities of the cervical spine include malformations of the craniocervical junction. Basilar invagination refers to the presence of the tip of the odontoid 5 mm or more above Chamberlain's line (drawn from the posterior margin of the hard palate to the posterior lip of the foramen magnum; see Chapter 33). Platybasia—marked by an angle between the clivus and the floor of the anterior cranial fossa greater than the normal 125 to 140 degrees—often accompanies this condition. Primary invagination is also associated with occipitalization (fusion of the atlas and occiput), whereas secondary lesions occur in osteoporosis, Paget disease, achondroplasia, fibrous dysplasia, and osteogenesis imperfecta. Os odontoideum is defined by the presence of an ovoid ossicle distinct from the body of C2 and may be difficult to

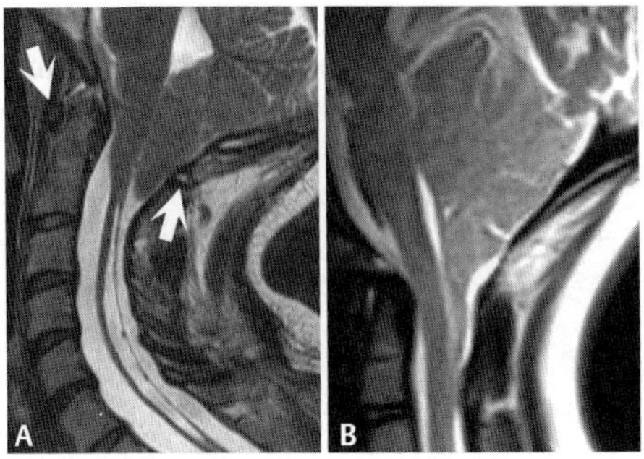

Fig. 29.1 (A,B)

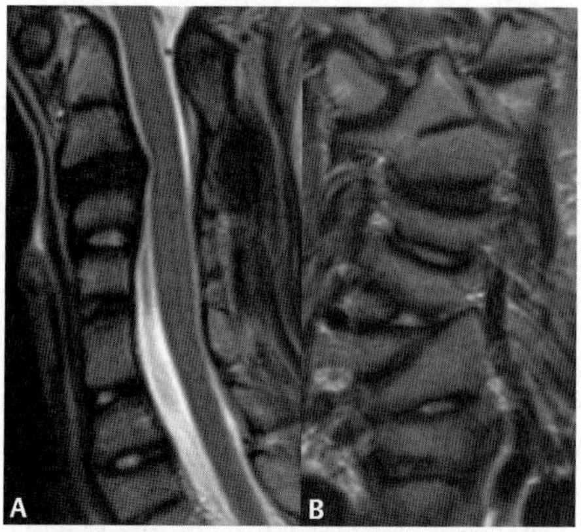

Fig. 29.2 (A,B)

distinguish from a traumatic odontoid fracture, although the former may also arise secondary to trauma. Hemi- and fused vertebrae are also commonly encountered congenital disorders. The most common fusion anomaly is simply the fusion of two adjacent vertebral bodies, seen not infrequently in the cervical spine. Typically, the two fused vertebral bodies have a small AP dimension, with the intervening disk space often only partially visualized. **Figures 29.2A and 29.2B** demonstrate multiple anomalies including right segmented hemivertebrae (C5, C6), fusions of the posterior elements (C1 to C2) and a wedge-shaped vertebral body (C7). As evident from this case, coronal imaging is essential for the proper evaluation of congenital abnormalities of the spine. The presence of hemivertebrae leads to a short, focal curve, often with severe scoliosis. Klippel-Feil syndrome is defined by the fusion of two or more cervical vertebrae in association with the clinical triad of a short neck with limited mobility and a low posterior hairline. Three types are defined to include extensive cervical and/or thoracic vertebral fusion (type 1), only one or two cervical fusions (type 2), or cervical in addition to thoracic and lumbar fusions (type 3). **Figure 29.3A** demonstrates hypoplastic, fused C2–C4 vertebral bodies lacking intervening disk spaces. In this particular case, the cervical spine was found to be fused from C1 to C6, and the case thus classified as Klippel-Feil type 1. Diastematomyelia—a symmetric or asymmetric longitudinal splitting of the spinal cord—is not uncommonly seen in Klippel-Feil (as in **Fig. 29.3B**). In **Fig. 29.3B**, the hemicords appear tethered together by a fibrous band and are enveloped by a single arachnoid-dural sheath (type 2). Type 1 diastematomyelia includes clefting of the meninges such that each hemicord is enclosed within its own dural sac, typically with an intervening bone spur between them. Both types of diastematomyelia are associated with multiple congenital and spinal abnormalities and consistently also with an overlying cutaneous patch of silky hair.

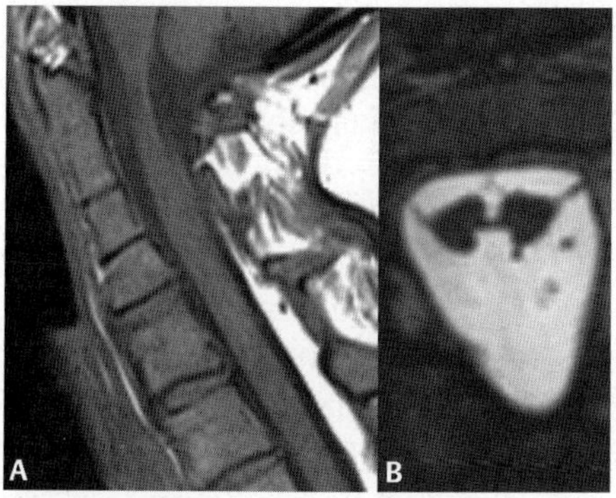

Fig. 29.3 (A,B)

30 Trauma

MRI offers superior evaluation of soft tissue and cord injuries and is preferred to CT for this purpose in the setting of trauma. The sagittal fat-saturated T2WI in **Fig. 30.1A** demonstrates compression of the cervical spinal cord by a small surrounding epidural fluid collection (*white arrows*). SI characteristics of this lesion on accompanying sequences helped identify it as an epidural hematoma. In the spine, these result from the tearing of the epidural venous plexus. The SI of these hematomas varies with the age of their constituent blood products. A traumatic disk herniation (*black arrow*) at the C6–C7 level is demonstrated in **Figs. 30.1B,C** on sagittal FSE T2WI and axial GRE T2WI, respectively. The axial image demonstrates a broad-based central and left paracentral disk herniation (*black arrow*), with associated mild cord flattening. Traumatic herniations may arise secondary to osseous injury as in the T2WI of **Fig. 30.2A**. Here the anterior subluxation of C4 relative to C5 has led to a disk protrusion with mild to moderate compression of the cord. A perched facet (*white arrow*) is also visible on the left parasagittal image in **Fig. 30.2B**. Occasionally, damage to the cord may occur without direct evidence of concurrent osseous or soft tissue injury. The T2WI of **Fig. 30.2C** demonstrates longitudinally extending cord edema (*black arrows*) with no other evidence of traumatic injury. In some cases, edema may result in cord enlargement, and distinguishing pure edema from a hemorrhagic lesion is crucial given the poor prognosis with the latter. The typical pattern consists of a spindle-shaped region of hemorrhage surrounded longitudinally by edema. The SI of the hemorrhagic component varies with blood product age (see Chapter 8), but with a markedly delayed progression versus that of blood products in the brain. Because of this delay, deoxyhemoglobin (low SI on T2WI) is the dominant acute species. GRE T2WI may aid in the detection of this and other blood products (as low SI) within the cord. In chronic cord injury, myelomalacic changes predominate with cystic necrosis—visualized as high and low SI on T2WI and T1WI, respectively—eventually progressing to syrinx formation and cord atrophy.

Specific osseous injuries to the cervical spine include atlanto-occipital dislocation, Jefferson fracture (a burst fracture involving the anterior and posterior arches of C1), hangman's fracture (a fracture of C2 and C3 that extends through the C2 pedicles), and clay shoveler's fracture (spinous process avulsion of C6 or C7). Odontoid fractures may affect the superior portion (type 1) or body (base) of the dens (type 2), or extend into the C2 body (type 3). A vertebral body may wedge anteriorly in flexion and break into

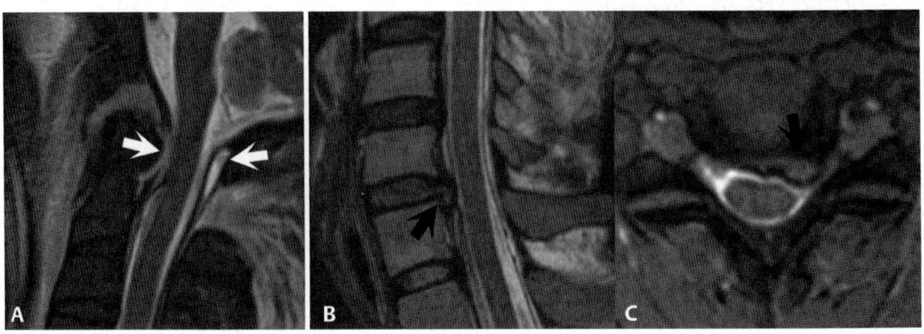

Fig. 30.1 (A–C)

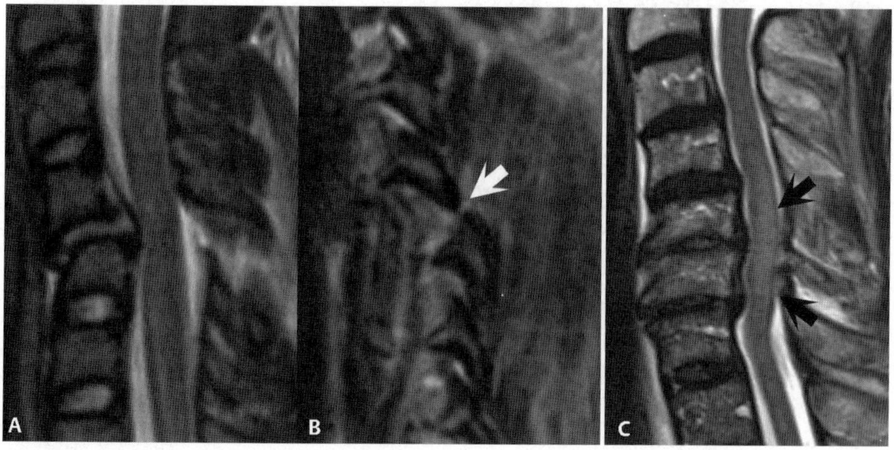

Fig. 30.2 (A–C)

fragments. Compression (burst) fractures, such as those resulting from excess axial load, are the most common traumatic injury in the thoracic spine. These may manifest as a loss of vertebral body height, as seen in the T3 vertebral body in **Fig. 30.3** (*lower white arrow*). Often, however, body height may be maintained, rendering visualization of these microfractures impossible on plain film or CT. With MRI, however, these fractures are clearly seen as an area of edema-like SI, as illustrated on the T1WI of **Fig. 30.3** involving C7 (*upper white arrow*).

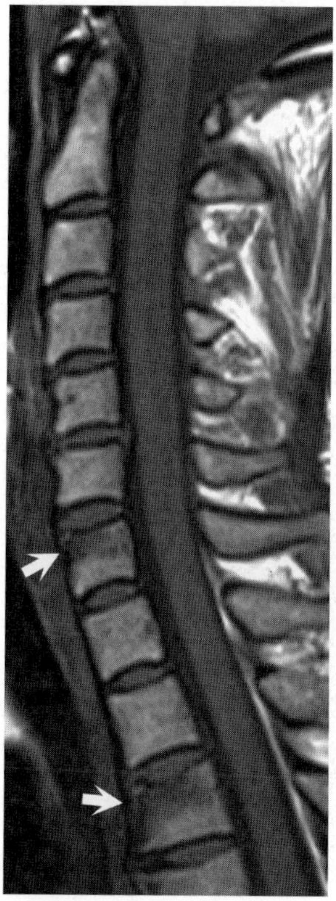

Fig. 30.3

MRI is the only modality allowing direct visualization of ligamentous injury. The dense avascular ligaments surrounding the spine appear as low SI on all pulse sequences. The anterior longitudinal ligament—commonly damaged in extension injury—is normally seen on sagittal images as a continuous thin band of low SI anterior to the vertebral bodies. Edema or discontinuity within this band signifies injury. In distinction, the posterior longitudinal ligament (PLL; which is also injured in extension) normally appears discontinuous due to variability in its width (thicker posterior to the disks but thinner posterior to the vertebral bodies). Flexion injury may damage the interspinous ligaments as in **Fig. 30.2A**, where there is edema posteriorly at the C4–C5 level and splaying of the spinous processes. The use of spectral fat saturation (with FSE T2WI) or STIR (see Chapter 34) improves the visualization of edema within the soft tissues. In the setting of spinal trauma, vascular structures—particularly the vertebral artery as it courses through the foramen transversum—must also be evaluated on MRI and MRA for the presence of dissection or occlusion.

31 Disk Herniations

Disk herniations (i.e., focal disk protrusions) in the cervical spine occur most frequently between the 4th and 7th vertebral bodies due to the greater mobility of the spinal column in this region. Optimal imaging technique is essential for detection of these and other cervical spine abnormalities, as the structures being evaluated are small and artifacts related to gross patient motion are common. Motion artifact (i.e., swallowing) is frequent, but correctable with saturation pulses or through changes in the direction of the phase encoding gradient. CSF pulsation artifact may be reduced by gradient moment nulling and cardiac gating. The small size of intervertebral disks warrants selection of a slice thickness of 3 mm or less, and for this reason imaging at 3 T—where a 3-mm slice thickness is standard—is imperative. Routinely acquired sequences for the evaluation of cervical disk herniations include sagittal and axial T1, sagittal FSE T2, and axial GRE T2WI. Whereas in the lumbar spine T1WI may detect the displacement of high SI epidural fat, indicating the presence of herniation, the lack of such fat in the cervical region renders this pulse sequence less useful. On FSE T2WI a herniated disk may mimic the low SI appearance of an osteophyte. Thus, (axial) GRE T2WI is the preferred sequence for evaluation of cervical disk herniations. GRE lacks the refocusing pulses present in spin and fast spin echo sequences and is thus more sensitive to T2* (magnetic susceptibility) effects. The high SI of the fluid-filled disk is thus well seen against the calcium-rich bone, which exhibits a very low SI.

Disk herniations are described in terms of their location, chronicity, and mass effect on the cord. **Figures 31.1A and 31.1C** demonstrate the typical appearance of a central cervical disk herniation (at C3–C4) on sagittal FSE and axial GRE T2WI, respectively. Mild cord flattening is present without any evidence of edema. The PLL and dura are apparent as a single rim of low SI along the perimeter of the herniated disk (**Fig. 31.1C**). Although clearly contiguous here, separation of the native and herniated portions of disk by the PLL—seen as an intervening band of low SI—indicates the presence of a disk fragment. The C5–C6 herniation in **Figs. 31.1B,D** not only exerts mass effect upon the cord, but also extends into the left neural foramina, impinging the exiting 6th cervical

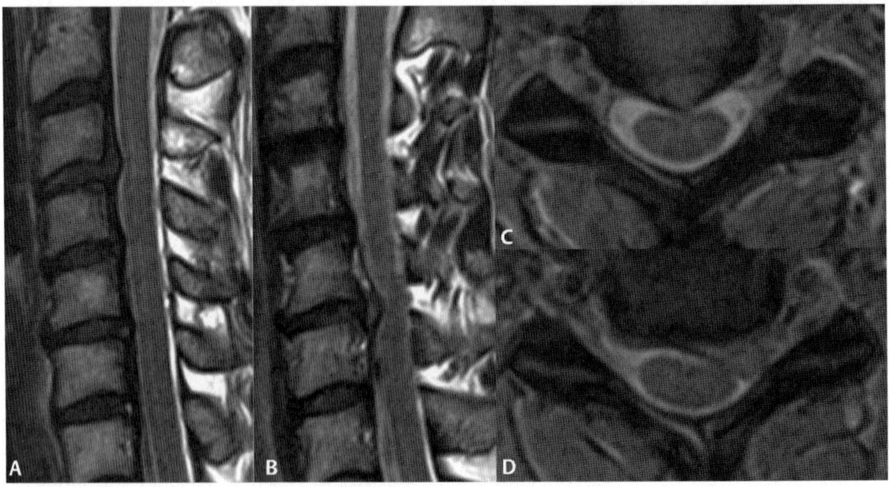

Fig. 31.1 (A–D)

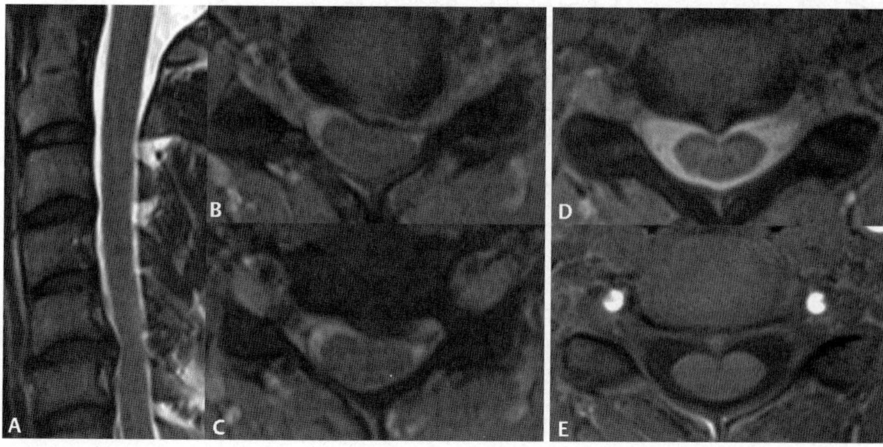

Fig. 31.2 (A–E)

nerve. Each cervical spinal nerve (eight in total) exits the spinal column above the correspondingly numbered cervical vertebral body (seven in total), except for the 8th nerve, which exits above the T1 vertebrae. Impingement of these roots causes radicular pain in the corresponding sensory dermatome. The C6 dermatome consists of the lateral arm, thumb, and index finger, the C7 of the central hand and middle finger, and the C8 of the fourth and fifth fingers along with the medial arm. A foraminal herniation may be difficult to identify, and specifically to distinguish from normal epidural venous plexus, as both are found in a similar location and exhibit slight hyperintensity on GRE T2WI.

Postcontrast T1WI can help delineate the brightly enhancing plexus from the nonenhancing disk. Contrast enhancement of a foraminal mass favors a nerve sheath tumor over a simple foraminal herniation. Enhancement is also seen in disk space infection and facet joint synovitis. All of the disk herniations in **Fig. 31.1** are acute, although this cannot be definitively proven on a single MRI. Clinically, acute herniations occur in active, middle-aged patients with new-onset pain often in precise dermatomal distributions. The presence of supra- or subjacent osteophytes implies herniation chronicity. **Figures 31.2A** and **31.2B** demonstrate a left foraminal herniation with **(B)** high SI disk surrounded by a low SI rim of ligament and dura on GRE T2WI. This herniation is flanked superiorly by an osteophyte that is visible on both **(A)** sagittal FSE T2WI and on **(C)** axial GRE T2WI as an area of uniformly low SI. PLL thickening (present somewhat here) and calcification may further compress the cord. A calcified herniation can appear similar to an osteophyte, confounding the diagnosis. Finally, **Figs. 31.2D,E** demonstrate a small central herniation on GRE T2WI and T1WI, respectively. The herniation effaces the ventral subarachnoid space, but does not contact the cord. Adjacent axial images demonstrated the presence of surrounding osteophytes, implying chronicity.

32 Degenerative Disease

Longstanding disk herniations or bulges may result in the formation of hypertrophic end plate spurs (i.e., osteophytes). The severity of symptoms resulting from osteophytes (which are typically asymptomatic) does not correlate with their imaging appearance. Osteophyte distribution within the cervical spine directly varies with spinal axis mobility: the mobile lower cervical spine is affected initially with superior spread as disease worsens. **Figure 32.1A** demonstrates a case of moderately advanced degenerative disease with disk osteophyte complexes at the C3–C7 levels. GRE T2WI aid in distinguishing osteophytes from similarly appearing disk herniations on FSE T2WI: the nucleus pulposus and inner disk annulus, due to their mucopolysaccharide matrix, demonstrate high SI on GRE T2WI, whereas susceptibility effects from calcium in osteophytes result in a very low SI appearance. The osteophytes in the FSE T2WI of **Fig. 32.1A** result in a mild degree of central canal stenosis—note the lack of CSF surrounding the cord at the involved levels. More severe stenosis is present on the FSE T2WI of **Fig. 32.1B** where an osteophyte compresses the thecal sac and flattens the cord at the C4–C5 level. The normal AP diameter of the cervical canal (best measured on axial FSE T2WI) is over 13 mm; a canal less than 10 mm in diameter is stenotic. Additional degenerative findings in **Fig. 32.1B** include disk space height loss at the C4–C5 and C5–C6 levels and a slight anterolisthesis of C2 on C3—both common degenerative findings. As osteophytes form around the uncovertebral joint (present from C2–C3 to C6–C7), neuroforaminal narrowing, most typically anteromedially, may occur. The uncovertebral joint is formed by the uncinate process of a given vertebral body extending superiorly to articulate with a depression in the adjacent end plate of the superior vertebral body. Foraminal narrowing may be exacerbated by disk space height loss. Stenosis of the foramen can compress the exiting nerve root resulting in radiculopathy. Foraminal caliber is often difficult to evaluate due to its small size relative to standard slice thickness (3–4 mm) and orientation oblique to the axial plane. Thin-slices, oblique sectioning, and 3D imaging—in which interslice gaps are eliminated—may

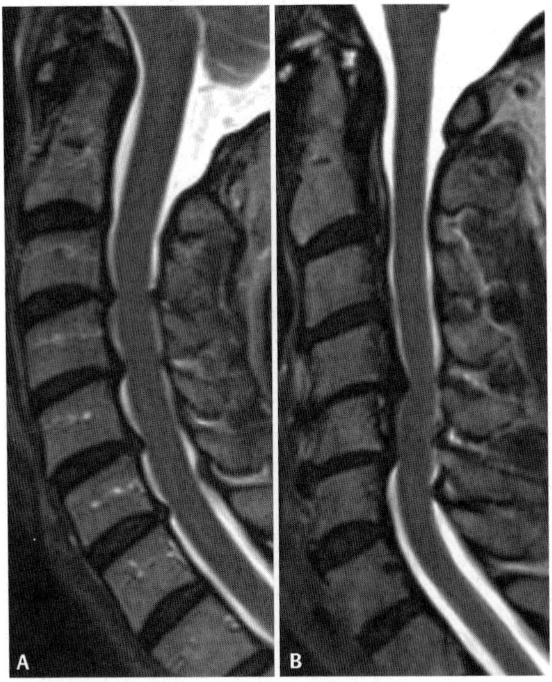

Fig. 32.1 (A,B)

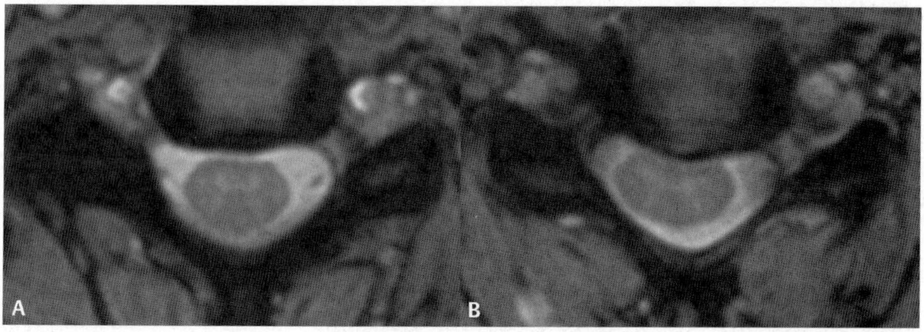

Fig. 32.2 (A,B)

improve visualization, although delineations between mild, moderate, and severe narrowing may still vary between readers. GRE T2WI—the mainstay for evaluating the neural foramen—in **Figs. 32.2A,B** demonstrate **(A)** moderate right neural foraminal narrowing in a patient with a **(B)** disk-osteophyte complex that also impinges the central canal, flattening the normal elliptical shape of the cervical cord. A disk herniation (see Chapter 31) may be superimposed on degenerative changes. The herniation seen on the FSE **(A)** and GRE **(B)** T2WI of **Fig. 32.3** severely narrows the neural foramen on the right. Moderate narrowing is present on the left. It is difficult to prove a herniation to be acute, although osteophytes were seen superior to the herniation in **Fig. 32.3**, implying a chronic process. In this image, the herniated disk deforms the cord, resulting in cordal hyperintensity likely correlating with edema or gliosis. Given the suspected chronicity of the lesion, the latter is more likely. As evident in this case, cord hyperintensity is typically more clearly seen with FSE than GRE T2WI.

Figure 32.4 demonstrates a particularly severe case of cervical spondylotic disease. **(A)** Central canal stenosis is present at multiple levels on sagittal FSE T2WI. Axial images at the most severely narrowed level (C2–C3) further highlight moderate to severe canal stenosis and marked cord flattening. Both the **(B)** axial GRE T2WI

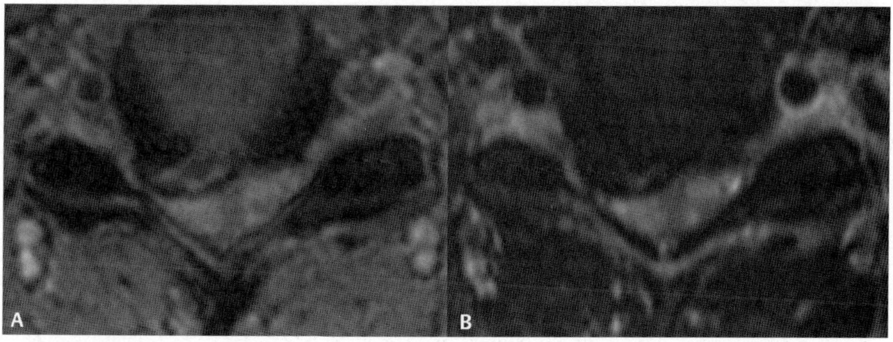

Fig. 32.3 (A,B)

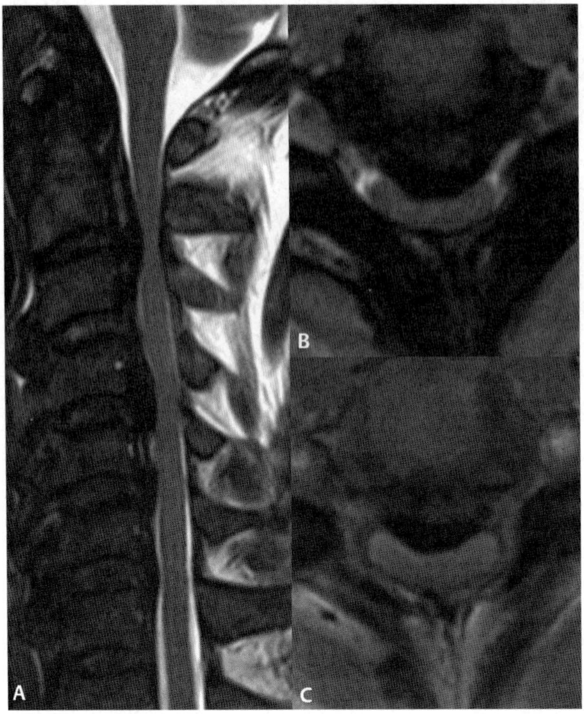

Fig. 32.4 (A–C)

and **(C)** T1WI also demonstrate a thick band of low SI posterior to the vertebral body. This represents dense calcium in the region of the PLL suggestive of PLL ossification. An ossified PLL is a fairly uncommon cause of spinal stenosis that typically involves the cord at multiple levels. Unless fatty marrow is present, it appears as low SI on T2WI due to the susceptibility effects of calcium. Patients with an ossified PLL are at higher risk of traumatic spinal cord injury.

33 Rheumatoid and Postoperative Changes

Rheumatoid arthritis exhibits a predilection for the cervical spine at the atlas and dens. Osteophytes are characteristically absent. Transverse ligament laxity and eventual atlantoaxial subluxation may occur. Such laxity is manifest as increased atlantoodontoid distance. Settling of the skull on the atlas is a severe complication and is demonstrated in **Fig. 33.1A**. In basilar invagination, by definition, the dens extends above Chamberlain's line (drawn from the posterior hard palate to the posterior lip of the foramen magnum) by >3 mm. This case also demonstrates a large, hypervascular pannus surrounding the dens (in particular anteriorly) and exhibiting high SI on **(A)** T2WI. A hypervascular pannus will brightly enhance, although minimally enhancing hypovascular and fibrous panni also occur, demonstrating intermediate and low SI on T2WI, respectively. Erosion of the dens is clearly seen on the **(B)** axial T1WI. Although such erosions may be better visualized on CT, MRI offers superior soft tissue evaluation, such as the rheumatoid-related cord compression in **Fig. 33.1A**. Sagittal images in flexion and extension may further aid in evaluation.

Ischemic cord damage resulting from chronic compression eventually warrants surgery to prevent further injury. An anterior approach is most common, whereby the disk is resected and replaced with bone graft. As seen with the anterior plate and screw fusion depicted on the sagittal T2WI image of **Fig. 33.2A**, the graft may initially demonstrate variable SI characteristics. After 2 years, successfully fused vertebral bodies should appear as contiguous marrow SI. Surrounding orthopedic hardware aids in the fusion, and appears as low SI due to the susceptibility effects of its constituent metal. Compared with FSE, GRE is inherently more prone to susceptibility artifact due to its lack of 180-degree refocusing pulses. Although the effects of susceptibility artifacts are greater at 3 T, SNR improvements at this field strength allow higher rates of bandwidth sampling and implementation of parallel imaging, which reduce such effects while preserving other benefits of imaging at 3 T. Sagittal FSE T2WI and axial FSE T1WI in **Figs. 33.2A,B**, respectively, demonstrate a central and left paracentral herniation just inferior to the fusion level with associated cord flattening and deformation. Surgical fusion predisposes to disk herniations superior and inferior to the operative level. The FSE T2WI of **Fig. 33.3A** demonstrates a less common, posterior approach to the correction of cervical spondylosis. Changes from a multilevel laminectomy are evident from the absence of posterior osseous structures, but degenerative changes persist, including severe C6–C7 canal stenosis and cord flattening. At this level, the cord also exhibits high SI—likely representative of gliosis in this setting. At C6–C7, an older style of vertebral body fusion

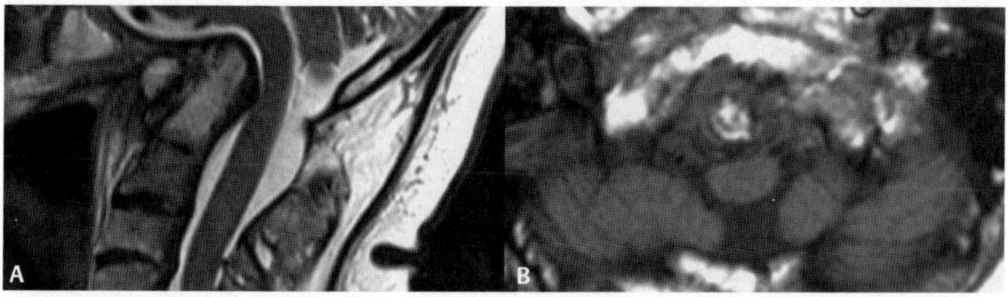

Fig. 33.1 (A,B)

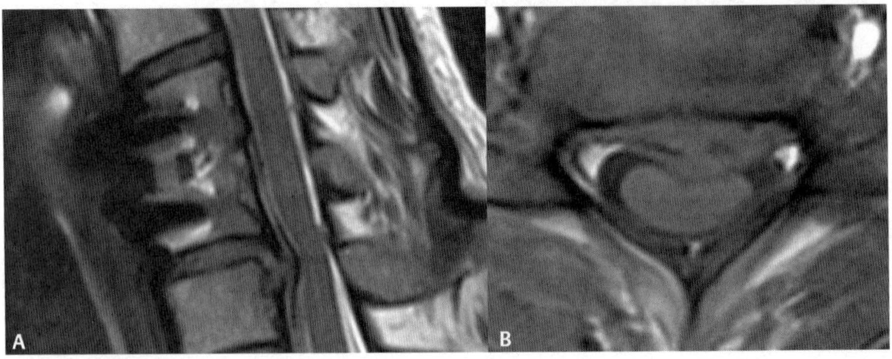

Fig. 33.2 (A,B)

surgery is evident from the incomplete disk space extending across that level. Such fusions utilized only bone graft within the disk interspace without additional orthopedic hardware. An osteophyte, clearly identified by its marrow-like SI, is also noted on the axial T1WI of **Fig. 33.3B** causing significant right-sided cord flattening.

In the postoperative spine, scar may mimic a disk herniation on MRI, although the former typically exhibits a lower SI on T2WI without mass effect. Images acquired immediately following contrast administration clinch the diagnosis as epidural scar tissue homogeneously enhances. Enhancement of the disk space itself is seen with infectious diskitis (see Chapter 48), a process favored by concurrent adjacent vertebral body or paravertebral soft tissue enhancement. Enhancement may also be seen in end plate degenerative changes as well, however. Diskitis will demonstrate intradiscal high SI with adjacent areas of vertebral end plate destruction, whereas degenerative disks should appear as low SI on T1 and T2WI. Degenerative disk disease must also not be confused with the normal changes of aging. With age decreasing glycosaminoglycans within the disk result in a slight decrease in SI on T2WI. Small concentric tears may occur with subsequent development of mucoid material or fluid within the torn space, identified by bands of high SI on T2WI. Although these changes are normal, significant changes in disk space SI or loss of disk space height suggest degeneration.

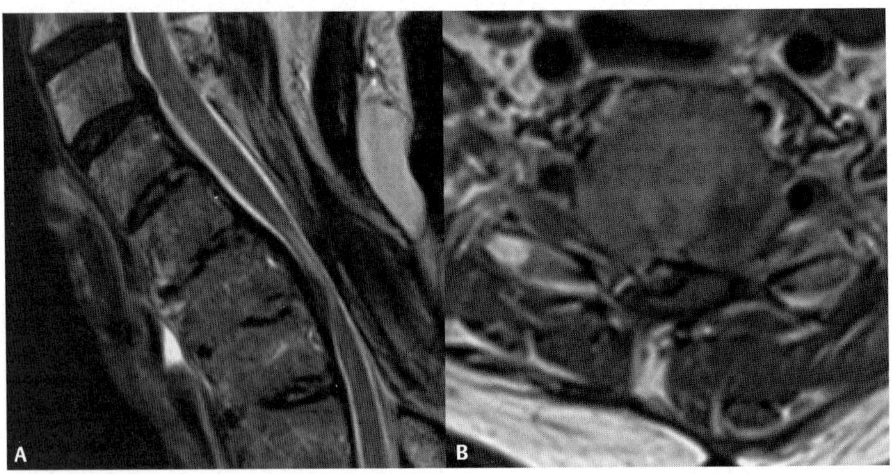

Fig. 33.3 (A,B)

34 Other Inflammatory/Infectious Diseases

At autopsy spinal cord involvement is seen in essentially all cases of MS. Cord lesions are also part of the consensus criteria for the MRI diagnosis of MS (see Chapter 18). Furthermore, isolated spinal involvement may occur in up to a quarter of cases, and suggestive lesions on spinal MRI are much more specific for MS than are hyperintensities on T2WI of the brain. Thus MRIs of the brain, cervical, and thoracic spine comprise a complete imaging evaluation of MS. MRI of the lumbar spine—where the spinal cord is absent—need not be performed. **Figure 34.1A** demonstrates an FSE T2WI of an MS plaque in the cervical spine with a focal area of high SI (*black arrow*) extending longitudinally within the cord. As is typical for MS, this lesion exerts little mass effect and it spans less than two vertebral body segments in length. Occasionally, edema above and below a plaque may result in a flame-like appearance on sagittal images. In **Figs. 34.1A,B,C** the lesion on sagittal MRI **(A)** is more subtle in appearance than in the axial GRE **(B)** and FSE T2WI **(C)**. The axial plane is preferred to sagittal imaging for the detection of MS in the spinal cord due in part to partial volume averaging—a term referring to the fact that the SI of a voxel on MRI represents an average of SI over a volume of actual tissue. Thus, in a longitudinally extending MS plaque of thin width, the SI of a voxel in the sagittal plane may contain SI contributions from both the plaque itself and also from normal cord, the average of the two contributing to a inconspicuous appearance of plaque on the final image. Lesions are typically not well-visualized on T1WI due to relative isointensity to the cord. In **Figs. 34.1B,C**, lesion conspicuity is also slightly

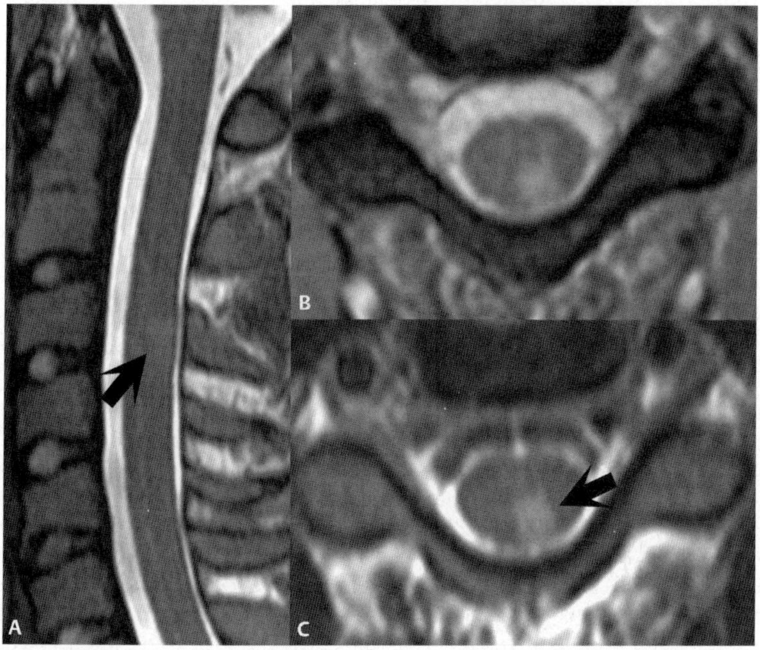

Fig. 34.1 (A–C)

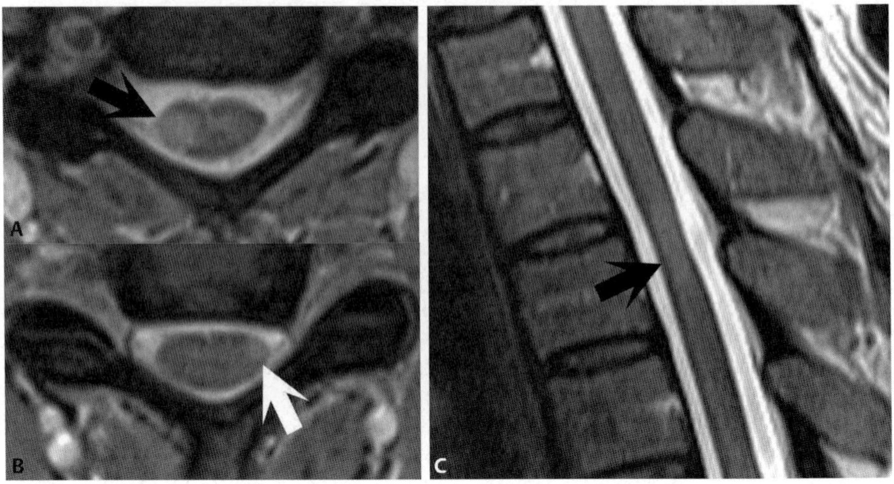

Fig. 34.2 (A–C)

greater on **(C)** the axial FSE (*black arrow*) than on the **(B)** GRE (note the extremely low SI of the osseous structures secondary to susceptibility effects) images in the same plane—a condition that holds true generally. **Figure 34.2A** (*black arrow*, GRE) demonstrates the tendency of cord plaques to indiscriminately affect gray and white matter, although the majority of cross-sectional cord area is spared even in this large lesion. There is also subtle mass effect, which is not uncommon. Small peripheral lesions (**Fig. 34.2B**, *white arrow*) may be difficult to detect even in the axial plane, emphasizing the need for optimal imaging technique. Changes in cord morphology due to a plaque may be appreciated and can manifest as focal atrophy (**Fig. 34.2C**, *black arrow*) or enlargement of the cord. The former correlates with increased clinical disability and chronicity, whereas focal enlargement is indicative of relapsing-remitting forms of MS.

As previously mentioned, optimal imaging techniques and pulse sequence selection are essential for the reliable detection of MS. For example, **Figs. 34.3A,B** demonstrate a lesion (**B**, *black arrow*) of the conus as seen on **(A)** FSE T2WI and **(B)** STIR (short tau inversion recovery)—the latter being a sequence in which an initial RF pulse is added with the purpose of suppressing signal from protons with a short T1, resulting in the nulling of SI from fat. For the detection of MS, STIR T2WI sequences are more sensitive than FSE in the cord, as evident from **Fig. 34.3A,B**, despite often being obtained at a lower spatial resolution (note the image blurriness). FLAIR T2WI, which have tremendous utility in brain MRI, consist of a similar initial pulse but one that is timed to suppress SI from protons with longer T1, specifically SI from CSF. FLAIR is less sensitive than either STIR or FSE T2WI for cord MS lesions. The use of FSE T2WI, though helpful in other settings, diminishes the conspicuity of MS lesions, impairing diagnosis. Motion and pulsation artifacts inherent to imaging of the thoracic spine may also hinder the detection of MS lesions occurring therein. Administration of IV contrast is another consideration as enhancement is frequently seen in symptomatic lesions and is indicative of plaque activity. **(C)** Sagittal and **(D)** axial images in **Fig. 34.3** demonstrate an elliptical-shaped enhancing lesion (*white arrow*). Because gadolinium chelates increase SI on T1WI by shortening the T1 (i.e., aiding relaxation) of nearby tissue protons, increased SI from contrast enhancement may not be visualized on postcontrast STIR sequences.

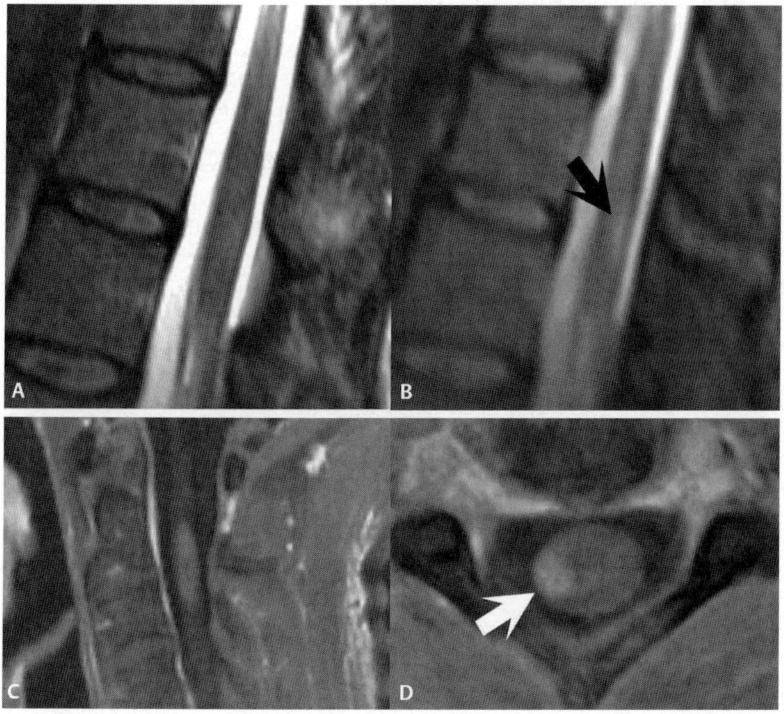

Fig. 34.3 (A–D)

Acute transverse myelitis may mimic MS both clinically and on MRI. Typical findings include a high SI focal abnormality on T2WI with fusiform cord enlargement. Unlike those of MS, lesions of transverse myelitis extend over several segments of vertebrae and occupy the majority of the cross-sectional cord area. Specific criteria have been developed for diagnosis. Inclusionary criteria ascertainable on MRI include the ruling out of compressive extraaxial etiologies as causes for neurologic findings and the presence of gadolinium enhancement, the latter indicative of cord inflammation. Without evidence of inflammation, which may also be obtained through CSF studies, close follow-up imaging and lumbar puncture are recommended. Intracranial findings suggestive of MS are exclusionary. **Figure 34.4** demonstrates a case of subacute combined degeneration—the spinal cord abnormality associated with vitamin B12 deficiency—in an individual with pernicious anemia. Areas of high SI on T2WI within the dorsal (as seen here) and lateral columns are the most common MRI findings.

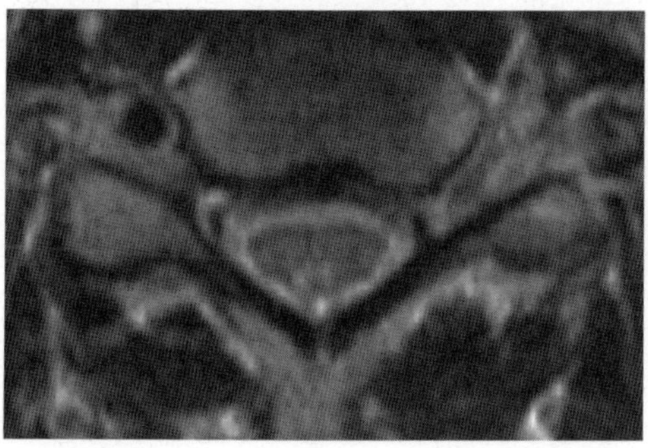

Fig. 34.4

35 Metastatic Disease

Of sites of skeletal metastasis, the vertebral column is the most common, and herein lung cancer is the most frequent culprit. Precontrast FSE T1WI is the preferred sequence for the detection of such metastases. As demonstrated in the sagittal images of **Fig. 35.1A**, infiltration of the vertebral body with tumor results in loss of the high SI of the fatty marrow. Typically, metastatic lesions will demonstrate SI equal to or less than the intervertebral disks on T1WI. This becomes especially important in cases of diffuse metastatic disease, whereby the vertebral body SI may be uniformly abnormal. Only by comparison with the disk SI can diffuse disease be diagnosed. An occasional hemorrhagic metastasis may appear as high SI on T1WI. Unfortunately, FSE T2WI do not typically display most vertebral body metastases well (**Fig. 35.1B**), due to the relatively high normal marrow SI (see Chapter 48). Even when fat suppression techniques are used, as in **Fig. 35.1C**, the high SI of metastases may be difficult to visualize against the suppressed fatty SI of the vertebral bodies. With the presence of a single vertebral lesion, reliable differentiation is not possible between metastasis and primary bone tumor. The presence of multiple lesions, however, strongly suggests metastatic disease. The most urgent complication from vertebral body metastases is compromise of the spinal canal and resulting cord compression. Because the hyperintensity of CSF on FSE T2WI allows excellent delineation of the subarachnoid space, this sequence is typically more useful for evaluation of canal compromise, as illustrated by a sagittal T2WI in **Fig. 35.2A**. Here, however, thecal sac compromise and cord compression are so severe to be well seen on (**Fig. 35.2B**) precontrast T1WI. As evident from **Fig. 35.2C**, axial imaging allows optimal evaluation of canal and cord compromise which is, in this case, severe.

In patients with uniformly diminished marrow SI—for example, children in which red marrow predominates or in patients with anemia of chronic disease or sickle cell (in which vertebral bodies are also classically H-shaped)—detection of metastatic lesions on T1WI may be problematic. Contrast administration in the setting of suspected vertebral body metastases, although not commonly performed, may nevertheless greatly improve tumor visualization. Although marrow SI is not diffusely abnormal in **Fig. 35.3A**, there is a large vertebral metastasis seen on the precontrast T1WI as an area of low SI against the

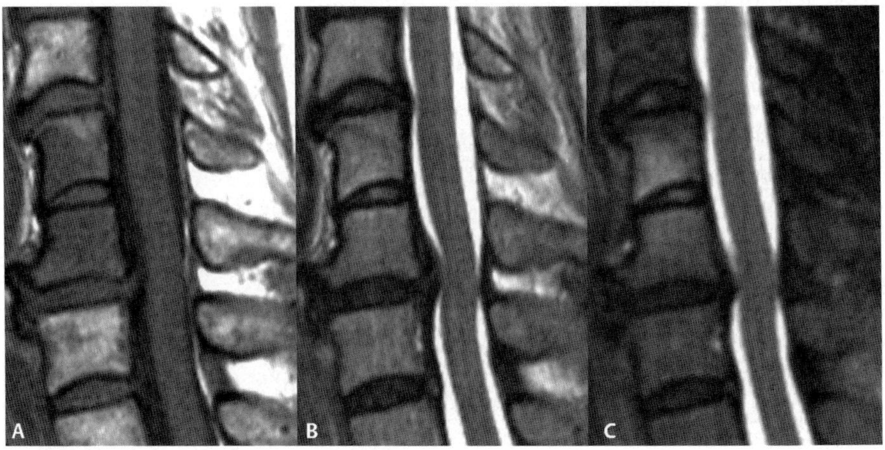

Fig. 35.1 (A–C)

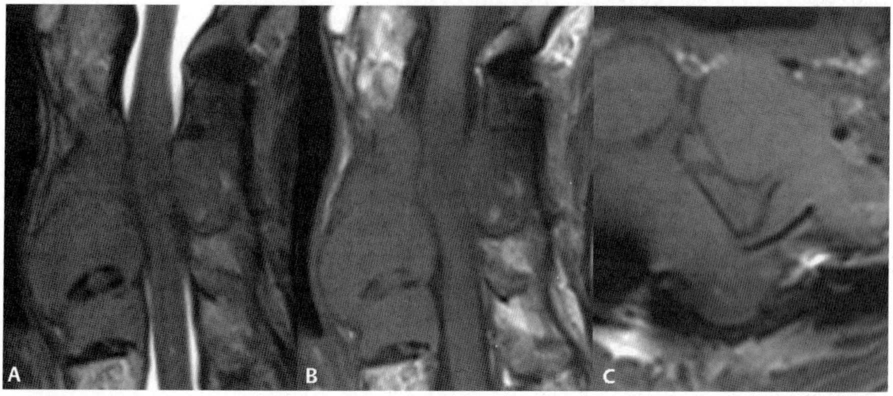

Fig. 35.2 (A–C)

higher SI fatty marrow of the T1 vertebral body. Visible, but much more subtle lesions are seen within the bodies of C7, T2, and the spinous process of T1. With contrast administration on **(B)** spectral fat suppressed T1WI, however, the visualization of these brightly enhancing lesions (*white arrows*) is greatly improved. Importantly, without some means of fat suppression, the enhancing tumor will not appear distinct from the high SI of surrounding marrow fat. Spectral fat saturation and STIR are discussed in more detail in Chapters 34 and 48, respectively; however, it is important to note that the inversion pulse used in STIR suppresses SI from tissues with short T1 comparable to that of fat. Gadolinium chelates diminish tissue T1, thus ordinarily increasing SI on T1WI. When STIR is utilized, however, often the reduced T1 obtained with gadolinium chelates is similar to that ordinarily suppressed through the inversion pulse in STIR. Thus, lesions that ordinarily enhance on T1WI may demonstrate lower (due to suppression) SI on STIR T1WI. A final clinical scenario in vertebral metastases involves distinguishing between fractures related to benign osteoporotic and neoplastic causes. This distinction is discussed in more detail in Chapter 43.

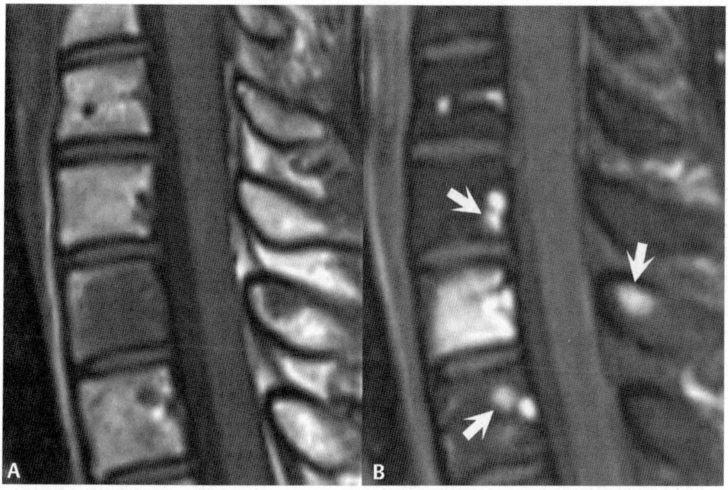

Fig. 35.3 (A,B)

36 Primary Neoplasms

Spinal neoplasias can be classified into lesions originating from the extradural, intradural extramedullary, and medullary spaces. Of the latter, astrocytomas are the most common in the cervical spine, frequently occurring in the thoracic spine as well. Astrocytomas classically span several vertebral segments in length and involve nearly the entire cross-section of the cord, the latter resulting in an expansile appearance on T1WI. Hyperintensity on T2WI reflects both the lesion and its surrounding edema. Enhancement is almost always present, to a degree, although some lesions and in particular more necrotic tumors may only enhance on delayed scans (30–60 minutes following contrast administration). Enhancement of the wall of cystic lesions aids in distinguishing them from otherwise similar appearing benign cystic lesions in the cord. Complex syrinxes too may mimic the appearance of an astrocytoma, although the walls of the latter are generally less distinct and CSF-pulsation artifacts absent. Contrast-enhanced MRI further aids in the distinction and should also be utilized in the initial workup of any syrinx without obvious cause (i.e., Chiari malformations).

Postoperatively, contrast administration is useful in differentiating nonenhancing postoperative changes from recurrent tumor, the latter almost invariably enhancing. In terms of differential diagnosis, an enhancing lesion of substantial craniocaudal extent could potentially represent cord ischemia or infarction, although this is very uncommon in the cervical spine. Unlike astrocytomas, ependymomas demonstrate a predilection for the lumbar spine; they are the most common tumor arising from the cauda equina and conus. Myxopapillary subtypes (see Chapter 51) in particular frequently originate in the lumbar spine. An example (in the cervical spine) of the more common cellular subtype is illustrated in the T2WI and contrast-enhanced T1WI of **Figs. 36.1A,B**, respectively. As shown here, ependymomas, unlike astrocytomas, are often heterogeneous on **(A)** T2WI. In this particular case, there is a **(B)** nonenhancing cyst at the most cephalad aspect of the lesion with edema extending from the lesion both rostrally and caudally as best seen on **(A)** T2WI. The cord is expanded, although somewhat more focally than would be expected with an astrocytoma, such expansion only spanning from C3–C4. Although cellular ependymomas are typically isointense to cord on precontrast T1WI, focal areas of hyperintensity secondary to subacute hemorrhage (on T1WI) or hypointensity due to hemosiderin deposition (on T2WI) may be seen. Astrocytomas hemorrhage less frequently. Ependymomas may contain foci of hypercellularity correlating with hypointensity on precontrast MRI sequences and tend to enhance more heterogeneously than astrocytomas. Involvement is also typically of a shorter segment of the cord than with an astrocytoma.

Turning to lesions that are typically smaller (and more focal), **Figs. 36.2A,B** demonstrate the appearance of a cavernous angioma on sagittal FSE T2WI and axial GRE T2WI, respectively. On the **(A)** sagittal image there is subtle cord expansion at the C2 level with the lesion demonstrating heterogeneous low SI on T2WI due to hemosiderin deposition. **(B)** The GRE T2WI, which is more sensitive to the susceptibility effects of blood products, exhibits the complete, hypointense hemosiderin rim typically associated with cavernous angiomas. Hemangioblastomas are another vascular lesion of the cervical and thoracic cord, although they are more common in the posterior fossa. Hemangioblastomas are discussed in greater detail in Chapter 51. Of intradural extramedullary lesions of the cervical cord, nerve sheath tumors and meningiomas (see Chapter 39 and 51) are most common. Like intracranial meningiomas, those of the spine tend to be found in adults. Purely extradural meningiomas may also

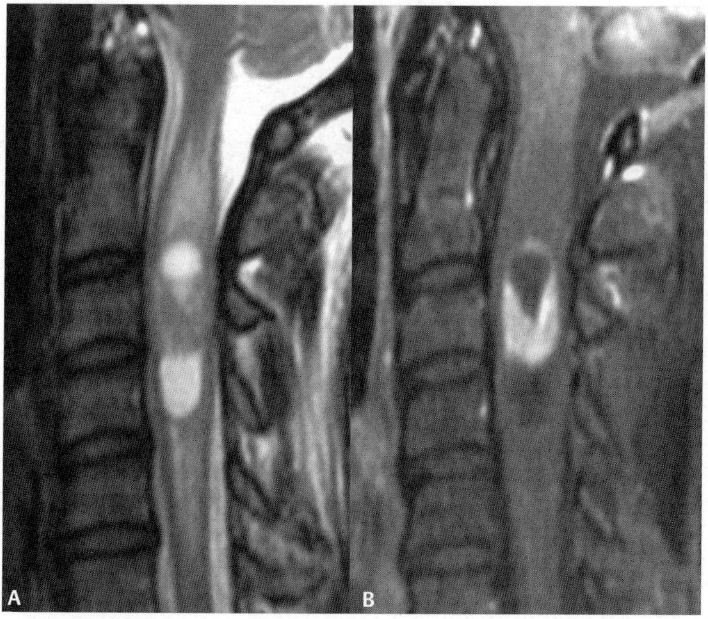

Fig. 36.1 (A,B)

occur and tend to be more aggressive. Meningiomas are typically solitary, although multiple lesions are associated with NF2. A typical appearance of a cervical cord meningioma is illustrated in the axial T2WI and contrast-enhanced T1WI of **Figs. 36.3A,B**, respectively. On the former, this well-delineated lesion clearly is arising within the dural space but outside of the spinal cord, somewhat compressing the latter posterolaterally and demonstrating slight hyperintensity to the cord on T2WI. Note also the broad dural base. The location of this tumor may be further elucidated on sagittal imaging where intramedullary extradural tumors demonstrate relative broadening of the subarachnoid space at its margin with the tumor as well as clear delineation of tumor from cord. As seen here, meningiomas characteristically enhance avidly and homogeneously postcontrast. Calcification is frequent, although not regularly

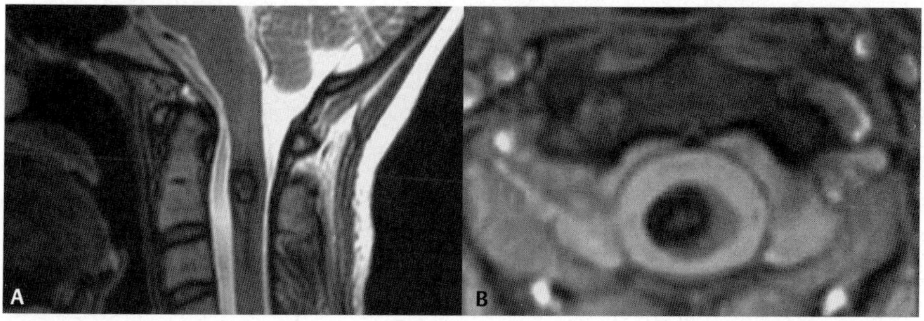

Fig. 36.2 (A,B)

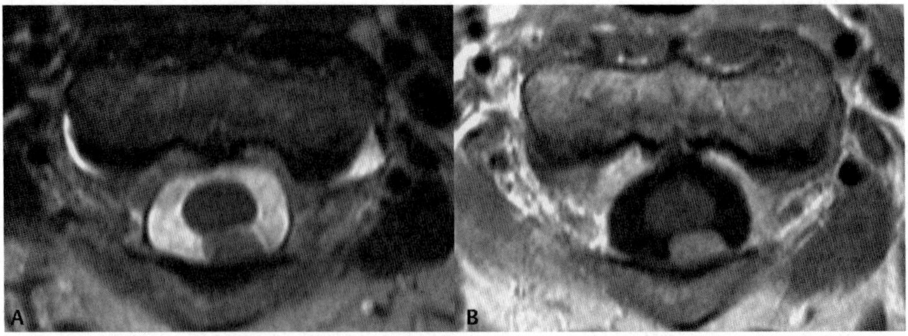

Fig. 36.3 (A,B)

appreciated on MRI, unless extremely dense (and then seen as a signal void). Points of distinction between spinal meningiomas and nerve sheath tumors as well as further differential considerations are covered in Chapters 39 and 51. Nerve sheath tumors are more frequently multiple in number, lack an enhancing dural tail, and may demonstrate foci of hypercellularity (Antoni A areas) correlating with low SI on T2WI in distinction to the normally homogeneous appearance of meningiomas.

37 Disk Herniations

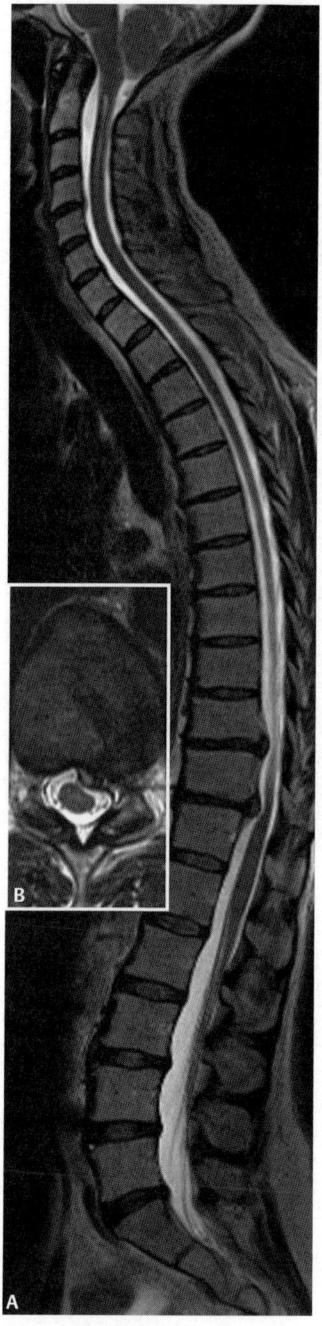

Fig. 37.1 (A,B)

Motion from CSF pulsation, respiration, and the beating heart complicate imaging of the thoracic spine. These effects can be minimized by the use of gradient moment nulling and saturation pulses. Proper evaluation of the thoracic spine begins with the acquisition of localizer sequences. Numbering begins from the dens, proceeding downward. Proper identification of lesions in this manner is necessary as the number of vertebrae in a given person is variable, owing most frequently to the presence of a sacralized L5 or lumbarized S1. **Figure 37.1A** is a standard localizing scan consisting of composed images of the cervical, thoracic, and lumbar spine. If the entire spine is being imaged during a single given session then, as seen here, high-resolution images can be used for the localizer image. Alternatively, a faster localization scan can be obtained by overlaying lower quality images to form the composed sagittal image. In this particular T2W localizer scan, pathology of the cervical spine is identifiable in this Chiari 1 patient, including occipital decompression (note the missing posterior arch of C1) and a small cervical syrinx. In the thoracic spine, two areas of herniation are present. **Figure 37.1B** more clearly demonstrates the herniation at T11–T12, which appears as a high SI protrusion outlined by the low SI PLL on this axial T2WI. Although the cord does not visibly contact the herniation itself on this image, with movement (such as bending), there can be contact and the cord can become deformed. As throughout the spine, acute and chronic herniations appear identical on MRI with adjacent osteophytes suggesting the latter. The disk herniation in **Fig. 37.2A** (at the upper of the two involved levels) thus appears to be chronic by virtue of its adjacent, superior osteophyte. This cord-deforming disk herniation appears as intermediate and low SI on T1 **(B)** and T2WI **(C)**, respectively. Generally speaking, smaller lesions than seen at

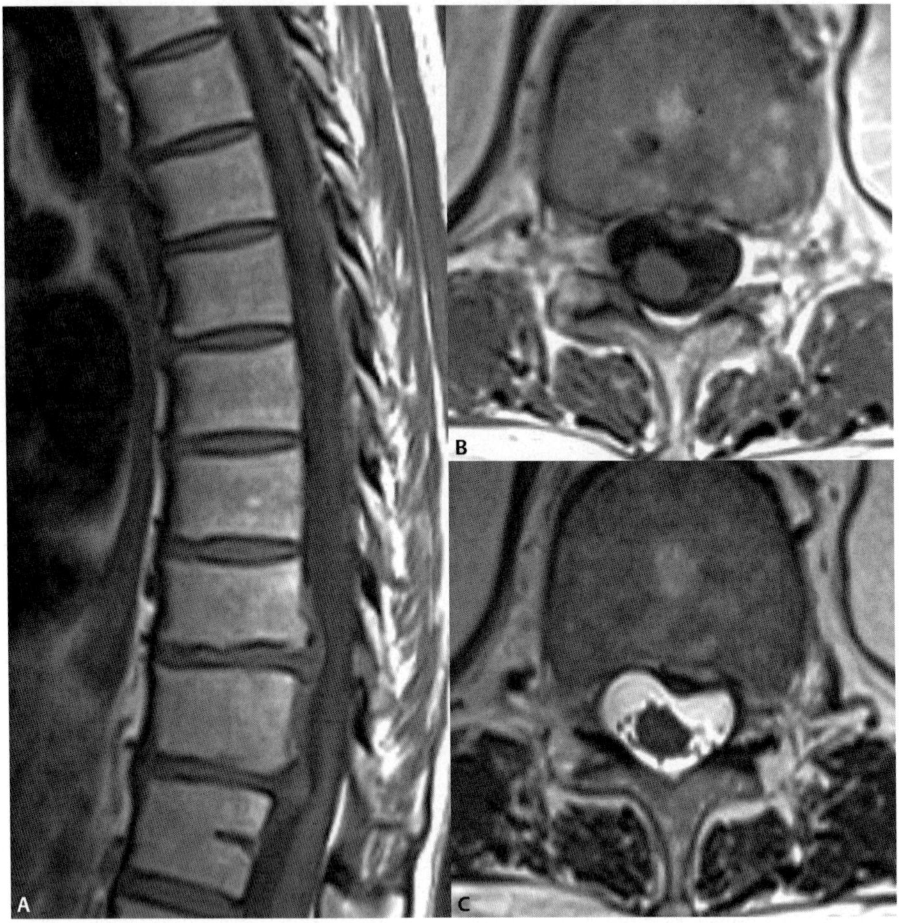

Fig. 37.2 (A–C)

other levels will impinge upon the thoracic cord due to its anterior position within the subarachnoid space. Such small disk herniations are optimally imaged with thin slices in the axial plane. With thinner slices, fewer protons are available within a slice to create signal, and SNR is reduced. With greater magnet strengths, however, more protons are recruited for signal creation; thus, imaging at 3 T allows routine acquisition of slices ≤3 mm thick on MRI. Such images are demonstrated in **Figs. 37.2 B,C**. Notably,

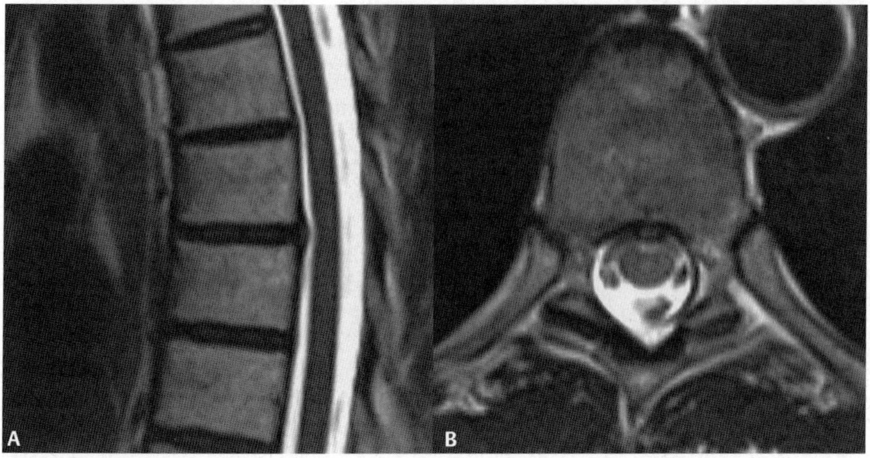

Fig. 37.3 (A,B)

sequences optimized for 1.5 T systems when performed at 3 T will result in poor image quality. The axial T1WI in **Fig. 37.2B**, for example, was not acquired with a traditional FSE sequence as would be used at 1.5 T, but rather a technique known as VIBE (volume interpolated breath-hold examination). CSF pulsation artifacts represent another dilemma in imaging the thoracic spine. **Figures 37.3A** and **37.3B** demonstrate the typical appearance of a small central disk herniation on sagittal and axial T2WI, respectively. On the latter, however, the additional areas of low SI within the hyperintense CSF obscure complete evaluation. Pulsatile motion within the CSF—greatest in the thoracic spine and in the young—has resulted in a flow void effect in this instance with resulting foci of decreased SI appearing within the normally high SI CSF.

38 Canal Compromise

The fact that compression fractures can be the result of metastatic involvement or benign osteoporosis was mentioned in Chapter 35 and is demonstrated in the precontrast T1WI of **Fig. 38.1A**. In this image, the SI of the T9 and T11 vertebral bodies is markedly higher than that of the normal T6, T7, and T12 vertebral bodies. In fact, vertebral bodies T8–T11 were irradiated to treat the metastatic tumor within T10. Within the first week of irradiation, edematous marrow changes lead to the appearance of high and low SI on T2WI and T1WI, respectively. However, just as ionizing radiation destroys metabolically active neoplastic lesions, so too does it kill active hematopoietic marrow cells within bone. Thus one week following radiation therapy, compensatory hypertrophy of the fatty elements of marrow begins to increase the SI on T1WI, eventually resulting in hyperintensity of these vertebral bodies when compared with normal. Structures irradiated with low doses of radiation may eventually return to a normal SI appearance. Unfortunately, radiation therapy in this case was not successful, and recurrence of metastatic disease within the T10 vertebral is seen. Related metastatic collapse has resulted in anterior compression of the spinal canal. As with any suspected compression, axial images should be examined to more accurately assess canal compromise. Finally, loss of anterior T8 vertebral body height suggests an additional compression fracture. With chronic fractures, the preservation of marrow signal intensity permits the diagnosis of an osteoporotic fracture; however, acute fractures due to osteoporosis and malignancy are difficult to distinguish on MRI because edema-like SI changes are present in both.

In this instance, a band of low SI edema is seen within T8 on **Fig. 38.1A**—a fracture favored to be osteoporotic due to the lack of a discrete metastatic foci. In **Fig. 38.1B**, involvement by metastatic disease has led to the expansion of the posterior elements

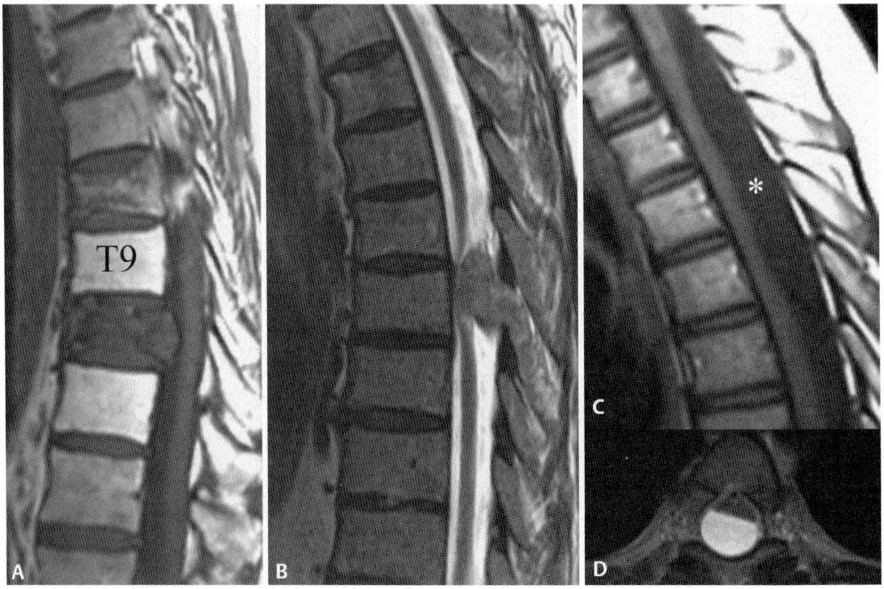

Fig. 38.1 (A–D)

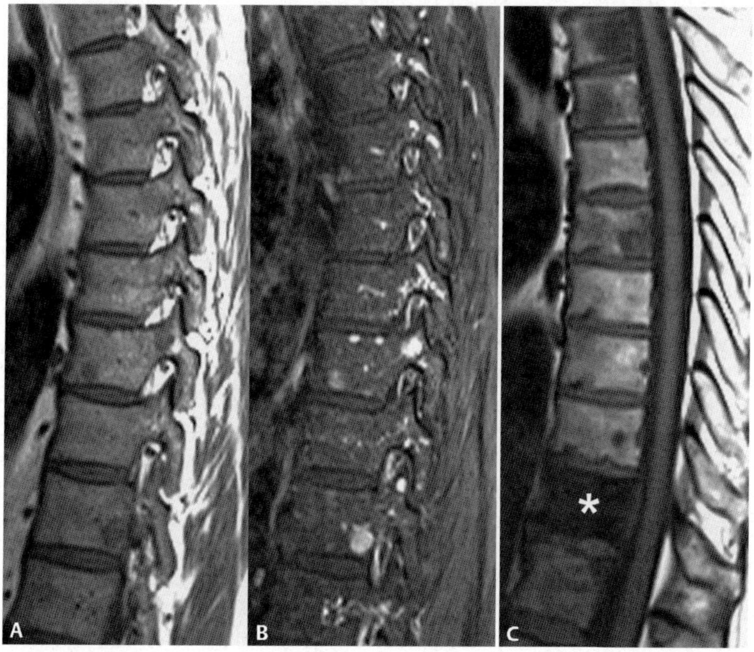

Fig. 38.2 (A–C)

of T7 with resultant compression of the cord. For reasons described in Chapter 38, the non-FS FSE T2WI shown fails to demonstrate the metastatic foci that were present on this slice in T3, T4, and T7 on the FSE T1 and FS T2WI. Not all lesions compressing the cord, of course, are metastatic (i.e., primary bone tumors like osteochondromas) or even neoplastic (i.e., epidural abscesses or osteoporotic compression fractures). An arachnoid cyst, as demonstrated in **Fig. 38.1C**, is another potential culprit. The SI of these lesions is characteristically that of CSF. As such they may only be detectable by noting spinal cord compression or nerve root displacement. Subtle distinction of the arachnoid cyst from normal CSF SI may be made due to differences in fluid mobility inside (*asterisk*) and outside of the cyst. As with any lesion impinging the cord, the degree of compression is best evaluated on axial images. The T2WI in **Fig. 38.1D** demonstrates marked compression of the normal low SI cord (displaced anteriorly) by the hyperintense arachnoid cyst.

In multiple myeloma, involved vertebral bodies may appear normal on MRI, or diffusely or focally infiltrated. The latter is the case in **Fig. 38.2A**, in which small low SI lesions are present, which are somewhat subtle on FSE T1WI. With the administration of contrast and saturation of fat SI, however (**Fig. 38.2B**), these lesions are much more obvious. Osteoblastic metastatic lesions, often found in prostate and breast cancer, appear as extremely low SI on T1WI and, as opposed to their lytic counterparts, T2WI. **Figure 38.2C** demonstrates a very low SI blastic metastasis (*asterisk*) among other, less hypointense lytic lesions on a sagittal T1WI.

39 Primary Neoplasms

Schwannomas and neurofibromas share a similar MRI appearance and are both common lesions in thoracic spine MRI. Schwannomas typically demonstrate heterogeneously high SI on T2WI with a moderate or low SI on T1WI. Foci of lower SI on T2WI may correlate with pathologically denser tissue in which there is a diminished amount of free water. In **Fig. 39.1A**, the extramedullary intradural mass—a location suggested by the relative broadening of the subarachnoid space at its margin with the tumor and the clear delineation of tumor from cord—compresses the spinal cord displacing it to the left. Both schwannomas and neurofibromas may occur less commonly extradurally or extend both intra- and extradurally leading to a dumbbell shape. As in the post-contrast T1WI of **Figs. 39.1A,B** these neoplasias often enhance heterogeneously, and small lesions may not be visible without contrast administration. The nonenhancing region of the tumor in **Fig. 39.1B** correlated with a region of high SI on T2WI, suggesting cystic degeneration and thus the diagnosis of schwannoma over neurofibroma. Other clues to distinguishing the two include the tendency of neurofibromas to be multiple and more homogeneous in their enhancement. They are also associated with NF1, although even the presence of a solitary neurofibroma makes an NF1 diagnosis likely. In contrast, spinal schwannomas are found more commonly, along with meningiomas, in NF2. Schwannomas also tend to arise eccentric to a given nerve, compressing it, whereas neurofibromas tend to enlarge the nerve itself. Malignant schwannomas may occasionally occur and demonstrate more infiltrative borders and a larger overall size than their benign counterparts.

Schwannomas and neuromas also comprise the most common cause of posterior mediastinal neoplasia along with—in increasing order of prognosis, age of onset, and degree of cellular maturation—neuroblastomas, ganglioneuroblastoma, and ganglioneuromas. The latter three entities are of neural crest cell origin, thus occurring along the sympathetic chain and within the adrenal medulla. Tumors arising at the former location may extend to involve the spine or surrounding structures. These tumors tend to affect patients younger than 20 years old with neuroblastomas pathologically classified as one of the small round blue cell tumors of childhood. Consequent hypercellularity may contribute to a lower SI on T2WI than that seen with nerve sheath tumors; although, this distinction is unreliable given the potential in the latter for areas of lower SI secondary to densely packed cellularity (termed Antoni A in schwannomas). Given its high and low SI on T2WI and T1WI, in **Figs. 39.1C,D** respectively, combined with its homogeneous enhancement with contrast (not shown), the posterior mediastinal mass in this figure (*asterisk*) could potentially represent any of the aforementioned entities with nerve sheath tumors representing statistically the most common pathology, especially in an older (83 years in this case) patient.

Meningiomas are the second most common intrathecal tumor after those of the neural sheath. As with intracranial varieties they tend to be histologically benign and slow-growing, demonstrating a broad dural base. Meningiomas tend to occur in an anterolateral location relative to the cervical spinal cord and posterolaterally at all other levels. Multiple paraspinal meningiomas (as with bilateral lesions involving the internal auditory canals) are nearly pathognomonic for NF2. Although multiple in this rare condition, meningiomas, like schwannomas and in contrast to neurofibromas, tend to occur as solitary lesions. With the latter two, dural adherence is less commonly seen. The meningioma in **Figs. 39.1E,F**, as is typical for this type of lesion, is

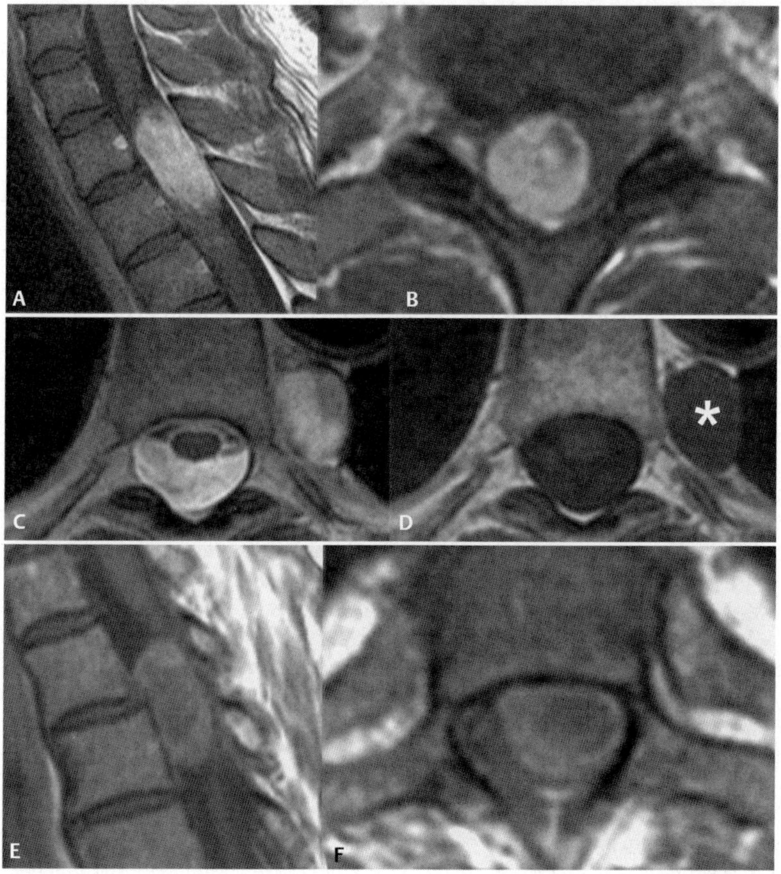

Fig. 39.1 (A–F)

intradural and extramedullary in location—which is again suggested by the broadened subarachnoid space near the tumor margin (well illustrated in this instance on the sagittal image, **E**)—displacing and compressing the spinal cord to the right **(F)**. Acquisition of the **(F)** provided post-contrast T1WI was delayed following contrast administration and because of this, lesion enhancement is less prominent than that typically seen with these highly vascular lesions. Also in this case, the central area of decreased SI seen on both sagittal (**Fig. 39.1E**) and axial (**Fig. 39.1F**) images was of similar low SI on all pulse sequences and correlated with an area of dense calcification on CT. The tendency to calcify is relatively characteristic of spinal meningiomas, occurring in approximately three-fourths of cases.

40 Vascular Abnormalities

Vascular pathology within the thecal sac includes structural abnormalities such as AVMs and arteriovenous fistulas (AVFs), in addition to ischemic and hemorrhagic disease resulting from these and other etiologies. AVMs are congenital lesions (associated with Osler-Weber-Rendu syndrome) that consist of a nidus of pathologic vessels between enlarged feeding arteries and draining veins. The nidus is typically located within the cord, and high flow into the nidus may result in aneurysms within the feeding spinal arteries. This increased flow may similarly result in ischemia of adjacent cord parenchyma through a steal phenomenon or venous hypertension. On MRI AVMs appear as multiple flow voids representing the nidus along with enlarged, extramedullary (often anterior) feeding vessels. T1WI and T2WI best identify lesions within the cord and CSF, respectively. CSF pulsation artifacts on T2WI may occasionally mimic an AVM, but because the enlarged draining veins of an AVM brightly enhance, contrast administration may aid in this distinction and also in the detection of smaller lesions. High cord SI on T2WI adjacent to an AVM on MRI may represent gliosis or edema resulting from the mechanisms above. Intramedullary hemorrhage may also be present, its MRI appearance varying with the stage of blood products. As opposed to the glomus AVM (intramedullary) discussed above, juvenile AVMs (extradural-intradural) are significantly larger, occupying the entirety of the canal at a given level.

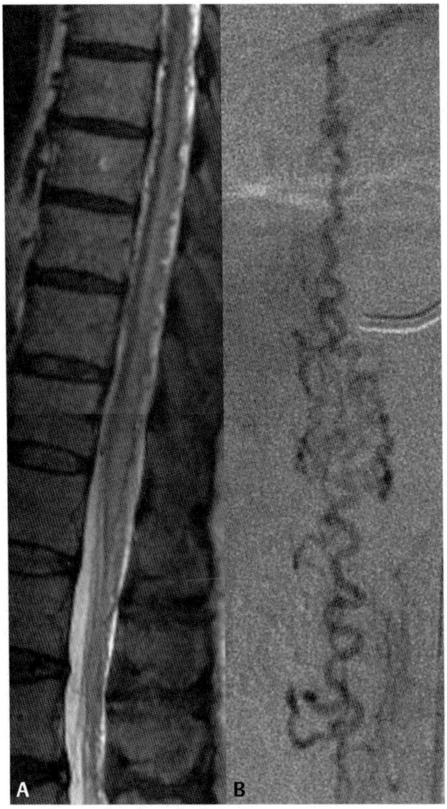

Fig. 40.1 (A,B)

In comparison to AVMs, AVFs are much more common and are acquired lesions favoring the lower cord. They consist of feeding arteries draining directly into enlarged veins. Two types of AVFs are defined in the spine: dural (most common) and cord AVFs. Dural AVFs lead to venous stasis and in some cases infarction. They occur along the dorsal aspect of the lower cord and conus and are fed by a single radicular artery through a dural branch. Secondary to increased venous flow, dural veins dilate, transmitting elevated venous pressures to cord veins, resulting in myelopathy and edema, which may both be visualized as high cord SI on T2WI (**Fig. 40.1A**). Typically, these SI changes involve the length of the cord from the conus to lower thoracic spine and are thus more diffuse than the SI changes present in demyelinating or inflammatory disorders. Even more suggestive of an AVF is the presence of dilated pial veins on T2WI as low SI flow voids against high SI CSF. In **Fig. 40.1A**, these serpiginous flow voids are present along both the ventral and dorsal aspects of the cord

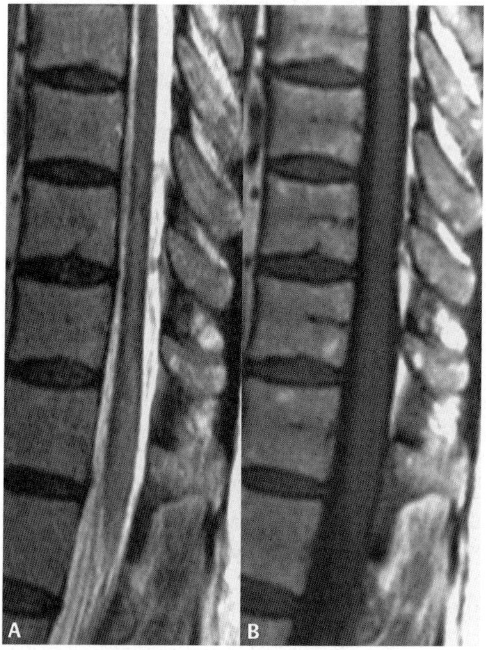

Fig. 40.2 (A,B)

in the lower thoracic spine and even within the cauda equina. CSF pulsation artifacts may mimic, in rare cases, such flow voids. Furthermore, the low SI appearance of the vasculature may be lost in areas of particularly slow venous flow as stagnant protons remain in-plane for the duration of the spin echo (see Chapter 12). In any case, contrast-enhanced T1WI as well as contrast-enhanced MRA reliably demonstrate enhancing, engorged pial veins. DSA provides the definitive diagnosis with identification of feeding and draining vessels: the dural AVF in **Fig. 40.1** was found on **(B)** DSA to be fed by a branch of the right T11 intercostal artery. In contrast to that of dural AVFs, the anomalous fistula of a cord AVF occurs within the cord and is fed directly by a spinal artery (most commonly the ASA). Cord AVFs also occur in a more ventral position. Cavernous malformations of the spinal cord—another important vascular abnormality—are discussed in Chapter 36.

Cord ischemia and infarction result from many causes, including atherosclerosis, vasculitis, embolism, infection, radiation, trauma, surgery, and spontaneous dissection. DWI is infrequently used in the spine due to marked susceptibility artifacts. T2WI demonstrate high SI within the cord (**Fig. 40.2A**) often confined to the metabolically active gray matter, and correlating with vasogenic edema. Differential considerations for this appearance are broad and include multiple sclerosis, transverse myelitis, neoplasia, and the venous hypertensive changes described above. Furthermore, on sagittal images, ischemic changes may not be apparent unless the cord is completely in-plane (that is, not oblique to the imaging plane) for its entire length. T1WI may only demonstrate focal cord enlargement (**Fig. 40.2B**), although enhancement may occur postcontrast. The key to diagnosing cord ischemia thus lies in the recognition of the longitudinal and cross-sectional distribution of the spinal arteries. The dorsal columns, in which isolated ischemia is rarely seen, are supplied by the paired posterior spinal arteries; however, the remainder of the cord is supplied by the single, midline anterior spinal artery (ASA). Although it is continuous, various radiculomedullary arteries feed the ASA at its major portions (cervicothoracic, midthoracic, and thoracolumbar), and full collateral flow between these portions does not occur. Because the midthoracic ASA and its portions from the low thoracic cord to the conus are both fed by single radicular vessels, these areas of the cord, along with watershed areas at the junctions of the major cord regions, are particularly prone to infarction. For example, the artery of Adamkiewicz (which typically arises from a left posterior intercostal artery) alone feeds the lower thoracic cord and conus. It is not uncommon for this artery to be damaged in abdominal aortic aneurysm repair.

41 Congenital Abnormalities

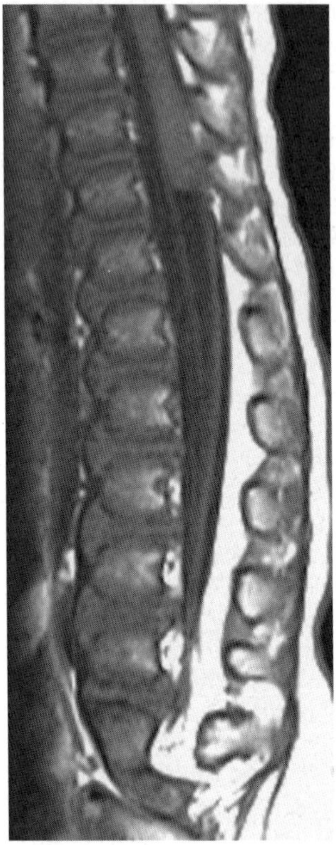

Fig. 41.1

Several congenital conditions affect the lumbar spine. Caudal regression refers to the absence of sacrococcygeal vertebrae with or without lumbar involvement. The typical appearance is illustrated in **Fig. 41.1**: on this sagittal T1WI portions of the sacrum are clearly absent and the conus demonstrates a wedge or hatchet-shaped terminal portion. Two groups have been described depending on whether the conus terminates rostrally (group 1) or caudally (group 2) to the inferior portion of L1, the latter exhibiting more frequent neurologic dysfunction. An abnormally low-positioned conus is referred to as a tethered cord, an entity with many additional (and more common) causes. These include a tight filum terminale, an intradural lumbosacral lipoma, and diastematomyelia. The typical tethered cord patient presents with progressive neurologic dysfunction. As such, most lesions are repaired at birth, but retethering may occur, as was the case of the lesion illustrated in **Figs. 41.2A,B**. Here, two adjacent sagittal T2WI demonstrate a retethered cord: the cord gradually tapers until reaching the end of the thecal sac without a distinctly identifiable conus—a typical appearance. Whenever a tethered cord is present, a reason for the tethering must be sought out. In this case a concomitant type 2 Chiari malformation (see Chapter 25) is to blame, demonstrating classic tectal beaking as well as partial callosal agenesis on the sagittal T1WI of **Fig. 41.2C**. Meningomyeloceles are almost uniformly associated with Chiari 2 malformations and

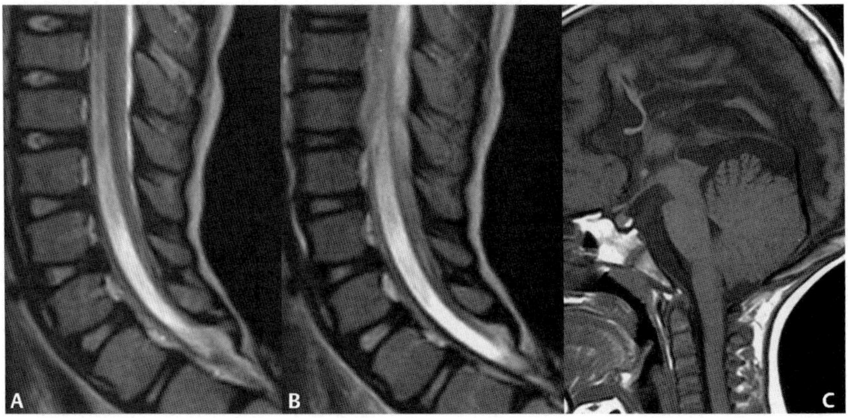

Fig. 41.2 (A–C)

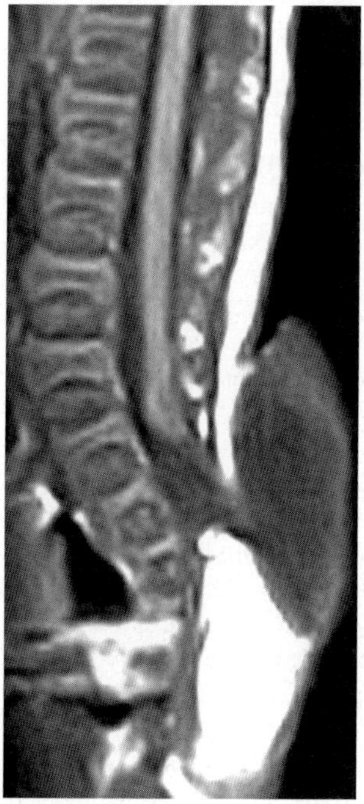

Fig. 41.3

may also be associated with a tethered cord as illustrated in **Fig. 41.3**. In contrast to spina bifida, meningomyeloceles consist of not only a posterior arch defect but also herniation of the meninges and neural structures through this arch. Here, the midline sagittal T1WI reveals a CSF-filled sac posteriorly in the lower lumbar region communicating with the normal thecal sac. Although not visible on this image, a single nerve was identified within this fluid-filled sac. The spinal cord extends to at least the level of the lumbosacral junction and dysraphic posterior osseous elements are present from L4 to S1. Abundant fatty tissue inferior to the defect manifests as high SI on T1WI. Note also the hypointensity of the vertebral bodies, typical for an infant (see Chapter 50). Following repair of a myelomeningocele retethering may occur: there is a limited amount of midline skin and dura, complicating closure over the cord and thecal sac and allowing adherence of the cord to the closure site. In postoperative retethering, the posterior cord will not be visible at the level of closure and the posterior subarachnoid space absent at this level as well. Dorsal dermal sinuses also fall within the spectrum of meningocele-type abnormalities. In this lesion, a midline epithelium-lined tract, with CSF-like SI characteristics, extends from the thecal sac to the skin surface. Half of such patients have an associated dermoid or epidermoid tumor at the tract's termination, and the tract will enhance in the presence of infection—a common complication. Lipomyelocele or lipomyelomeningocele are additional considerations and are similar to myelocele or myelomeningocele except the lipoma is firmly attached to the dorsal surface of the neural placode (cord terminus) which herniates through the dysraphic spinal canal, the lipoma merging with the subcutaneous fat. Lipomas may also occur in the absence of dural defects, as illustrated in **Figs. 41.4A,B,C,D**. Here, the lipoma appears essentially isointense to the vertebral bodies on **(A)** T2WI but demonstrates high SI consistent with fat on **(B)** T1WI. Confirming the presence of fat, the lesion loses SI on **(C)** contrast-enhanced FS T1WI, and as would be expected in a lipoma, does not enhance. Notable in all of these images, and best demonstrated in the axial T1WI of **Fig. 41.4D** is the undisrupted passage of nerve roots through the lipoma. As such these lesions are typically asymptomatic, not requiring treatment.

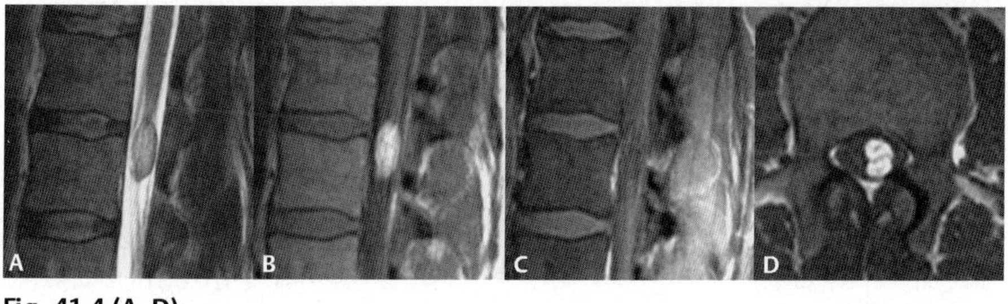

Fig. 41.4 (A–D)

42 Common Incidental Findings

Benign vertebral body hemangiomas are a common incidental finding in the spine. Larger lesions may bleed, expand to compress the spinal canal, or weaken the vertebral body leading to fracture, although all of these complications are very rare. Hemangiomas consist of adipose and angiomatous tissue. As illustrated in **Fig. 42.1**, the fat within these lesions results in a high SI appearance on both **(A)** FSE T2WI (sagittal) and **(B)** T1WI (axial). An **(C)** axial T2WI further illustrates this high SI, whereas **(D)** contrast-enhanced T1WI shows the enhancement expected with such a vascular lesion. Trabecular bone, if sufficiently prominent within a hemangioma, leads to vertical low SI striations (i.e., a so-called jail bar appearance). The major differential consideration with vertebral body hemangiomas is focal fatty deposition (which is extremely common), the pathogenesis of the latter consisting of marrow ischemia followed by fatty replacement. Fatty deposits are illustrated in **Figs. 42.2A,B** where **(A)** sagittal T1WI demonstrates a high SI lesion with SI dropout on **(B)** FS T2WI. In distinction, the high SI of a hemangioma often persists on FS T2WI, secondary to signal from its vascular components. Schmorl nodes can be differentiated from these lesions due to their low SI on both T2WI and T1WI. This typically asymptomatic entity results from prolapse of the nucleus pulposus through the end plate and into the medullary vertebral body space as a result of axial loading. Due to their discal origin such lesions, as shown in **Figs. 42.3A,B**, thus have low SI on both **(A)** T1 (sagittal) and **(B)** T2WI (coronal). Granulation tissue at the periphery of Schmorl nodes may result in peripheral lesion enhancement on contrast-enhanced imaging, whereas acute (i.e., recently prolapsed) lesions may appear hyperintense on FS T2WI due to surrounding edema. Type 1 end plate degenerative changes may mimic this appearance but will appear less focal, with the associated edema eventually being replaced by fat (type 2). A focal metastatic lesion may mimic a Schmorl node; the latter, however, should be contiguous with and isointense to the intervertebral disk.

Tarlov cysts (and more generally extradural meningeal cysts of all types) and synovial cysts are common incidental cystic lesions. The latter, most common in the lower lumbar spine, are associated with degenerative facet disease and may occasionally be symptomatic, resulting in nerve root compression and radicular pain. MRI readily identifies such lesions, often indistinguishable from disk herniations on CT, by their CSF-like SI and close association with a facet joint.

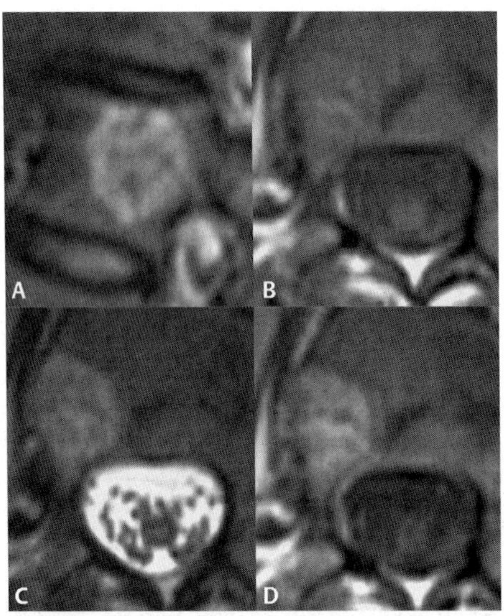

Fig. 42.1 (A–D)

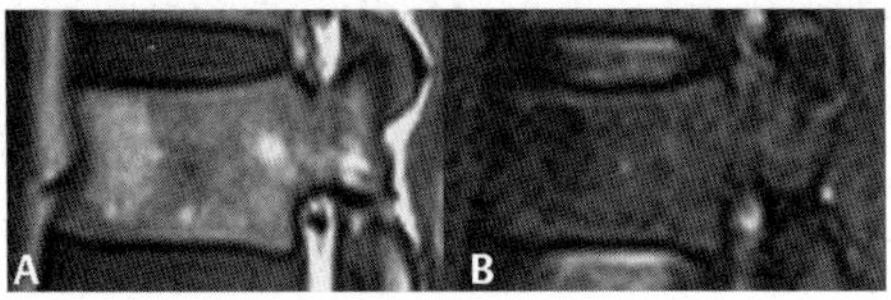

Fig. 42.2 (A,B)

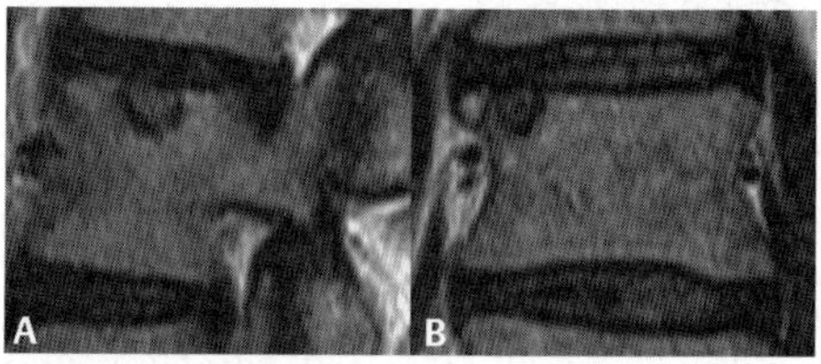

Fig. 42.3 (A,B)

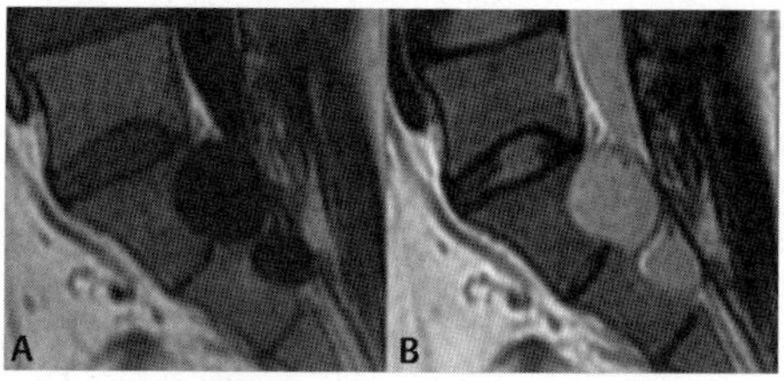

Fig. 42.4 (A,B)

These lesions may, however, acquire any combination of SI appearances on T1 and T2WI owing to variability in cystic contents. The cyst capsule typically enhances. Extradural meningeal cysts consist of lesions that do not contain nerve root fibers (type 1) versus those that do (type 2) as well as intradural cysts (type 3). Of these, Tarlov cysts—a type 2 lesion—are most commonly encountered in routine practice. Such lesions typically involve the sacral nerve roots, and demonstrate CSF SI on all pulse sequences, as shown in the respective sagittal T1WI and T2WI of **Figs. 42.4A,B**. As evident in these images, associated foraminal enlargement and posterior scalloping of the vertebral bodies may be present. Lumbosacral nerve root anomalies are also a frequent incidental finding, particularly at the L5–S1 level. These are crucial preoperative findings. Several types of conjoined roots are possible, from those arising from a single root sleeve but exiting separately in the appropriate foramina (the most common type) to those with a connecting anastomotic root, to those in which two conjoined roots exit through a single foramen. **Figures 42.5A** through **42.5C** illustrate T1 depicting conjoined left L5 and S1 nerve roots within the left L5–S1 neural foramen. In the lumbosacral spine, T1WI readily depicts hypointense nerve roots against the surrounding high SI fat. The sections chosen for illustration show the two nerve roots on the left **(A)** just after separation, **(B)** on the slice just caudal to this, and then **(C)** on a final more caudal axial slice where relative symmetry of right and left has been reestablished. Similar to Tarlov cysts, these lesions may be associated with enlarged neural foramina or diminutive pedicles. Unlike with Tarlov cysts, however, such changes are rare and generally mild in degree. Nerve sheath tumors may exhibit similar SI to portions of a conjoined nerve root at a given level, the former being distinguished by their bright contrast enhancement. Only the dorsal root ganglia of conjoined nerve roots, in distinction, enhance. Disk herniations and synovial cysts are also differential considerations, but in both cases all identifiable nerve roots should exit from the thecal sac at their normal levels.

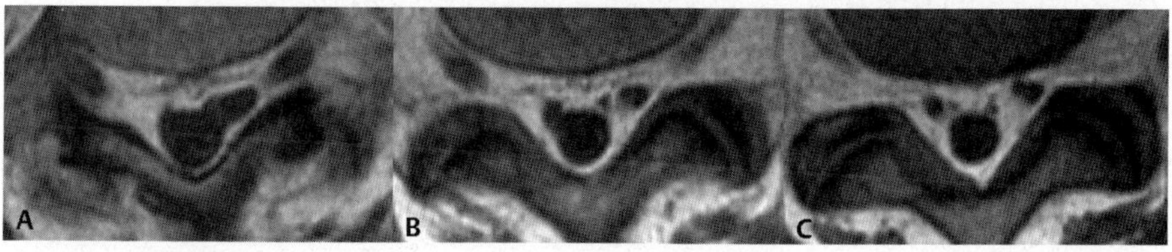

Fig. 42.5 (A–C)

43 Compression Fractures

The typical MRI appearance of an acute, osteoporotic compression fracture is illustrated in **Figs. 43.1A,B**. On **(A)** sagittal FS T2WI, high SI edema is present throughout the vertebral body, while the normal high vertebral SI on **(B)** T1WI is replaced by low SI edema. Superior end plate compression deformity and resultant height loss is also present. **Figures 43.2A** through **43.2D** illustrate a less common appearance of such fractures. Here, the T12 vertebral body demonstrates height loss, low SI within the marrow due to edema, and a pocket of low SI fluid on **(A)** T1WI. Due to the use of FSE technique, vertebral body SI appears almost normal in the T2WI of **Fig. 43.2B**, although the fluid pocket is better visualized. On **(C)** FS T2WI the fluid pocket is again well seen, together with the edema within the adjacent marrow. **(D)** Contrast-enhanced FS T1WI show the fluid pocket as low SI surrounded by avidly enhancing tissue, the latter likely correlating with damaged, leaky capillaries resulting from the fracture present. Chronic, benign fractures lack edema and may be somewhat subtle (reflected by height loss alone). The L5 vertebral body in this case had demonstrated a loss of height, from end plate to end plate, since the prior examination, and exhibits reduced height versus the other vertebrae in **Fig. 43.2**—findings consistent with an interval but chronic, benign compression fracture. Acute compression fractures can involve just the end plate or a portion thereof, leading to confusion with end plate degenerative changes or edema-like SI associated with a Schmorl node (as in the inferior L5 vertebral body in **Fig. 43.2**).

The presence of corresponding end plate SI changes in the immediately adjacent vertebra favors the latter two entities. In **Fig. 43.2**, a nodular lesion is also incidentally noted within the cauda equina, with considerations including ependymoma (i.e., myxopapillary type), schwannoma, neurofibroma, and metastatic lesions. This particular lesion was stable over several years, and in this postoperative patient was felt to represent a surgical granuloma. Fractured vertebrae may be injected with polymethylmethacrylate—a type of cement often infused into fractured vertebrae during minimally invasive interventional procedures aimed at relief of pain from benign and malignant fractures. The compound quickly (<1 hour) polymerizes from a liquid to solid state upon injection. The solidified cement appears black (an absence of SI) on T1WI and T2WI. Rare complications from vertebroplasty are generally better visualized on CT, although related infectious or soft tissue processes are better evaluated with MRI. Sacral insufficiency fractures may also occur in osteoporotic patients. These are at times overlooked on sagittal MRI of the lumbar spine as they are located within the lower portion of the viewed images, and often only on

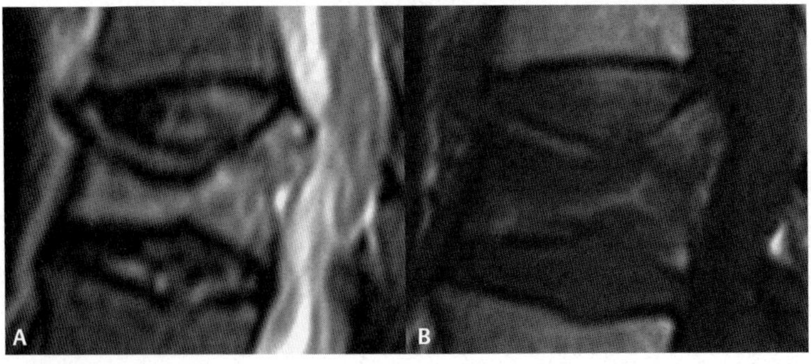

Fig. 43.1 (A,B)

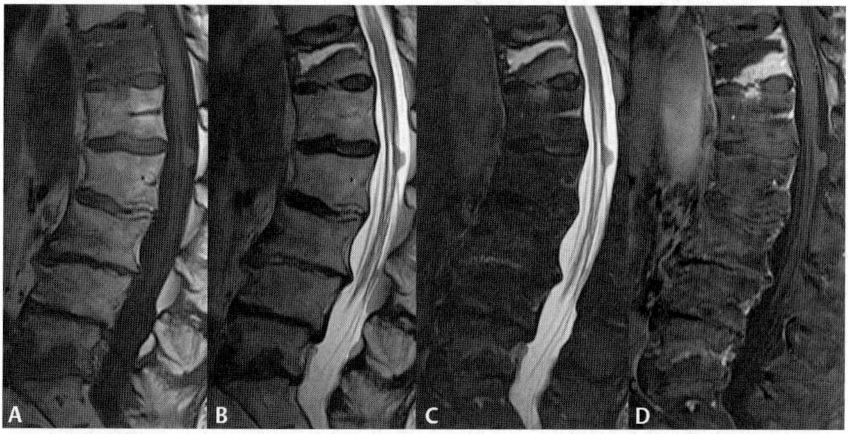

Fig. 43.2 (A–D)

the end slices (away from midline). Nevertheless, when attention is paid to this area, such lesions are readily visualized as, seen in **Fig. 43.3**, **(A)** hyperintensity on STIR (or FS T2WI) and **(B)** hypointensity on T1WI. The lesion in **Fig. 43.3** involved the bilateral sacrum, which is common, as illustrated by bilateral marrow hypointensity in **(C)** axial T1WI.

The crucial consideration in evaluation of any compression fracture is whether its etiology is benign (i.e., osteoporotic) or malignant (i.e., pathologic). The acute compression fracture involving the L1 vertebral body in **Fig. 43.1** was benign in etiology. On T1WI however, extensive edema replacing the high SI fatty marrow may be confused with the appearance of metastatic tumor. As such, the distinction between benign and malignant acute fractures is not reliably made on conventional MRI. The presence of an adjacent soft tissue mass or substantial posterior extension of abnormal soft tissue signifies a malignant etiology. Chronically, the vertebral body SI abnormalities associated with benign vertebral body fractures resolve, whereas abnormal marrow SI remains present in malignant fractures due to underlying tumor. Other, nonfractured vertebral bodies may be infiltrated with tumor in the latter case, making diagnosis more certain. Diffusion weighted imaging (DWI) has shown promise in discriminating between benign and metastatic vertebral body fractures, although such images are not routinely acquired for this purpose and techniques utilized for such imaging vary. The theoretical basis of DWI is that water protons undergo random (Brownian) motion, and restrictions in such motion lead to increased SI on images acquired to provide contrast on this basis. Edema associated with benign fractures is freely diffusable and thus of low SI on DWI, whereas water protons within hypercellular, malignant fractures are restricted, demonstrating lower values on ADC maps and high SI on DWI.

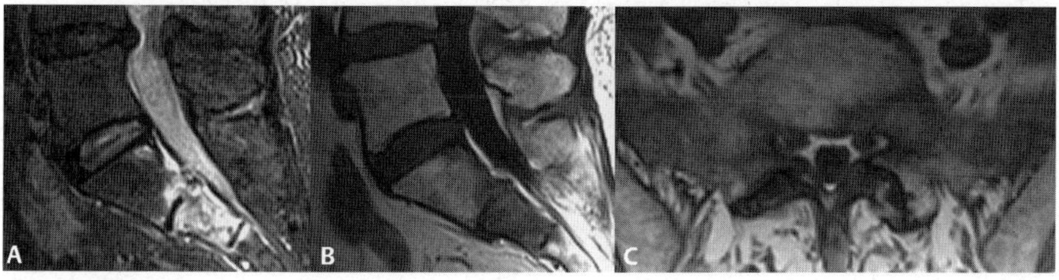

Fig. 43.3 (A–C)

44 Disk Herniations

Pathologic extensions of the intervertebral disk beyond the vertebral end plate margin are categorized as bulges, protrusions, extrusions, or free fragments. A disk bulge results from laxity of and tears within the annulus fibrosis that allow nonfocal extension of the nucleus pulposus posteriorly, with the posterior disk margin forming a smooth, curvilinear contour. Disk bulges are broad-based, circumferential, and may narrow the spinal canal and neural foramen. A disk protrusion, in distinction, is a focal extension or herniation of disk material beyond the posterior end plate margin. Disk protrusions and extrusions are similar but distinct entities, extrusion referring to a protrusion of the nucleus pulposus in which no intact annular fibers remain. This distinction cannot reliably be made on MRI, and thus the term disk protrusion is generally reserved for a small herniation and extrusion for a large herniation. It is imperative to distinguish whether a disk herniation is central, paracentral, or foraminal in location. **Figures 44.1A** and **44.1B** demonstrate a disk extrusion at the L4–L5 level on sagittal T2WI and axial T1WI, respectively. Herniations at L4–L5 and L5–S1 comprise 90% of lumbar herniations. This particular extrusion migrates inferiorly on **(A)** sagittal imaging, and is isointense to the native disk. In the setting of herniation, the native disk may demonstrate a lower than normal SI on T2WI, owing to desiccation and occasionally intradiscal gas. **(B)** Axial T1WI localize this extrusion to a right paracentral location. Note the preserved hypointensity of the left L5 nerve within high SI epidural

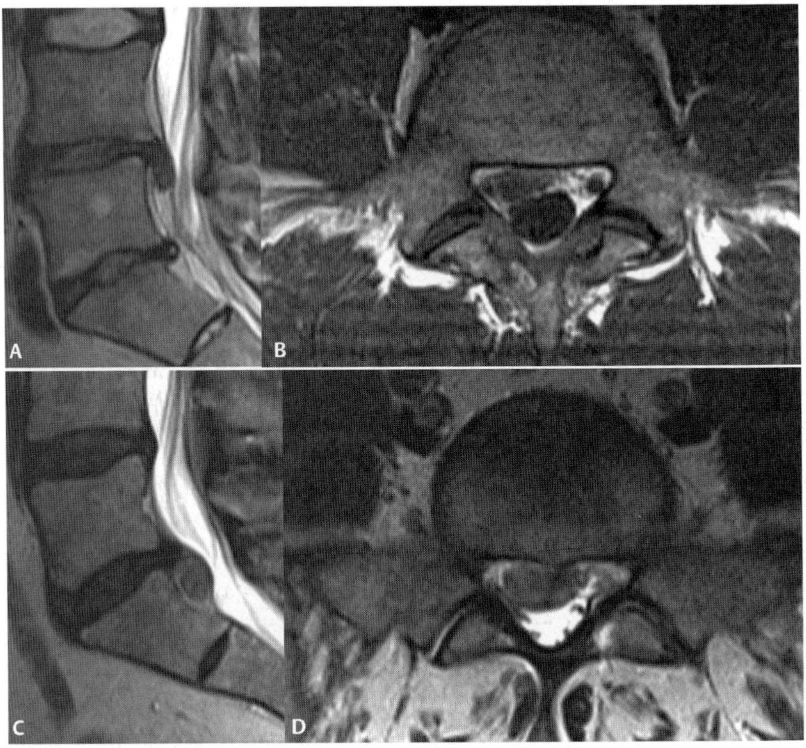

Fig. 44.1 (A–D)

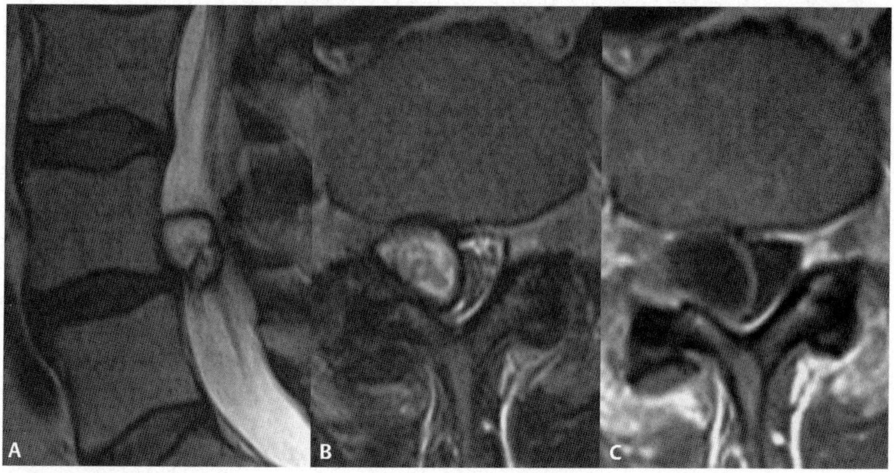

Fig. 44.2 (A–C)

fat, having just exited from the thecal sac. The right epidural fat and L5 nerve, in distinction, are obliterated by the paracentral herniation.

Examination of the epidural fat, more prominent in the lumbar spine, allows for the detection of subtle disk herniations on axial T1WI. Paracentral herniations tend to impinge the exiting nerve root, whereas foraminal herniations compress the ganglion or nerve root in the foramen. Thus, while the paracentral herniation in **Figs. 44.1A,B** compresses the exiting L5 nerve root, a foraminal herniation at this vertebral level would involve L4. Acutely compressed nerves may exhibit high SI edema on T2WI and enhance, although contrast-enhanced imaging is not routinely acquired in this patient population. Central herniations less commonly result in radiculopathic symptoms. A right paracentral central disk extrusion at L5–S1 is illustrated in **Figs. 44.1C,D**. Note that again the herniated disk has migrated somewhat inferiorly on **(C)** sagittal T2WI, while **(D)** axial T2WI demonstrate impingement of the exiting right S1 nerve root. Also note that this herniation is hyperintense to the native disk on these images. Although the hyperintense inferiorly extending portion of the extrusion is in apparent contiguity with the native disk, this change in SI is suggestive of a disk fragment—an important finding preoperatively. Large disk herniations also commonly demonstrate rim enhancement postcontrast. A synovial cyst, illustrated in **Figs. 44.2A,B,C**, may mimic a disk herniation in appearance and symptomatology. **(A)** Sagittal T2WI demonstrates a lesion isointense to CSF with a low SI outline. The SI of synovial cysts is variable, depending on cyst contents, but such cysts are generally isointense to CSF on T1WI and T2WI. The **(B)** axial T2WI localizes the lesion to predominantly the right side of the spinal canal and demonstrates its association with a severely degenerated right facet joint—an association present in most cases of symptomatic synovial cysts and a key feature in their differentiation from disk herniations. The cyst displaces the thecal sac to the left and obliterates the right lateral recess. Finally, **(C)** contrast-enhanced T1WI demonstrates rim enhancement typical of a synovial cyst. Conjoined nerve roots may also be confused for herniations on CT, but are readily distinguished on MRI by their isointensity to CSF. Metastases to the epidural space are infrequently centered at the disk level and demonstrate homogeneous contrast enhancement, permitting easy differentiation from disk herniations and synovial cysts.

45 Postoperative Lumbar Spine

Gadolinium chelate contrast agents are routinely utilized in the MRI evaluation of the postoperative spine to distinguish epidural fibrosis (scar) and recurrent disk herniations—both important etiologies of failed back surgery syndrome. There is good specificity for this distinction utilizing contrast-enhanced scans acquired less than 20 minutes following contrast administration at 3 months or more after surgery. **Figures 45.1A** through **45.1F** illustrate this use. On sagittal **(A)** T1 and **(B)** T2WI there is a defect in the right L5–S1 lamina as a result of prior posterior decompression surgery. In addition, a low to moderate SI focus of soft tissue protrudes posteriorly at the level of the L5–S1 disk. On the basis of these images alone, such a finding, which appears to extend from the desiccated, compressed L5–S1 intervertebral disk, might be mistaken for a disk herniation. **(C)** Contrast-enhanced FS T1WI, however, shows this soft tissue focus to enhance uniformly following contrast administration—an appearance consistent with epidural fibrosis or scar. Axial **(D)** T1, **(E)** T2, and **(F)** FS contrast-enhanced T1WI more clearly demonstrate the partial right-sided facetectomy and laminectomy, with scar extending from the defect to the anterior epidural fat, crossing the midline to contact the left S1 nerve root. Sagittal contrast-enhanced T1WI illustrates envelopment of the low SI right S1 nerve root by the enhancing epidural fibrosis. The rationale for the enhancement of fibrotic tissue relates to extravasation of gadolinium chelates through leaky tight junctions in the vascular endothelium, leading to accumulation of such agents within the extracellular space. Fat may be grafted in the laminectomy bed to reduce epidural scarring with MRI findings accordingly appearing as high SI foci on T1WI within the region of the posterior elements. In distinction to epidural fibrosis, a recurrent disk herniation will not enhance uniformly. **Figures 45.2A** through **45.2F** illustrate sagittal and axial images from a patient that, in addition to the degenerative findings present, has undergone bilateral L3–L4 laminectomies. A large low SI lesion is present within the spinal canal on **(A)** T1 and **(B)** T2WI. The latter clearly illustrates marked narrowing of the central canal. Although such an appearance could represent epidural fibrosis, the pattern of enhancement on **(C)** sagittal contrast-enhanced T1WI is diagnostic for a recurrent, inferiorly migrated disk extrusion at the site of prior surgery.

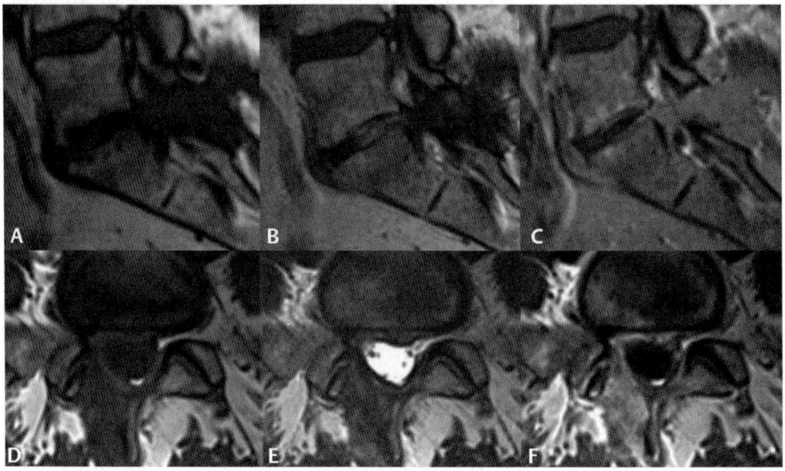

Fig. 45.1 (A–F)

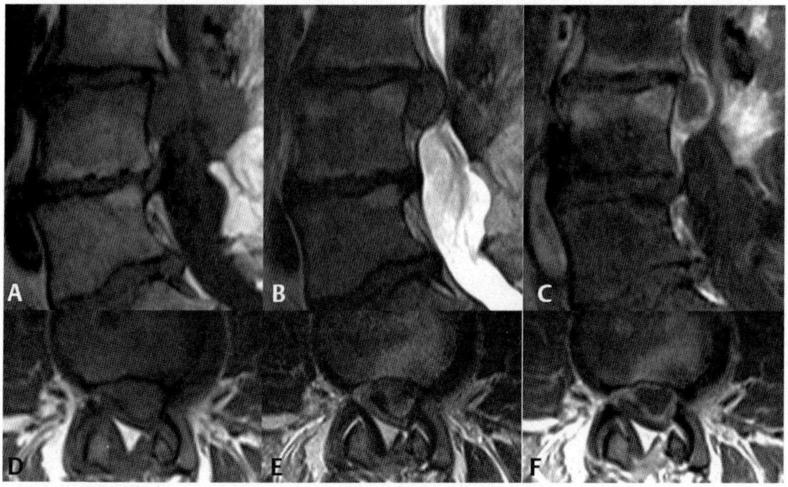

Fig. 45.2 (A–F)

Axial **(D)** T1WI and **(E)** T2WI illustrate the postoperative posterior element defect and localize the extrusion to a left paracentral location. **(F)** Contrast-enhanced T1WI illustrates rim-like enhancement of the disk herniation, correlating with surrounding scar tissue.

Early postoperative imaging of the spine must be performed with caution due to prominent soft tissue edema present immediately (<6 weeks) following surgery. Characterization of operative procedures can often be made on MRI. Findings associated with vertebroplasty are discussed in Chapter 43, while a laminectomy consists of removal of the ligamentum flavum along with the portions of the neural arch. Discontinuity in the low SI ligamentum flavum is often useful in detecting a site of operative intervention. In a laminectomy, the entire spinal lamina is removed along with the ligamentum flavum. Defects from diskectomy may also be seen as may osseous spinal fusions of articular processes. Additional complications of lower back surgery include arachnoiditis (see Chapter 48), radiculitis, postoperative infection, and pseudomeningocele. Radiculitis is apparent on MRI as postoperative spinal nerve root enhancement. This may be confused with normal enhancement seen in the dorsal root ganglia, which lack an intact blood–neuron barrier. Findings of postoperative infections within the spine are similar to those described in Chapter 48. In the postoperative patient, however, a concurrent paravertebral infection will often be present. Such pathology is well depicted on STIR or FS T2WI as hyperintense, and on contrast-enhanced T1WI as heterogeneously enhancing, soft tissue. Because similar changes may be seen as a result of normal inflammation in the early postoperative patient, MRI must be interpreted with caution in this setting. A pseudomeningocele is a nonenhancing, CSF SI fluid collection communicating with the thecal sac but not lined with meningeal tissue. In the presence of ferromagnetic orthopedic hardware, evaluation of the spine may be limited due to susceptibility artifacts. Susceptibility is an intrinsic physical property referring to the ability of an object to become magnetized thus resulting, in the context of MRI, in inhomogeneity of the main magnetic field, leading to the appearance of artifact. If all other scan parameters are equal, effects from susceptibility result in greater artifact at 3 T than at 1.5 T. Gains in SNR at 3 T, however, allow utilization of techniques that diminish artifacts from susceptibility while preserving SNR levels equal to or above that achievable at 1.5 T, and thus diagnostic quality postoperative spine MRI is well-performed at both field strengths.

46 Degenerative Disk Disease I

Techniques for the MRI evaluation of the lumbar spine differ from those implemented in the cervical and thoracic regions. For axial imaging in the cervical region, GRE T2W techniques are obtained due to potential problems from CSF pulsation and the small size of cervical spinal structures warranting thin slice imaging (2–3 mm). In distinction, slice thicknesses of 3 to 4 mm are acceptable in imaging of the lumbar spine where less prominent pulsation artifact also favors the acquisition of FSE T2WI. A thick coronal saturation slab is also routinely placed over the prevertebral tissues to eliminate artifacts from the aorta and vena cava, as well as abdominal motion. FSE has other advantages over GRE, including—due to its additional 180-degree refocusing pulse—diminished artifacts arising from differences in tissue susceptibility. Such artifacts play a role clinically, not only in postoperative patients wherein ferromagnetic implants may limit the diagnostic utility of GRE sequences, but also with respect to evaluation of spinal canal and neuroforaminal narrowing. With the latter, susceptibility effects from bone may exaggerate canal or foraminal narrowing depending upon the selection of imaging parameters. Tissue contrast with FSE T1WI of the lumbar spine is derived from differences in SI between high SI epidural fat versus the low SI thecal sac contents and intervertebral disk. This contrast is lost somewhat on FSE T2WI due to the preservation of hyperintense fat signal on such sequences.

The MRI appearance of the intervertebral disk changes with age. The intervertebral disk of a neonate is of moderate and high SI on T1WI and T2WI, respectively, the latter due to cartilaginous ground substance. The rim of the disk is of low SI as cartilage in this region is denser (i.e., containing less ground substance). With time, such cartilage comes to comprise the outer annulus and equator, resulting in a similar low SI. The collagen of the inner annulus remains of high SI on T2WI, isointense to the nucleus pulposus. Such SI is related to the presence of mucopolysaccharides with strong, fixed negative charges that attract free water into the disk. With normal aging, various factors may contribute to loss of such molecules and thus of intradiscal free water. The annulus may, for example, tear as illustrated in **Figs. 46.1A,B**. Here, sagittal **(A)** FSE T2WI demonstrates a disk bulge with a radial annular tear that has allowed high SI fluid and mucoid material (*white arrow*) to fill the resulting gap. **(B)** Axial T2WI illustrate mild resulting narrowing of the central spinal canal from the disk bulge, along with the aforementioned high SI (*white arrow*) material along the posterior disk margin. This hyperintense region typically enhances on contrast-enhanced T1WI. Concentric tears run parallel to the vertically oriented collagenous fibers of the disk, while transverse tears, resulting from the disruption of the attachment (i.e., Sharpey fibers) of the annulus to the cartilaginous vertebral body end plate, run perpendicular to the peripheral collagenous fibers. Nociceptive neural receptors are present within the outer annulus, and thus annular tears, even if an isolated finding, constitute a potential cause of back pain. Although some loss of disk SI occurs normally with age, desiccation is the hallmark of degenerative disk disease. Disk desiccation occurs due to proteoglycan loss within the nucleus pulposus resulting in a diminished ability of that structure to attract water.

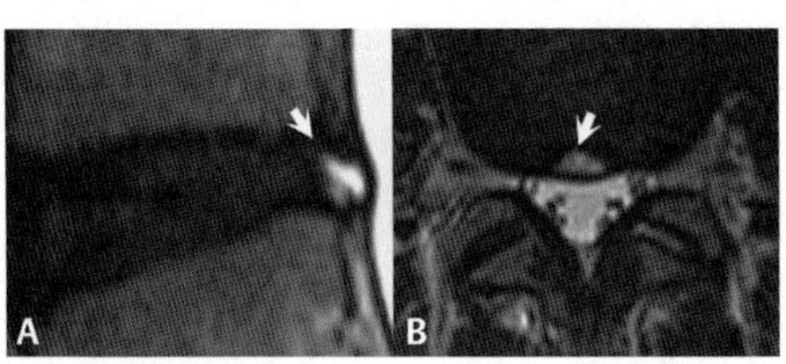

Fig. 46.1 (A,B)

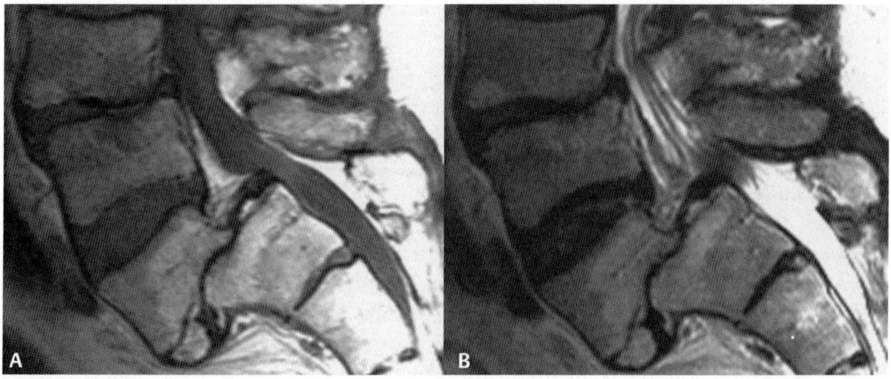

Fig. 46.2 (A,B)

A relatively normal L2–L3 disk is illustrated in **Figs. 46.2A,B**: **(A)** sagittal T1WI demonstrate preservation of intervertebral disk height, whereas **(B)** FSE T2WI illustrate a relatively normal hyperintense nucleus pulposus surrounded by the low SI annulus. Note as well, the normal low signal intensity intranuclear cleft. In distinction, the L3–L4 intervertebral disk demonstrates marked loss of height and SI, the latter evident by the uniformly low SI on **(B)** FSE T2WI. Severely degenerated disks may contain foci of gas, contents suggested in this case by the linear hypointensity within the disk on **(A)** T1WI. The lack of mobile protons within these likely nitrogen-containing gas pockets results in low SI on both T1WI and T2WI. **Figures 46.2A** and **46.2B** also illustrate mild end plate degenerative changes at L3–L4 (see Chapter 47) as well as a grade 3 anterolisthesis of L5 on S1. Grading of anterolisthesis is based upon the degree of anterior displacement of the superior vertebral body. Grade 1 lesions consist of displacement less than 25% of vertebral body length, grade 2 lesions of displacement between 25 and 50%, and grade 3 lesions of displacement greater than 50%. The anterolisthesis in **Figs. 46.2A,B** was associated with bilateral pars interarticularis defects—a finding better visualized on CT and present bilaterally in nearly all patients with grade 2 or 3 listhesis. Pars defects are likely related to prior trauma, although a congenital etiology has also been suggested in the past. In the absence of pars defects, spondylolisthesis is typically accompanied by marked bilateral facet arthropathy. The L5–S1 intervertebral disk in **Figs. 46.2A,B** rests superior to the posterior portion of S1 despite the anteriorly displaced L5 vertebrae. This portion of the disk does not extend significantly beyond the posterior border of S1 but appears to result in AP narrowing of the central spinal canal—a phenomenon known as a pseudo bulge. An anterolisthesis will also lead to elongated neural foramina in the AP dimension, narrowing them in the craniocaudal dimension. Although axial imaging is typically obtained with slices parallel to the intervertebral disk—to facilitate evaluation of disk protrusions and associated canal stenoses—nonangled imaging planes (with acquisition of a continuous slice block) may aid in visualization of pars interarticularis defects.

47 Degenerative Disk Disease II

Spondylolisthesis is but one cause of central canal stenosis. The sagittal FSE T2WI of **Fig. 47.1A** illustrates a normally hydrated intervertebral disk at L5–S1, with desiccated disks at all other levels. Despite this, no significant disk bulges or protrusions are present, although the canal is, nevertheless, of small (<11.5 mm) AP diameter. Congenitally shortened pedicles—the etiology of this finding—is evident in the axial T2WI of **Fig. 47.1C**. A congenitally narrow canal will amplify the severity of any degenerative findings that might develop. The canal in **Figs. 47.1B,D** is also narrowed. Here, a (**B**) FSE T2WI demonstrates loss of disk SI at all visualized levels except S1–S2. Loss of vertebral body height at L5–S1 suggests loss of discal SI secondary to degenerative changes rather than normal aging. A prominent disk bulge is also present at L4–L5, which together with ligamentum flavum hypertrophy at this level, results in moderate to severe central canal stenosis—a finding best appreciated on the axial T2WI of **Fig. 47.1D**. Other structures surrounding the spinal canal can similarly lead to canal stenosis. Degenerative changes of the spine are present in **Fig. 47.2** including disk bulges or disk-osteophyte complexes at all visualized lumbar levels as well as disk space height loss at L3–L4 and L4–L5. Modic type 2 degenerative changes (with the signal intensity of fat) are present at L4–L5. Proliferation of the epidural fat is, however, in this case the most salient contributor to spinal canal stenosis, particularly at the L5–S1 level. Epidural lipomatosis occurs most frequently in the lower thoracic and lumbar spine and is often associated with exogenous steroid administration. A subacute epidural hematoma may exhibit similar SI, but is not suppressed on STIR or FS imaging.

Degenerative changes of the intervertebral disk do not occur in isolation and often result in discogenic sclerosis of the adjacent vertebral body end plates. End plate degeneration involves the L5–S1 vertebral body end plates in **Fig. 47.1B**. Here, FSE T2WI demonstrates abnormal end plate hyperintensity. Such changes are consistent with Modic type 1 or type 2 degenerative disease. Type 1 changes consist of edema-like SI (low SI on T1WI) at the end plates, believed to correlate with increased vascularity. Type 2 changes occur chronically and represent fatty infiltration, exhibiting high SI on both T1 and FSE T2WI. Type 3 changes are associated with development of sclerotic bone, manifesting as low SI on both T1 and T2WI. Distinction among the different types of end plate disease is significant as Modic type 1 changes appear similar to findings in infectious diskitis. End plate enhancement is seen with both entities, further complicating the diagnosis. Disk SI tends to be low in degenerative disease, secondary to desiccation; the disk in infection is marked by high SI fluid/edema. In addition, normal or degenerated intervertebral disks do not

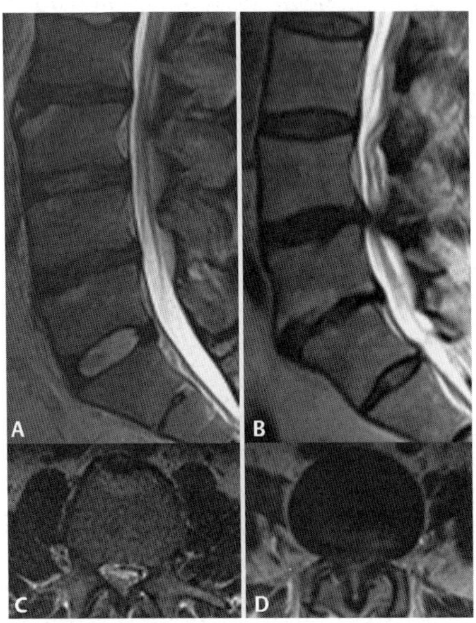

Fig. 47.1 (A–D)

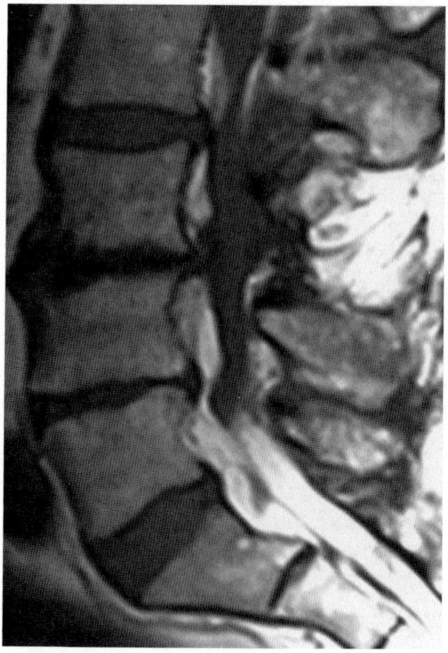

Fig. 47.2

enhance or enhance only peripherally, while discal enhancement in diskitis may be diffuse.

Strain induced by Sharpey fibers upon the vertebral disk end plate may result in development of osteophytes that can narrow the central canal or neural foramina, the latter illustrated in **Fig. 47.3A,B**. In the lumbar spine, high SI epidural fat outlining the low SI nerve roots allows for accurate evaluation of neuroforaminal stenosis on sagittal T1WI. This appearance is illustrated in **Fig. 47.3A** at the level superior to the white arrow. The caliber of the neural foramen at this level is not, however, normal as the normal foramina should have the appearance of a keyhole. In this case, as is typical, the inferior portion of the foramina, consisting of veins and fat, is narrowed while the superior portion, which contains neural tissue, is spared. At the subjacent level, a disk osteophyte complex—isointense to the vertebral body—is present, compromising the foramen and obliterating the fat surrounding the nerve root (*white arrow*). **(B)** Axial images confirm severe narrowing of the right neural foramina and illustrate as well normal facet joint anatomy. The facet joint is the articulation between the inferior and superior articular processes of vertically adjacent vertebrae and can be normally filled with high SI synovial fluid as in **Fig. 47.3B**. As shown, the ligamentum flavum comprises the joint's anteromedial border. Degenerative changes of the facets consist of joint space narrowing, cartilaginous obliteration, as well as osseous erosions and osteophytosis. In contrast to facet arthropathy, facet synovitis is marked by hyperintense signal on FS or STIR T2WI. Both sterile and infectious synovitis enhance, rendering their distinction difficult on MRI. Arthropathy of the superior facets in particular may narrow the lateral recess—the region between the anteromedial superior facet and the posterior border of the vertebrae—resulting in compression of the nerve root prior to its entrance into the neural foramen.

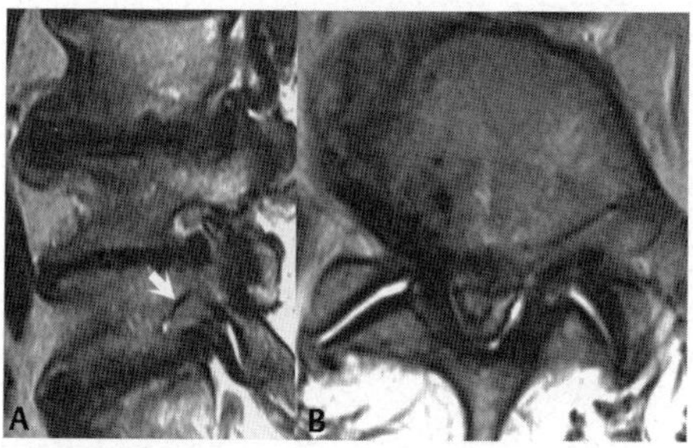

Fig. 47.3 (A,B)

48 Infections

MRI is the most sensitive imaging modality for the detection of spondylodiskitis. **Figures 48.1A through 48.1C** present such a case, with a typical disk space fluid pocket (at L3–L4), seen as high SI on **(A)** FSE T2WI. Adjacent vertebral bodies are completely involved in this severe infection, but edema in milder cases may be limited to a fraction of the vertebrae adjacent to the disk space–an appearance which, in the absence of disk SI changes or irregularity, appears similar to type 1 degenerative end plate changes. The **(A)** T2WI and **(C)** contrast-enhanced T1WI were obtained with spectral FS. On conventional SE T2WI (with one or two refocusing pulses and large echo spacing), the standard T2 sequence in years past, fat is low signal intensity (due to J-coupling) and thus marrow edema was easily visualized. However, with FSE T2WI, the approach most often used today, J-coupling is negligible and the signal intensity of fat high. Thus without FS (or alternatively the use of STIR), high SI edema is not well-visualized on T2WI against the moderate SI fatty marrow. Because fat and water protons resonate at different frequencies, spectral FS is possible, a technique in which an RF pulse is applied to saturate the spins of protons resonating at the frequency of fat, diminishing their SI contribution. Spectral FS must similarly be applied to contrast-enhanced T1WI, to permit visualization of abnormal enhancement, against the background of normal fatty marrow. (**C**) FS T1WI clearly demonstrates enhancement of the L3 and L4 vertebral bodies with sparing of the discal fluid pocket. Epidural and prevertebral enhancement (infection) is also present.

This case was attributable to methicillin-resistant *Staphylococcus aureus* and demonstrates findings that would be otherwise unusual: the infection extends to involve the superior portion of L5, and while the L4–L5 disk space enhances, the T2WI does not suggest the presence of a fluid pocket. Another infectious focus is seen within the superior portion of L2, with abnormal low SI on (**B**) the precontrast T1WI. More common pyogenic etiologies may be distinguished from tuberculosis by the involvement of three or more levels, relative disk sparing, and a disproportionately large soft tissue mass, all typically seen in the latter. Regardless of etiology, because MRI findings lag clinical resolution, follow-up imaging should be obtained only after several months.

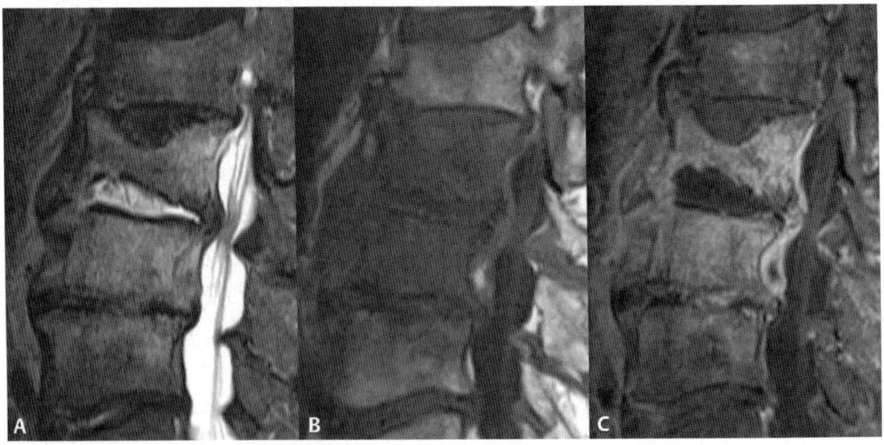

Fig. 48.1 (A–C)

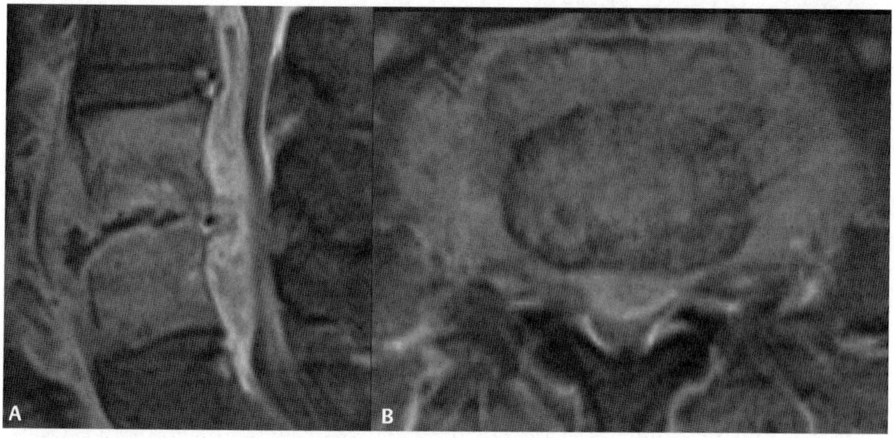

Fig. 48.2 (A,B)

Contiguous spread of spondylodiskitis is common, as in the contrast-enhanced FS T1WI of **Figs. 48.2A,B**, where an L4–L5 disk space infection involves adjacent vertebral bodies, the epidural space, and the pre- and paravertebral soft tissues. Paravertebral enhancement is well seen on both **(A)** sagittal and **(B)** axial images, compression of the thecal sac by the enhancing epidural infection being evident on the latter. Epidural infections may be subtle on T2WI, emphasizing the need for contrast administration. Epidural abscesses may enhance either homogeneously or in a rim-like pattern (**Figs. 48.3A,B**). Abscesses with a higher fluid content may appear as high SI on T2WI (**Fig. 48.3A**), thus confusing their appearance with that of the CSF. FLAIR-like sequences (and contrast-enhanced T1WI, **Fig. 48.3B**) may aid in this distinction.

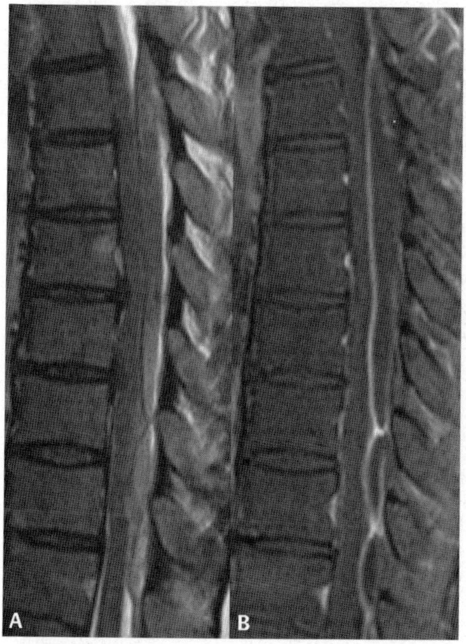

Fig. 48.3 (A,B)

Arachnoiditis refers to pial and arachnoid mater inflammation resulting in clumping and apparent thickening of nerve roots. This can relate to surgery, infection, intrathecal injections, or hemorrhage. In mild cases, clumped nerve roots lie centrally within the thecal sac or adherent to its periphery—the latter making the sac be empty. Clumping of nerve roots can also be seen with spinal stenosis. In severe arachnoiditis, the sac fills with abnormal soft tissue, obscuring individual nerve roots. Root enhancement indicates acute meningitis. Arachnoiditis sequelae include subarachnoid cysts and syringomyelia.

49 Metastatic Disease

Metastatic disease at other levels of the spinal column and its effects on the central spinal canal has been previously discussed (see Chapters 35 and 38). The lumbar spine is the second most common location of vertebral metastases (after the thoracic spine), and renal, GI, and prostate cancer demonstrate a predilection for the lumbosacral region. The rationale for the SI changes associated with metastases to the vertebral bodies was described in Chapter 35. Essentially in an adult, there is a majority of fatty compared with hematopoietic marrow, and as such, vertebral bodies demonstrate high SI on T1WI, due to the relatively short T1 of fat. Note that this appearance is largely absent in the vertebral bodies illustrated in **Fig. 49.1A**. Confluent metastases have resulted in the replacement of high SI marrow fat, resulting in the majority of the lumbar vertebrae, in addition to S1, demonstrating a low SI on T1WI. Higher SI vertebrae or portions thereof as in L5 and S2 reflect normal fatty marrow. FS FSE T2WI (**Fig. 49.1B**) demonstrates these lesions as more focal-appearing hyperintensities against the suppressed fat SI in the involved vertebral bodies. Edema associated with metastatic disease, as has been previously discussed, is difficult to detect on FSE T2WI without fat suppression. A hemorrhagic metastasis may occasionally prove an exception to the above principles, presenting as hyperintensity on T1WI. In addition, sclerotic and hypercellular metastases tend to demonstrate low SI on FS T2WI. As previously discussed in Chapter 38, metastatic multiple myeloma—the most common primary bone tumor—may demonstrate a variety of appearances on MRI including normal (no detectable abnormality). Diffuse and multifocal lesions are also seen, the latter illustrated in **Figs. 49.2A,B** on pre- and postcontrast T1 and FS T1WI, respectively. On the nonenhanced scan, there is involvement of the most inferiorly displayed vertebral body—L5. This vertebral body partially enhances in **Fig. 49.2B**. Additional small hypointense metastases are seen on the precontrast images, but are more easily visualized after contrast administration (*black arrows*). Contrast-enhanced imaging must be performed with FS, to allow clear depiction of enhancing lesions against the suppressed SI of vertebral bodies. As the bodies contain greater amounts of marrow compared with the remainder of the vertebrae, they are more commonly sites of metastatic vertebral involvement. The posterior elements must, however, also be scrutinized for the presence of metastatic disease. In **Fig. 49.2B**, the metastatic lesion within the S1 spinous process is very subtle, but enhances brightly with contrast administration along with the other smaller vertebral body lesions (*black arrows*). Concomitant

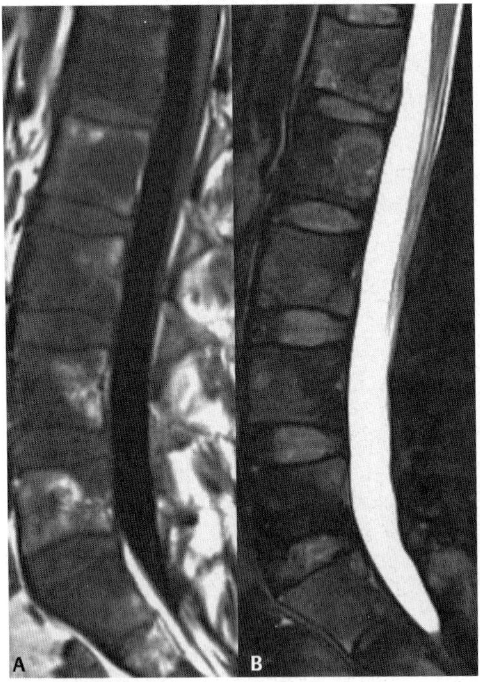

Fig. 49.1 (A,B)

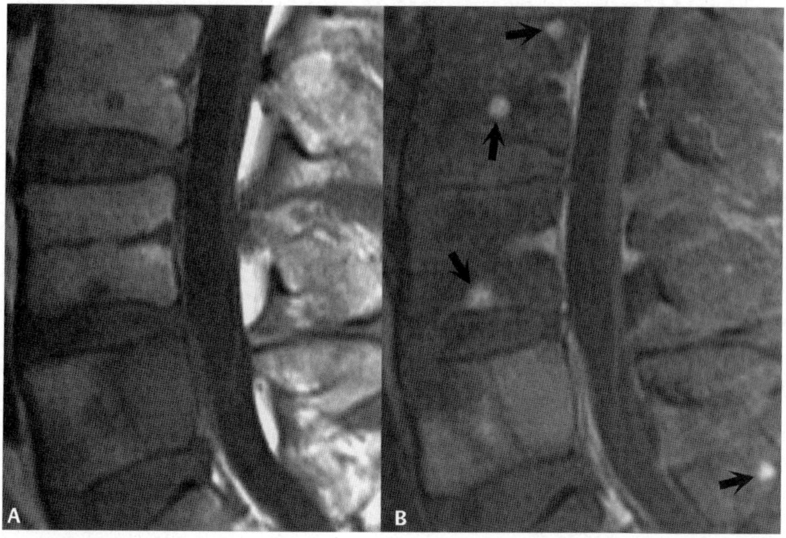

Fig. 49.2 (A,B)

involvement of the anterior body and posterior vertebral elements is illustrated in **Figs. 49.3A,B**. Sagittal T1WI reveals loss in height of the L5 vertebral body compared with L4 and diffuse hypointensity within the former, consistent with replacement of normal vertebral body fat. Although compression of the thecal sac and posterior extent of this mass are clearly identifiable on these images, more precise characterization of the tumor's extent and resulting canal compression is possible with (**B**) the axial T1WI. Evident here is obliteration of the left L4 lamina, pedicle, and transverse process. The compressed spinal canal itself is hypointense to this large mass and displaced posterolaterally to the right, posterior to the remaining hyperintense epidural fat. Contiguous spread of this metastatic lesion extends posterior to involve the paraspinal musculature on the left and laterally to displace the nearby left psoas muscle anterolaterally. This extensive metastatic lesion was found to be secondary to a ganglioneuroblastoma primary.

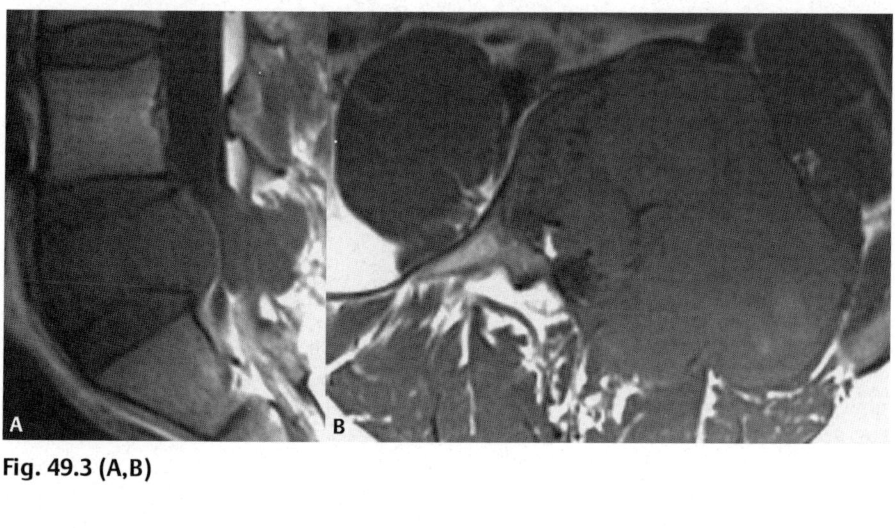

Fig. 49.3 (A,B)

50 Disorders of Marrow

As discussed in the previous chapter, the MRI appearance of multiple myeloma in the vertebral axis is variable, ranging from a normal imaging appearance to one indicating focal, multifocal, or diffuse involvement. Within the myeloma spectrum also is the diagnosis of plasmacytoma, which refers to plasma cell proliferation within only a single focus and likely represents an early stage of multiple myeloma. The diffuse pattern involvement in multiple myeloma is illustrated in the sagittal T1WI of **Fig. 50.1A**. Note that in this case the homogeneous appearance of the vertebral bodies may be misleading—the lack of a focal lesion hindering the detection of abnormality. Thus, it is essential when evaluating sagittal T1WI of the spine to compare the SI of the vertebral bodies to that of the intervertebral disks. Normally, fat content within the vertebral bodies will render them hyperintense to the disks on T1WI. In the present case, however, the vertebral bodies and intervertebral disks are essentially isointense, raising a concern for diffuse marrow pathology. Differential considerations for this appearance include marrow replacement, as in myeloma or metastatic disease, as well as marrow reconversion to a hematopoietic dominance. Lymphoma is another cause of marrow replacement and is illustrated in **Fig. 50.1B**. Note that this appearance is indistinguishable from that of myeloma (**Fig. 50.1A**) and that of acute lymphocytic leukemia (**Fig. 50.1C**). Proliferation of other cell line precursors, such as red blood cells in polycythemia rubra vera, may lead to a similar appearance. Analogously, treatment with chemotherapeutic agents designed to stimulate cell-line precursors may stimulate

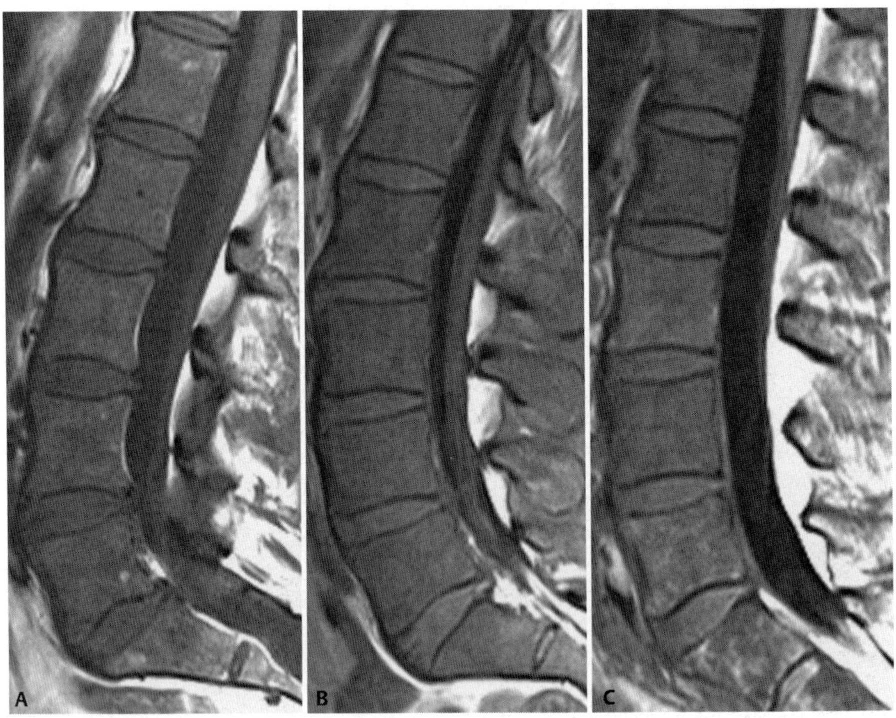

Fig. 50.1 (A–C)

growth of hematopoietic elements in marrow, leading to a predominance of hematopoietic marrow and diffuse low SI on T1WI. Examples of such agents include granulocyte and erythrocyte stimulating factors. In the late stages of polycythemia rubra vera, myelofibrosis may occur resulting in fibrous replacement of marrow, yielding a low SI appearance on T1WI and T2WI.

In the absence of a supportive history, other causes for diffuse vertebral marrow hypointensity on T1WI must be considered. In particular, interpretation of marrow SI must be made within the context of the patient's age. At birth, the percentage of hematologically active marrow is much greater than that of a normal adult. Thus, diffuse low SI marrow on T1WI is normally seen in children, with the SI increasing with age. As this conversion to fat-predominant marrow progresses, hematopoietic marrow is completely replaced within the appendicular skeleton. Within the vertebral column and axial skeleton, however, the latter persists, but in lesser percentage than fatty marrow. Due to this persistence, reconversion of yellow to red marrow is more likely to occur in the axial skeleton. This may at times be a normal finding secondary to chronic hypoxemia in endurance athletes, obese smokers, and in the setting of heart failure. Such reconversion is thought to be mediated by erythropoietin. In distinction to malignant conditions replacing the marrow, like multiple myeloma and metastatic disease, foci of enhancement are often not seen with physiologic marrow reconversion, although hematopoietic marrow may normally exhibit faint enhancement. Red marrow predominance may also be distinguished from tumor infiltration by superparamagnetic iron oxide (SPIO) contrast-enhanced imaging: hematopoietic marrow will accumulate SPIO, the susceptibility effects from which result in a markedly diminished SI on STIR and T2WI. Ancillary findings such as associated compression fractures and paravertebral tumor extension favor a diagnosis of neoplastic marrow replacement. Chronic anemias like sickle cell (see Chapter 96) and thalassemia are also frequent causes of diffuse marrow hypointensity on T1WI. In sickle cell, additional findings include H-shaped vertebral bodies due to infarctions leading to central vertebral body collapse with peripheral height maintenance.

Characteristics of an acute infarct include the presence of irregular areas of marrow edema manifesting as high SI on T2WI. Serpentine enhancement is also characteristic, as opposed to enhancement with osteomyelitis—which may also occur in sickle cell—which is typically more rounded or diffuse. Secondary findings of bone infarct and infection are less common in thalassemia than in sickle cell, but in both conditions frequently administered blood transfusions may lead to an accumulation of iron within tissue including the vertebrae. Associated susceptibility effects lead to a markedly diminished SI on FSE and GRE T2WI. In diseases such as thalassemia, hereditary spherocytosis, and myelosclerosis extramedullary hematopoiesis may also occur as a compensatory response to insufficient marrow red blood cell production. Favored sites include the spleen, liver, and lymph nodes. Thoracic involvement is rarer, but may be appreciated on imaging as a paraspinal mass resulting from extrusion of proliferating marrow from vertebral bodies to a subperiosteal location. This will appear on MRI, along with diffuse low SI vertebral marrow on T1WI, as multiple, smoothly marginated, paraspinal masses without bone erosions. In thalassemia in particular, these masses may grow large enough to compress the spinal canal. These masses typically demonstrate isointensity to vertebral body marrow on T1WI and T2WI, and may enhance to varying degrees, confusing the overall appearance with one of multiple myeloma, metastatic disease, or lymphoma.

51 Primary Neoplasms

As with spinal cord neoplasms in other regions, neoplasms of the lumbar spine are classified as extradural, intradural extramedullary, and medullary. If an extradural lesion contacts the cord, the subarachnoid space will be present at the interface. In the lumbar spine, extradural lesions predominantly consist of vertebral body tumors and metastatic disease (see Chapter 49). Neural sheath tumors and meningiomas comprise the major neoplasms in the intradural extramedullary space. The major nerve sheath tumors are schwannomas and neurofibromas, the imaging appearances of which were discussed in Chapter 39. These lesions are somewhat less common in the lumbar spine as compared with the thoracic. Frequently affecting the nerve roots within the intervertebral foramina in the cervical and thoracic spine, schwannomas within the lumbar spine may also involve the roots of the cauda equina. Such an appearance is demonstrated in the T2WI and CE T1WI of **Figs. 51.1A,B**, respectively. Schwannomas and neurofibromas are difficult to distinguish, even on MRI, although a heterogeneous appearance on T2WI (as in the rather lobulated lesion of **Fig. 51.1**) tends to favor the former. Schwannomas also occur peripheral to the nerve, tending to compress rather than enlarge it, more commonly exhibit cystic degeneration, and tend to be solitary rather than multiple. **Figures 51.2A** through **51.2C** (T2WI, T1WI, contrast-enhanced T1WI) demonstrate a neurofibroma scalloping the posterior margin of the L2 vertebral body and widening the neural foramina in a patient with NF1. Based on the illustrations presented here, this lesion could represent a schwannoma or neurofibroma, however, in this case two additional enhancing intrathecal lesions were seen, favoring the latter. Although cystic degeneration is seen on T2WI **(A)** as an area of central high SI, a more characteristic appearance is that of a target-like configuration on T2WI with a bright rim surrounding a center of low SI. A nerve sheath tumor in this location may be distinguished from a foraminal disk herniation by the presence of bright contrast enhancement. A plexiform neuroma—pathognomonic for NF1—may occasionally be seen involving the sacral plexus as a bulky, multinodular, enhancing mass.

Meningiomas are a further differential consideration with an intradural extramedullary mass. Unlike in the cervical spine, these tend to involve the posterolateral aspect of the canal. The widened subarachnoid space above and below the lesion in **Figs. 51.3A,B,C** localizes it to the intradural extramedullary space. As with the aforementioned lesions, this meningioma demonstrates isointensity to the cord on precontrast T2WI **(A)** and T1WI **(B)**, most well-visualized on the former against the high SI CSF. **(C)** Contrast administration reveals characteristic bright, homogeneous enhancement due to tumor vascularity. Occasionally, flow voids on FSE T2WI may be seen along the periphery of particularly well-vascularized meningiomas. Dense calcification, resulting in low SI on all imaging sequences, is also common. The axial images of **Fig. 51.3D** demonstrate this meningioma to extend within the right neural foramina.

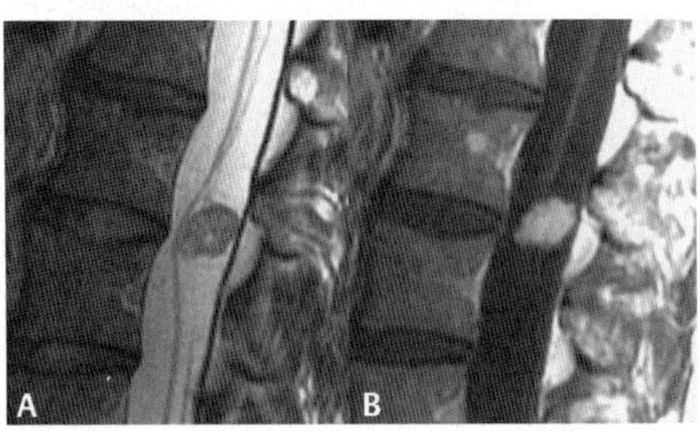

Fig. 51.1 (A,B)

Unlike the other predominately intramedullary tumor—astrocytomas—ependymomas frequently involve the lumbar spine and are the most common tumor of the conus, cauda equina, and

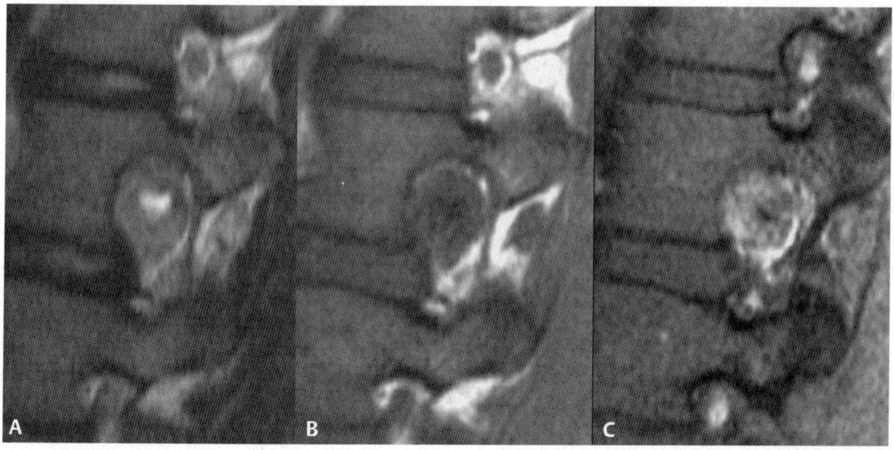

Fig. 51.2 (A–C)

filum terminale. Their central, intramedullary location reflects their origin in the ependymal cells which line the CSF-containing central canal throughout the spinal cord. The lesion in **Figs. 51.4A,B** extends from L1 to L3, nearly filling the spinal canal and resulting in nerve root displacement. Its iso- to slight hyperintensity with the cord is punctuated by small foci of lower SI, which may represent hemorrhagic components or areas of hypercellularity. Calcification may have a similar appearance on T2WI, although this is much less common in spinal ependymomas versus those of the brain. Further, the lack of corresponding low SI on postcontrast T1WI (**B**) makes calcification

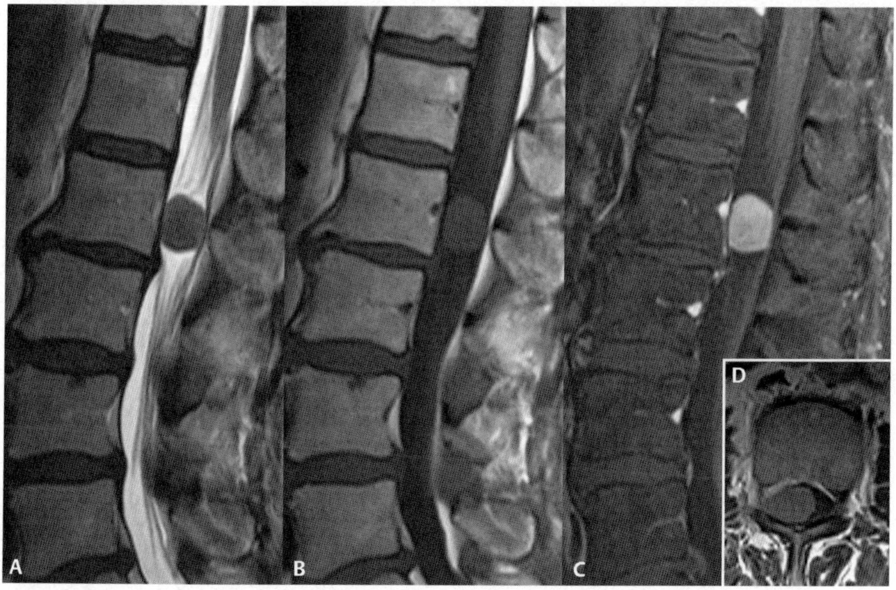

Fig. 51.3 (A–D)

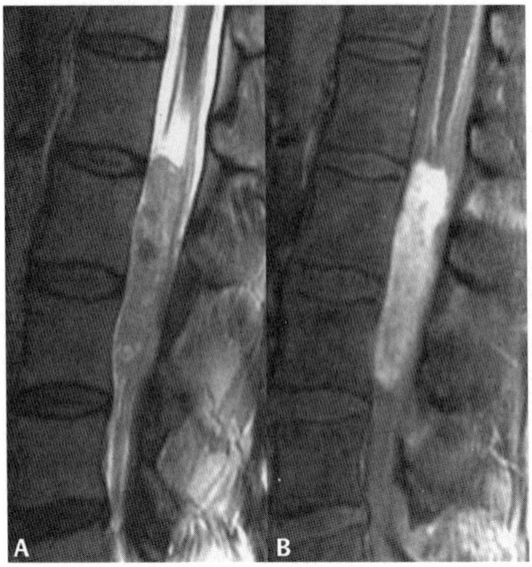

Fig. 51.4 (A,B)

unlikely. The SI of this lesion on T2WI is actually slightly greater than that seen with the typical cellular-type of ependymoma. In fact, within the lower cord and especially in the area of the filum (90%), the myxopapillary subtype is more common, and the abundant mucinous secretions within the myxopapillary ependymoma in **Figs. 51.4A,B** have resulted in a high SI appearance on T2WI. Similarly, myxomatous lesions appear of higher SI than isointense (to the cord) cellular ependymomas on T1WI. Myxomatous lesions also tend to be larger and hemorrhage more frequently than their cellular counterparts. Both myxomatous and cellular subtypes enhance avidly, but nonuniformly with such enhancement potentially outlining cystic areas of tumor, which often appear isointense to CSF on other sequences. In this specific patient case, the enhancement surrounding the conus in **Fig. 51.4B** was felt likely to represent metastatic spread. At surgery, this was confirmed, along with involvement of and adherence to the nearby nerve roots. In addition to the aforementioned characteristics, ependymomas are distinguished from astrocytomas by their propensity to hemorrhage, to contain regions of low SI hypercellularity, and to have more precisely demarcated borders.

Like the lesions above, hemangioblastomas also tend to be intramedullary, although they occur more frequently in the cervical and thoracic regions and are fairly rare in the spinal cord overall. Multiple cord hemangioblastomas are pathognomonic for VHL (see Chapter 28). They may be solid or cystic in appearance, the latter more common in intramedullary lesions and demonstrated in **Figs. 51.5A,B**. The SI of the cystic component varies, depending upon proteinaceous content. Although a large cystic metastasis could have a similar appearance, the presence of flow voids from dilated

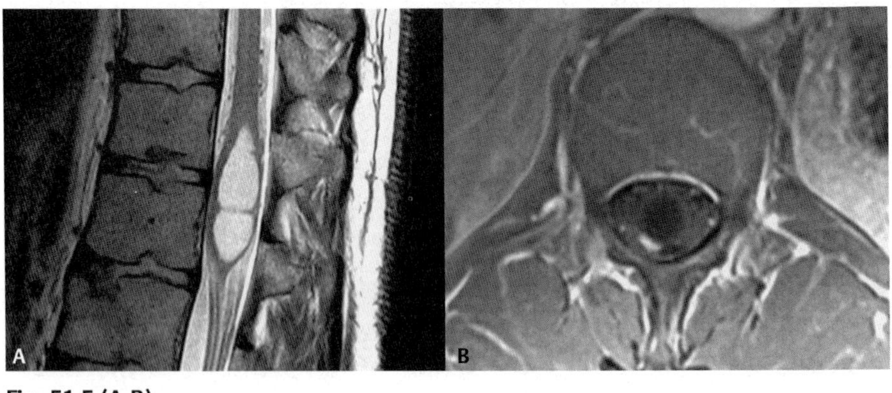

Fig. 51.5 (A,B)

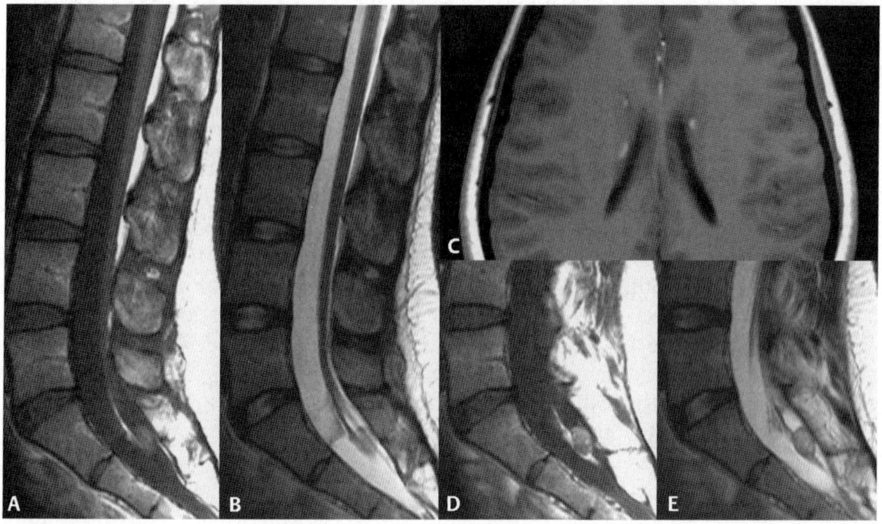

Fig. 51.6 (A–E)

meningeal veins on FSE T2WI is nearly pathognomonic for hemangioblastoma. No nidus was readily identifiable on precontrast sequences in the patient case illustrated. On **(B)** axial postcontrast T1WI, a brightly enhancing nidus is visible posterolaterally to the cystic component, emphasizing how small this area may be compared with the cystic component. Although not seen here, the association of hemangioblastomas with significant cord edema may further complicate their distinction from metastatic lesions.

As demonstrated in **Figs. 51.6A–E**, a dermoid (or epidermoid) is a benign entity that may also appear as an intramedullary mass, most frequently in the lumbosacral region. In this case (as best seen in **Figs. 51.6A,B**), the lesion is associated with a tethered cord—a congenital abnormality in which the conus is held in an abnormally low position. The appearance of this lesion, located at the termination of the thecal sac, on the respective T1WI and T2WI of **Figs. 51.6A,B** is nonspecific, but areas of subarachnoid lipid SI on axial T1WI of the brain (**Fig. 51.6C**) and additional sagittal spine images (**Figs. 51.6D,E**) clinch the diagnosis of a ruptured dermoid. Unlike an epidermoid, these lesions contain dermal appendages such as hair and sebaceous glands, secretions from the latter leading to the appearance of fat-like SI within the lesion. Fat particles are present as foci of high SI within the ventricles of the brain on (**C**) T1WI, indicating dermoid rupture. The fat within the dermoid is seen as high SI on both the T1 and fast spin echo T2WI of **Figs. 51.6D,E**. A dermoid is reliably distinguished from a lipoma due to the relative absence of nonfat SI in the latter.

52 Leptomeningeal Carcinomatosis

The presence of metastatic disease to the leptomeninges is a poor prognostic indicator, occurring most commonly with primary CNS neoplasms—so-called drop metastases most frequently from medulloblastoma, glioblastoma, ependymoma, and pineal tumors. Non-CNS culprits include most frequently primary breast followed by lung cancers. Due to the effects of gravity, the lumbar spine is most commonly involved. The appearance of such lesions is variable on MRI. Findings in a patient with primary breast carcinoma are illustrated in **Figs. 52.1A,B,C**. Sagittal T2WI **(A)** demonstrates small moderate SI nodules involving the cauda equina. **(B)** Axial contrast-enhanced T1WI just above the level of termination of the conus demonstrates brightly enhancing lesions, typical of metastases to this structure. At the **(C)** level of the tip of the conus, axial contrast-enhanced T1WI display brightly enhancing small nodules surrounding but sparing the conus. More superiorly in the cord, in the cervical spine of the same patient, an enhancing intramedullary lesion is seen on the contrast-enhanced T1WI of **Figs. 52.1D,E** (*white arrow*). Enhancement indicative of involvement of the dorsal pia-arachnoid is present as well both on (**D**) sagittal and (**E**) axial contrast-enhanced T1WI. Whether this particular tumor represented a primary metastasis to the dura now involving the cord or alternatively a primary intramedullary metastasis now involving the dura remains indeterminant.

Figures 52.2A and **52.2B** demonstrate a case of lymphoma metastatic to the epidural space on axial T2WI and contrast-enhanced T1WI, respectively. Marked compression of the thecal sac by this **(B)** enhancing process is present, as is extent to the bilateral neural foramina. In addition to intramedullary and extradural metastases, subarachnoid spread of metastases may occur. This is shown in **Figs. 52.3A,B**: on contrast-enhanced FS T1WI of the **(A)** cervical spine, a nodular enhancing lesion is evident at the C3–C4 level (*white arrow*); however, in addition, there is diffuse subarachnoid spread of the tumor more inferiorly, leading to an appearance of "icing" of the cord (*black arrows*). Unenhanced MRI is particularly insensitive to this pattern of leptomeningeal involvement with contrast administration greatly improving diagnostic sensitivity. Images in the **(B)** lumbar spine of this patient demonstrate a large intrathecal lesion of moderate SI on T2WI. Associated nerve

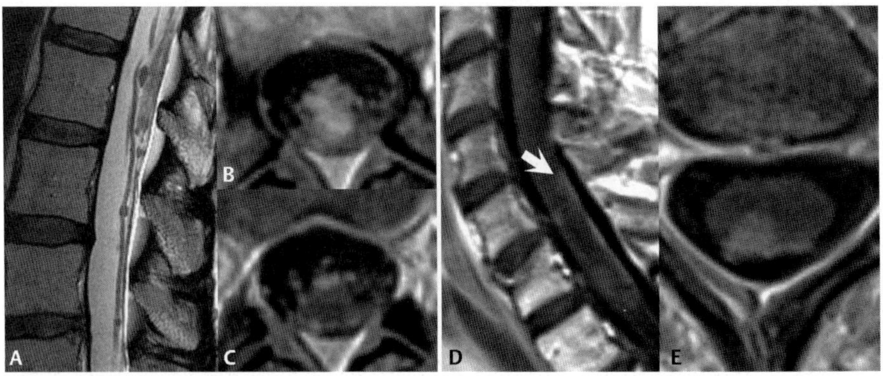

Fig. 52.1 (A–E)

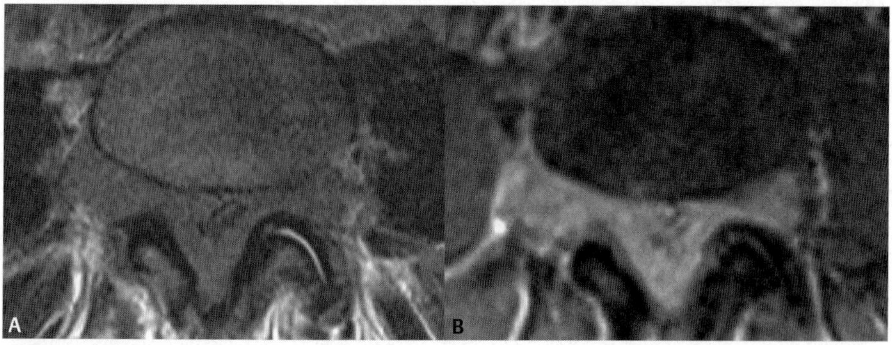

Fig. 52.2 (A,B)

root thickening is present from the level of the mass to the conus, findings also evident from the bright nerve root enhancement present on contrast-enhanced T1WI (not shown).

The differential diagnosis of nerve root enhancement includes benign infectious and inflammatory conditions, in addition to leptomeningeal metastatic disease. The presence of nodularity should suggest neoplastic involvement. Guillain-Barré syndrome classically demonstrates preferential involvement of the ventral nerve roots, as illustrated in the axial contrast-enhanced FS T1WI of **Fig. 52.4**. Chronic inflammatory

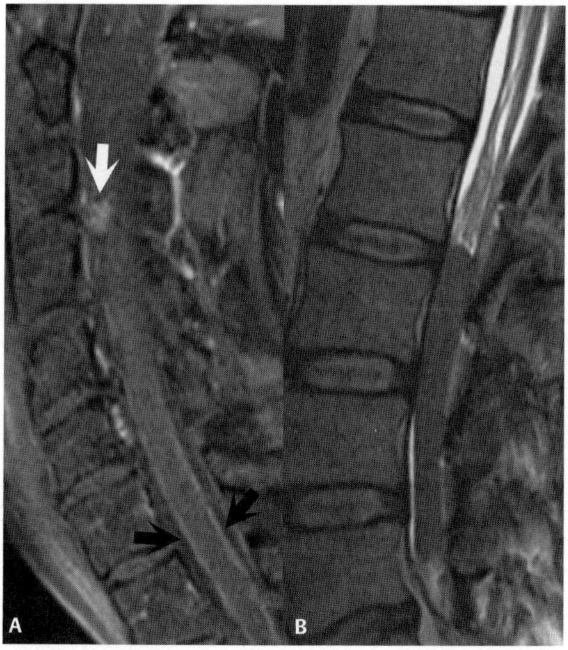

Fig. 52.3 (A,B)

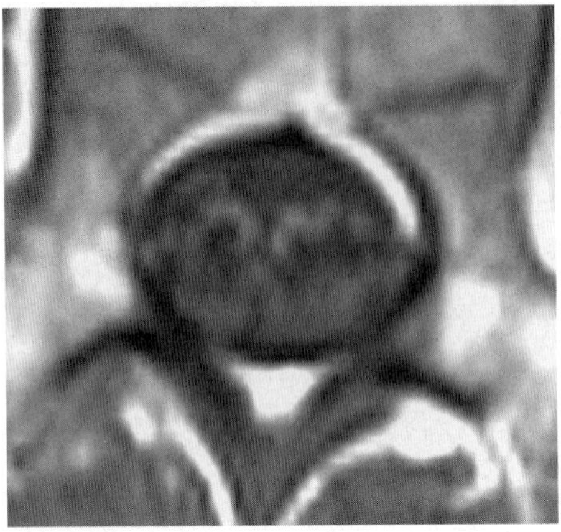

Fig. 52.4

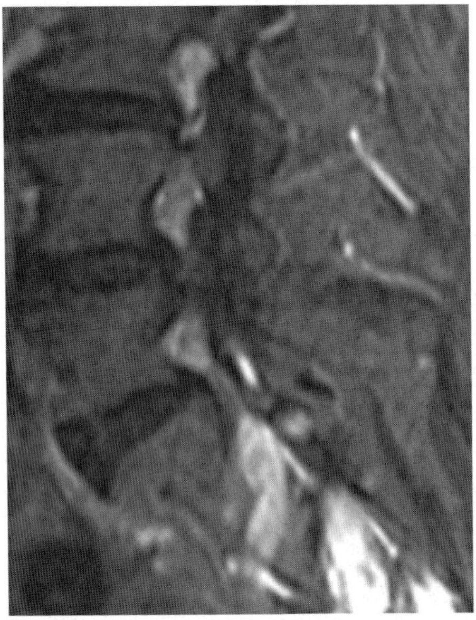

Fig. 52.5

demyelinating polyneuropathy (CIDP) presents with enlargement and hyperintensity on T2WI of nerve roots, ganglia, and peripheral nerves, as illustrated on the STIR image in **Fig. 52.5**. Hereditary motor-sensory neuropathy, better known as Charcot-Marie-Tooth disease, is essentially indistinguishable except via genetic testing. In the presence of appropriate clinical findings, neural sheath tumors and plexiform neuromas—associated with NF1—are another consideration. Cystic dilatation of nearby structures may appear similar on unenhanced MRI, but are distinguished from the lesions above by a lack of enhancement. A lateral meningocele or a perineural root sleeve cyst, for example, will demonstrate a bright CSF-like SI on T2WI. Associated widening of the neural foramina from thinning of the adjacent pedicles may occur.

53 Common Incidental Findings

Incidental findings within the sinuses are commonly seen on head and neck MRI performed for other reasons. Mucous retention cysts most commonly occur in the maxillary sinuses and are asymptomatic unless they disrupt mucociliary clearance. The typical appearance is illustrated in **Figs. 53.1A,B** where bilateral lesions exhibit high and low SI on **(A)** axial T2WI and **(B)** contrast-enhanced T1WI, respectively. A large lesion can be confused with an air-fluid level, leading to a false diagnosis of sinusitis. The nondependent location of the retention cysts in **Figs. 53.1A,B** aids in this distinction, but dependent mucous retention cysts are more problematic: a convex border with surrounding air suggests a retention cyst versus the concave up borders of an air fluid level. Evaluation of the lesion in multiple planes can further aid in differentiation. Polyps are also typically asymptomatic and exhibit variable SI based on their relative protein content. Such lesions are not reliably distinguished from mucous retention cysts by their MRI appearance. Mucosal thickening is often asymptomatic, and is defined as thickening of the lining of the maxillary and ethmoid sinuses greater than 4 and 2 mm, respectively. **Figures 53.2A and 53.2B** demonstrate left maxillary sinus mucosal thickening: compared with the right sinus wall, added moderate and high SI is present on the left in **(A)** T1WI and **(B)** T2WI, respectively. Such findings correlate with inflammatory edema or hyperplasia. Abnormal SI within the ethmoid air cells has been shown to alternate from the left to right side over the course of the day as part of a normal nasal cycle.

Sinusitis, further discussed in Chapter 56, constitutes the major differential consideration with the findings above, air fluid levels being the most reliable marker of acute disease. Clinically, acute sinusitis is symptomatic for less than 4 weeks and subacute between 4 and 12 weeks. On a subacute or chronic basis, secretions may become inspissated—a finding correlating with hyperdensity and proliferative bone formation (i.e., osteitis) on CT. Inspissation increases the protein content of contained sinusoidal fluid, leading to alterations in MRI SI. Increases in fluid protein concentration up to 25% aid T1 relaxation, manifest as increased SI on T1WI. This appearance is illustrated in **Figs. 53.3A,B,C** in a patient who had undergone resection of a pituitary macroadenoma, with fat placed during surgery within the sphenoid sinus. On the **(A)** T1WI, high SI

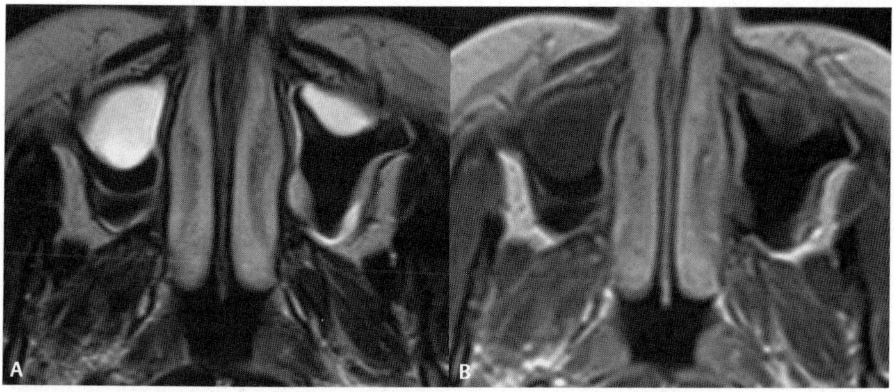

Fig. 53.1 (A,B)

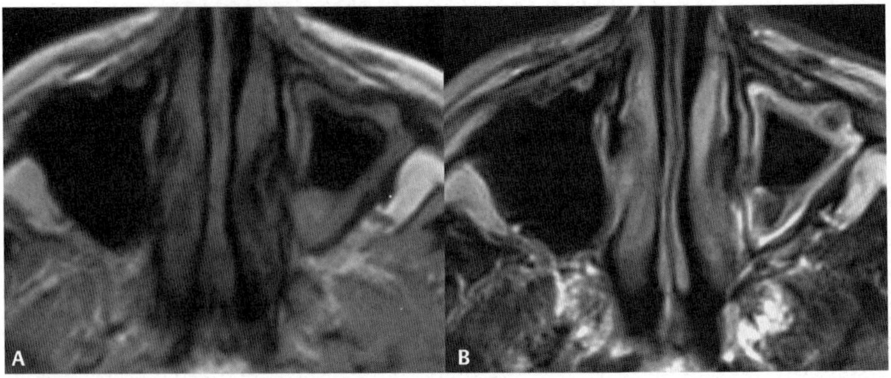

Fig. 53.2 (A,B)

material (*white arrow*) predominates posteriorly within the left sphenoid retention cyst, correlating with increased protein concentration. Hypointensity remains on the left more anteriorly, correlating with lower protein content. With increasing protein concentrations, SI of sinusoidal secretions on T2WI initially remains high; however, concentrations eventually become so high so as to facilitate proton-proton interactions, aiding T2 relaxation. As such, the proteinaceous area of the inspissated secretions in **Fig. 53.3A** correlates with a low SI on the **(B)** axial T2WI, with the surrounding low protein content fluid exhibiting expected hyperintensity. An additional, similar appearing, inspissated secretion containing, retention cyst (*white arrow*, **Fig. 53.3B**) is also present. The protein concentration in the periphery of this smaller lesion is actually low enough to not alter significantly the T1WI of this fluid, allowing partial SI suppression by the inversion recovery pulse utilized to obtain **(C)** FS FLAIR images. This is not the case with the peripheral fluid within the larger lesion that remains hyperintense. Protein concentrations greater than 25% result in macromolecular crosslinking, the resulting rigid structure inhibiting T1 relaxation with resulting hypointensity on both T1WI and T2WI—an appearance similar to that of a normally aerated sinus.

Tornwaldt cysts, arising from the notochordal remnant in the posterior nasopharyngeal vault along the midline, are common incidental findings in the parapharyngeal space. As in **Figs. 53.4A,B** these lesions tend to exhibit homogeneous hyperintensity on (**A**, axial) T2WI. This lesion also exhibits high SI on **(B)** sagittal T1WI, a finding correlating with its

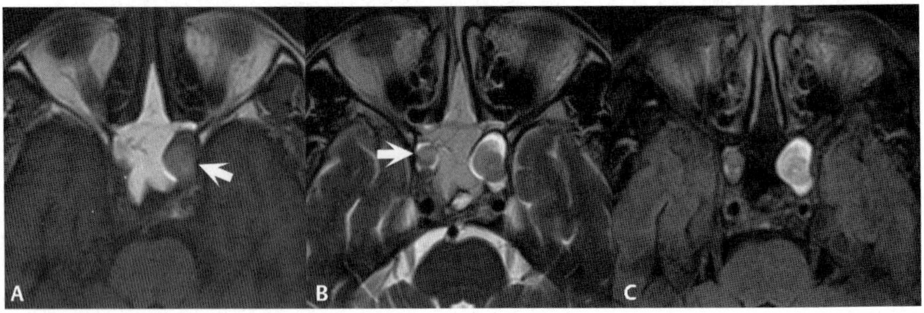

Fig. 53.3 (A–C)

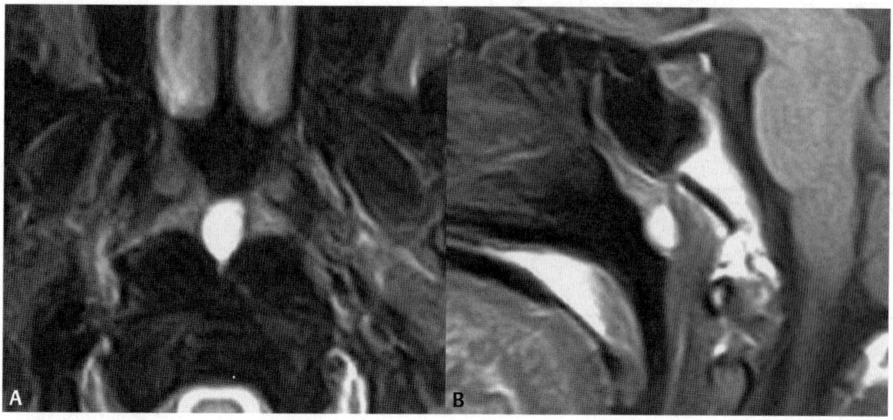

Fig. 53.4 (A,B)

increased protein content. SI on T1WI of these lesions is variable, and lesions often exhibit faint wall enhancement. Differential considerations include pharyngeal space mucosal retention cysts—which may be multiple or occur laterally but do not enhance—and cystic adenoidal hyperplasia. Of neoplastic entities in this space, squamous cell carcinoma is by far the most common, followed by minor salivary gland tumors and lymphoma. Infectious entities like tonsillitis as well as locally extending or remote metastatic lesions are additional considerations for mass lesions in this region.

54 Neoplasia I

Squamous cell carcinomas are the most common head and neck cancer, arising from the sphenoid sinus in **Figs. 54.1A,B**. This lesion extends to the nasal cavity and middle cranial fossa, demonstrating a heterogeneous appearance on **(A)** GRE T1WI. On GRE T1WI, arterial structures demonstrate high SI, highlighting mild compression of the left internal carotid in this instance. **(B)** Coronal contrast-enhanced T1WI reveals enlarged (short axis >1 cm) enhancing bilateral lymph nodes suspicious for metastatic involvement. Low central nodal SI is consistent with necrosis—a finding suggestive of neoplastic involvement regardless of size. Other malignant features include lack of hilar fat SI, rounded appearance, marginal blurring, infiltration of surrounding fat, or low ADC values. Benign mass-like lesions of the nasopharynx and paranasal sinuses expand rather than invade bone and do not enhance diffusely. An expansile ethmoid mucocele is illustrated in **Figs. 54.2A,B,** demonstrating fluid-like SI on **(A)** T2WI and **(B)** CE T1WI. **(B)** Faint peripheral enhancement correlates with active mucoperiosteum. If thicker, such enhancement signifies a mucopyocele. Allergic fungal sinusitis and sinonasal polyposis both exhibit similar MRI appearances, but typically involve multiple sinuses. The latter is of inflammatory rather than atopic etiology and is associated with polyps, although these may be seen with allergic fungal sinusitis as well. Such polyps enhance only peripherally.

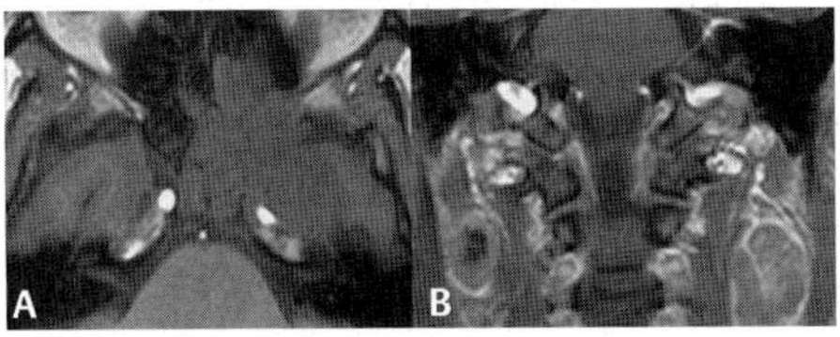

Fig. 54.1 (A,B)

Antrochoanal polyps involve both the maxillary sinus and nasal cavity. These dumbbell-shaped lesions arise from the maxillary antrum, extending into the adjacent nasal cavity. SI on unenhanced images is characteristically fluid-like, although on T1WI SI may increase with greater protein content. Inverted papillomas are benign but may be locally aggressive. The most common presentation is that of an enhancing mass centered in the middle meatus, with local bone remodeling and sinus obstruction. A small percentage degenerate into or coexist with squamous cell carcinoma. The lesion illustrated in **Figs. 54.3A,B** extends posteriorly into the nasopharynx and superiorly into the ethmoid air cells, as seen on axial **(A)** T2 and coronal **(B)** contrast-enhanced T1WI. Ostiomeatal obstruction, which is typical, has resulted in fluid accumulation in the right maxillary sinus. Faint circumferential enhancement correlates with inflamed mucosa. Juvenile nasal

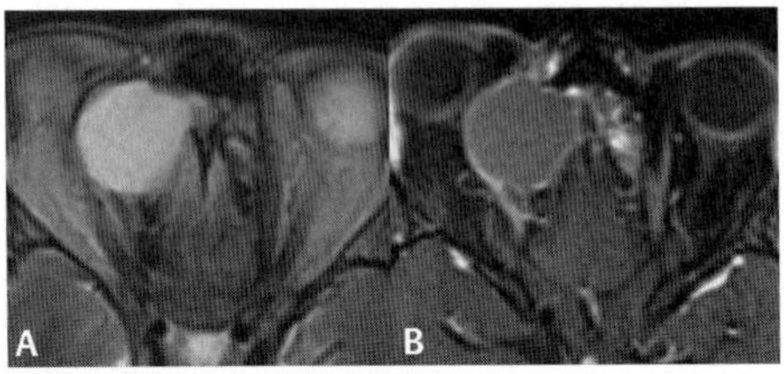

Fig. 54.2 (A,B)

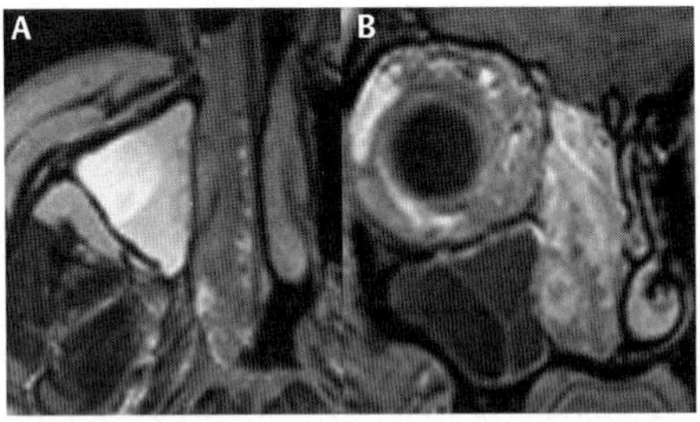

Fig. 54.3 (A,B)

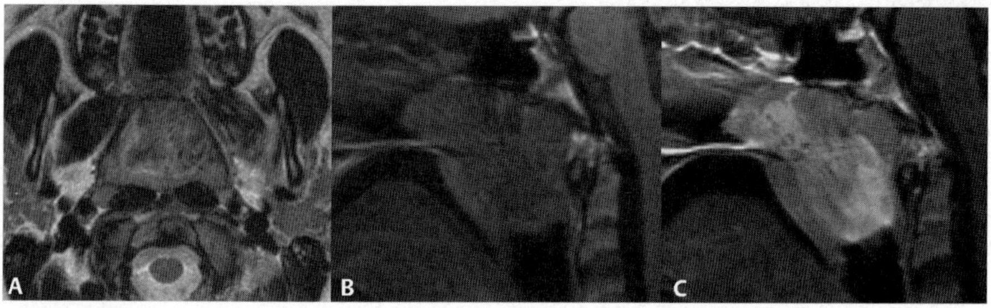

Fig. 54.4 (A–C)

angiofibromas arise specifically at the nasopalatine foramen, occurring most frequently in adolescent boys. As illustrated in **Figs. 54.4A,B,C** (images courtesy of H. Kramer), these infiltrative but benign tumors exhibit **(A)** multiple flow voids, resulting in heterogeneous high SI on T2WI. Pre- and postcontrast T1WI in **Figs. 54.4B,C**, respectively, illustrate avid lesion enhancement, due to high vascularity, with flow voids also present in both images. Both hemangiomas and prominent adenoidal soft tissue in this area do not enhance as brightly and differ in presentation.

Squamous cell carcinoma is the most frequent cancer of the lower face, tongue, oropharynx, and larynx. Evaluation of adjacent spaces is critical for surgical planning and well-assessed on MRI. The masticator space, also a site of spread for intracranial tumors via the foramen ovale, may become involved. Accessory parotid glands are another common mass-like entity in this region. Mandibular involvement presents as a loss of normal marrow hyperintensity on T1WI. This appearance is distinct from that of the usual cystic inflammatory lesions (i.e., periapical and dentigerous cysts) arising in this area. Congenital lesions of the lower face also tend to be cystic, including ranula, cystic hygromas, thyroglossal duct, and branchial cleft cysts. Cysts of the second branchial cleft are a differential consideration for parapharyngeal space masses, as are other benign entities like schwannomas, minor salivary gland pleomorphic adenomas, meningoencephaloceles, and infectious processes. Salivary rest carcinomas, plasmacytomas, and, in children, rhabdomyosarcomas constitute the malignant concerns in this space. Other primary neck tumors and those of the skull base frequently spread to the parapharyngeal space. Of skull base processes, metastatic disease, lymphoma, infection and meningiomas, as well as primary tumors of bone can involve any of its portions. Sinonasal carcinomas and esthesioneuroblastomas frequently involve the anterior base, whereas sella, pituitary tumors, chordomas, and chondrosarcomas—arising centrally and off laterally respectively—involve the central skull base. The importance of MRI in the skull base is on delineation of lesion extent rather than determination of tissue type. Contiguous and perineural spread of tumors to the skull base frequently occurs, the latter most typically by adenoid cystic carcinoma spreading through the cavernous sinus or Meckel cave along the trigeminal nerve.

55 Neoplasia II

A wide variety of other neoplasias may affect the head and neck. In the parapharyngeal space, these include neural tumors (see Chapter 39), salivary tumors, and paragangliomas. Glomus jugulare (**Fig. 55.1**) and carotid body (glomus) paragangliomas are distinguished by their location, the former arising from the jugular fossa and the latter at the carotid bifurcation. Glomus vagale tumors also occur. All tend to demonstrate a characteristic salt and pepper pattern on MRI, attributable to several factors. In the precontrast GRE T1WI of **Fig. 55.1A**, the fibrotic, hypointense tumor ("pepper") arising from the jugular bulb is contrasted against the hyperintense regional vascular structures ("salt"). Alternatively, tumor hyperintensity may represent hemorrhagic foci with interspersed hypointensity from vascular flow voids on FSE T2WI. This highly vascular tumor also demonstrates intense enhancement on (**Fig. 55.1B**, *black arrow*) contrast-enhanced FS T1WI. As seen in this figure, extension to the internal carotid artery, and even displacement, may occur. Anterior displacement is characteristic of glomus and neural tumors, whereas tumors of the salivary glands tend to displace these vascular structures posteriorly. Medial disruption of the parapharyngeal fat plane suggests a deep parotid tumor, along with characteristic waist-like narrowing as tumor passes between the styloid process and the mandibular condyle. The parotid gland is the most common origin of salivary tumors with pleomorphic adenomas being the most common culprit. Visualization of usually benign, low SI pleomorphic adenomas is aided by the high SI of normal, fatty parotid on T1WI. Although such lesions may (falsely) appear cystic, they tend to enhance brightly and uniformly. Malignant entities (i.e., mucoepidermoid and adenoid cystic carcinoma) cannot be differentiated from benign salivary gland tumors on MRI. A nonenhancing unilateral parotid lesion is likely a Warthin tumor (with 20% multicentric); a truly cystic lesion likely represents a brachial cleft malformation.

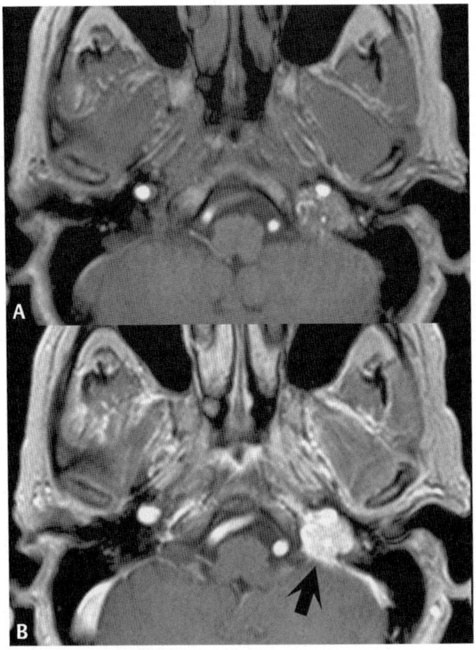
Fig. 55.1 (A,B)

Ocular melanoma is the most common malignant intraocular malignancy in adults, arising from the uveal structures. Paramagnetic effects of melanin (which occur due to the unpaired electrons of stable free radicals) shorten T1 and T2. Thus, ocular melanoma appears hyper- and hypointense on T1WI and T2WI, respectively, compared with vitreous fluid. Melanoma may be distinguished from surrounding fluid or hemorrhage with contrast-enhanced T1WI as a melanoma will brightly enhance. Retinoblastomas may demonstrate similar MRI SI characteristics to melanoma due to hemorrhage, necrotic elements, or calcification therein. Detection of the latter—limited on

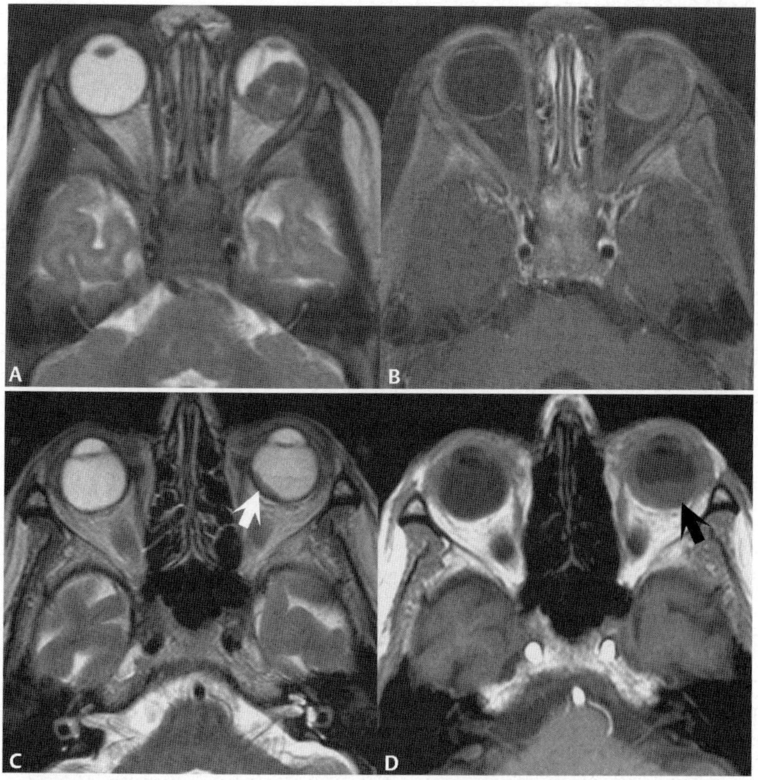

Fig. 55.2 (A–D)

MRI—on CT distinguishes retinoblastoma from melanoma, as does patient age as retinoblastoma is found almost exclusively in children. The presence of trilateral retinoblastoma (bilateral in the orbits and a third pineal or suprasellar lesion) is well-evaluated on MRI. The retinoblastoma in **Figs. 55.2A,B** demonstrates characteristic low SI appearance on **(A)** T2WI, and although not shown, was slightly hyperintense on T1WI. Enhancement is present on **(B)** contrast-enhanced FS T1WI. FS images were obtained in this case to suppress high SI from retrobulbar fat, which would otherwise obscure evaluation of optic nerve enhancement indicative of contiguous tumor spread. Such involvement is seen most frequently in exophytically spreading lesions, which may cause retinal detachment, correlating with the moderate SI linear structure anterior to the mass in **Figs. 55.2A,B**. Amelanotic melanoma and metastatic neoplasias generally lack the relaxivity enhancing properties of the tumors above, and thus appear as high and low SI on T2 and T1WI, respectively. Exceptions to this include mucinous and hemorrhagic adenocarcinomas, the former demonstrated in **Figs. 55.2C,D**. The lesion is best identified as hypointensity on the **(C)** T2WI (*white arrow*), but appears as subtle, moderate SI on **(D)** T1WI. Resulting retinal detachment is best seen as intermediate SI on the **(D)** T1WI (*black arrow*). Due to its vascularity, the uveal tract is the most frequent site of metastatic disease to the orbit.

56 Infections

Of the inflammatory conditions affecting the head and neck, the most commonly observed on MRI is sinusitis. The respective sagittal and axial T1 and T2WI of **Figs. 56.1A,B** demonstrate a band of low to moderate and high SI, respectively, surrounding the periphery of the maxillary sinuses, bilaterally. This finding correlates with mucosal thickening, which alone does not indicate the presence of a sinus infection. In this case, however, the **(B)** bilateral dependent areas of high SI fluid with resulting air-fluid levels and associated mucosal thickening clinch the diagnosis of sinusitis. Sagittal images, as in **Fig. 56.1A**, can be used to confirm that the fluid is dependant, aiding in differentiation from a retention cyst. The variance in MRI SI characteristics of sinusoidal fluid is described in Chapter 20. Contrast administration helps to distinguish the enhancing, inflamed mucoperiosteum in acute sinusitis from the nonenhancing contents of a retention cyst, mucocele, or retained secretions. Mucoceles—most commonly occurring in the frontal sinuses—are benign, slow-growing, cystic, expansile masses that develop secondary to obstruction of the sinus ostium. The SI of mucoceles also vary directly with protein content such that especially proteinaceous lesions mimic the high SI appearance of hemorrhage (more frequently seen in coagulopathy or the setting of trauma) on T1WI. Desiccation over time results in a lower SI on both T1WI and T2WI. The SI evolution of sinusoidal blood products is similar to that described for intraparenchymal blood in Chapter 8, although a delay in course may be observed due to overall poor oxygenation. Sinusitis associated with Wegener's granulomatosis is

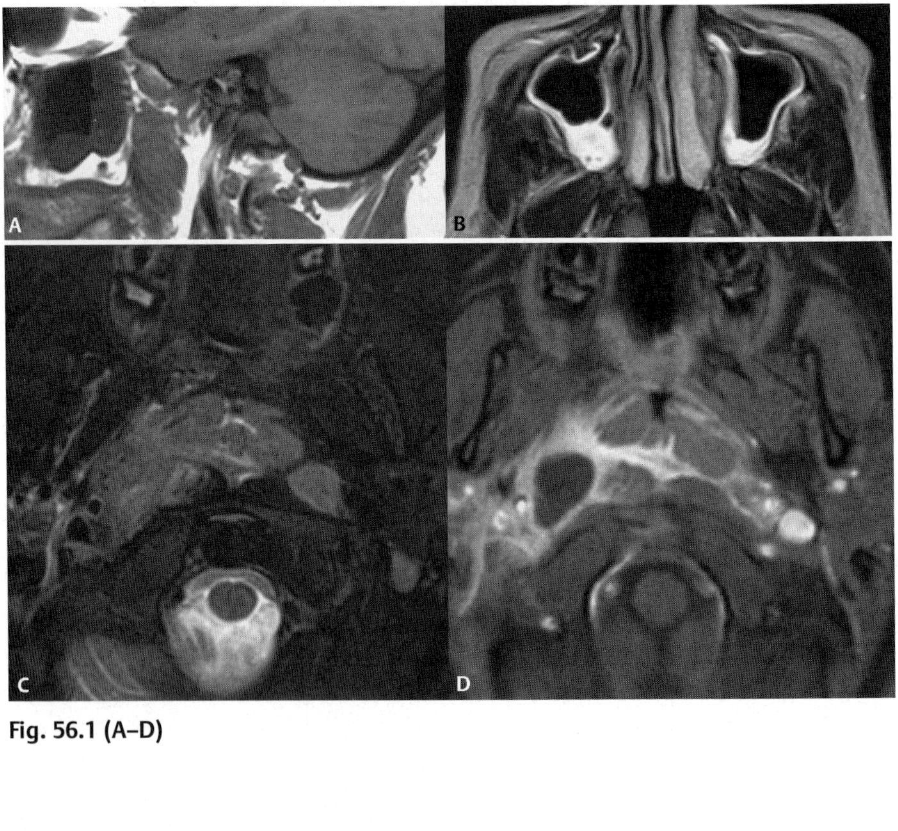

Fig. 56.1 (A–D)

identifiable by osseous destruction out of proportion to mucosal involvement. In an immunocompromised patient or one in which a sinus infection has not responded to antibiotic therapy, a superimposed fungal infection must be considered. The signal intensity of secretions within the involved sinus is variable, although fungal elements may lead to low SI on T2WI. These organisms also frequently invade sinusoidal emissary veins to extend intracranially or into the cavernous sinus via the cortical veins or dural venous sinuses, respectively. Enhancement or loss of the normal signal void within the dural venous sinus is an ominous finding. Orbital extension may also occur, initially visualized as edematous SI changes within the eyelid. Progression of orbital cellulitis results in chemosis, formation of subperiosteal phlegmon, then abscess, and finally infiltration of the peri- and retroorbital fat. Idiopathic orbital inflammatory disease (pseudotumor) is a similarly appearing inflammatory condition, marked by a poorly marginated enhancing soft tissue mass within any area of the orbit, and is a diagnosis of exclusion.

Other infections within the head and neck take a multitude of forms. Although seldom obtained for acute otitis media or mastoiditis, MRI readily demonstrates fluid within the middle ear or mastoid air cells. Likewise cholesteatomas—associated with chronic middle ear infections—are most commonly evaluated by CT, although MRI allows differentiation of the nonenhancing lesion from any surrounding enhancing, inflammatory granulation tissue. Fat within a cholesterol granuloma, meanwhile, lends it a high SI on T1WI, distinguishing it from the two previous entities. Within the external auditory canal, malignant otitis externa appears as high SI on T2WI, potentially eroding the undersurface of the temporal bone and extending intracranially. Subsequent parenchymal or dural involvement is best visualized on postcontrast scans. On the other hand, osteomyelitis—which more commonly occurs in the mandible secondary to infected teeth—is more sensitively detected as low SI on precontrast T1WI. Infections may spread to the parapharyngeal space via the petrous bone or tonsils. A peritonsillar abscess is demonstrated, respectively, on the FS T2 and contrast-enhanced FS T1WI of **Figs. 56.1C,D**. On the former, enlarged, inflamed lymph nodes and tonsillar tissue appear distinct from muscle as high SI. Encasement of the internal carotid artery—appearing as a dark flow void—constitutes a surgical emergency, whereas compromise and leftward shift of the nasopharyngeal airway are also present. The illustrated abscess also characteristically demonstrates a nonenhancing, necrotic center encased by a large region of peripheral enhancement (**Fig. 56.1D**). As opposed to postcontrast scans, precontrast T1WI are best obtained without FS to allow for identification of normal fat planes and their destruction. Abscesses within the salivary glands appear similar, mimicking malignancy in this area; symmetric, bilateral gland enlargement suggests inflammation related to autoimmunity. Ductal calculi—a common cause of sialadenitis—may be seen as signal voids (due to dense calcification), but are more reliably imaged by CT or sialography. MR sialography may, however, eventually replace the latter for evaluation of chronic sialadenitis, allowing noninvasive assessment of the ductal system and gland parenchyma. Finally, causes of inflammatory thyroiditis are not reliably distinguished on MRI, although periglandular extension of hyperintensity on T2WI distinguishes an infection from autoimmune entities like Graves disease. The latter may appear concomitant with extraocular myositis, which demonstrates diffuse muscular enlargement and occasional optic nerve compression on MRI. The fibrosis of Reidel thyroiditis correlates with low SI on T1WI and T2WI, while Hashimoto thyroiditis appears as prominent areas of high SI separated by fibrotic areas of low SI on T2WI.

57 Cardiomyopathy

Motion from the beating heart poses a particular challenge to acquiring high-quality MR images, one often solved by prospective triggering or retrospective electrocardiographic gating. In prospective triggering, image acquisition is triggered by the R wave of the electrocardiogram (ECG) or the peak of the pulse wave, allowing for imaging during relatively quiescent diastole. In retrospective gating, MR images are acquired along with an ECG, allowing visualization of the heart within the context of the cardiac cycle. Normal motion from respiration is also problematic, although breath holding may be employed. The short acquisition time of the steady-state free precession (SSFP) sequence makes it ideal for evaluation of cardiac function and blood flow via cine images. On these intermediately T1WI and T2WI, blood demonstrates high SI, and thus SSFP is also known as a bright blood sequence. In distinction, prospectively triggered sequences obtained during diastole are best utilized for evaluation of peri- and myocardial morphology. Flowing blood within the cardiac chambers and great vessels appears as signal void, and these sequences are thus known as black blood sequences. With ultrafast GRE sequences first-pass perfusion imaging after application of contrast media is feasible and may depict reduced myocardial perfusion at rest or during physical or pharmacologic stress. Myocardial SI may be suppressed by applying a preliminary IR pulse analogous to that used in STIR. Combining this with contrast-enhanced T1WI allows for assessment of myocardial viability. Residual enhancement after 10 to 15 minutes implies nonviable tissue, consistent with myocardial scarring (i.e., fibrosis and inflammation). Images in various planes are often acquired in cardiac MRI, including short axis (**Figs. 57.1A,B**), three-chamber (**Fig. 57.1C**), and horizontal long axis or four chamber (**Fig. 57.1D**) views.

MRI is frequently utilized to distinguish constrictive pericarditis, which warrants surgical treatment, from restrictive cardiomyopathy, which is managed medically. The normal parietal pericardium is best seen during systole on T1WI as low SI less than 2 mm in thickness. The pericardium is often incompletely visualized in MRI. This makes diagnosing agenesis difficult, although a posteriorly, leftward shifted heart is suggestive. The short-axis, contrast-enhanced IR T1WI in **Fig. 57.1A** demonstrates a thickened (>4 mm) pericardium, enhancing superiorly and inferiorly with a small effusion posteriorly. As evident here, the motion-induced flow voids of simple effusive fluid leads to a low SI on SE T1WI. Such effusions demonstrate high SI on cine sequences. In restrictive cardiomyopathy, the pericardium is seldom thickened, while the atrium and right-sided venous structures may be dilated. Endomyocardial fibrosis and amyloidosis are two potential causes of restrictive cardiomyopathy. The cardiac wall may enhance in both. The myocardium in amyloidosis often demonstrates low SI on T1WI and T2WI. Dilated cardiomyopathy may also be detected on MRI, thinning the walls of both ventricles, despite an overall increased myocardial mass. Asymmetric wall thinning or subendocardial enhancement may implicate ischemia as the underlying cause. Myocarditis-related fibrosis may also cause dilated cardiomyopathy. Acute (and as is typical, viral) myocarditis is demonstrated in the short axis contrast-enhanced IR images of **Fig. 57.1B**. Here, patchy myocardial enhancement involves the subepicardium and mid-myocardium as opposed to the subendocardial enhancement pattern in ischemia. Dilated cardiomyopathy from hemochromatosis is distinguished by its low SI appearance on T1WI and T2WI due to susceptibility effects from iron deposition. Hypertrophic cardiomyopathy is a potential cause of sudden death and is best assessed on three-chamber (inflow-outflow) views as in **Fig. 57.1C**. Here cine SSFP sequences

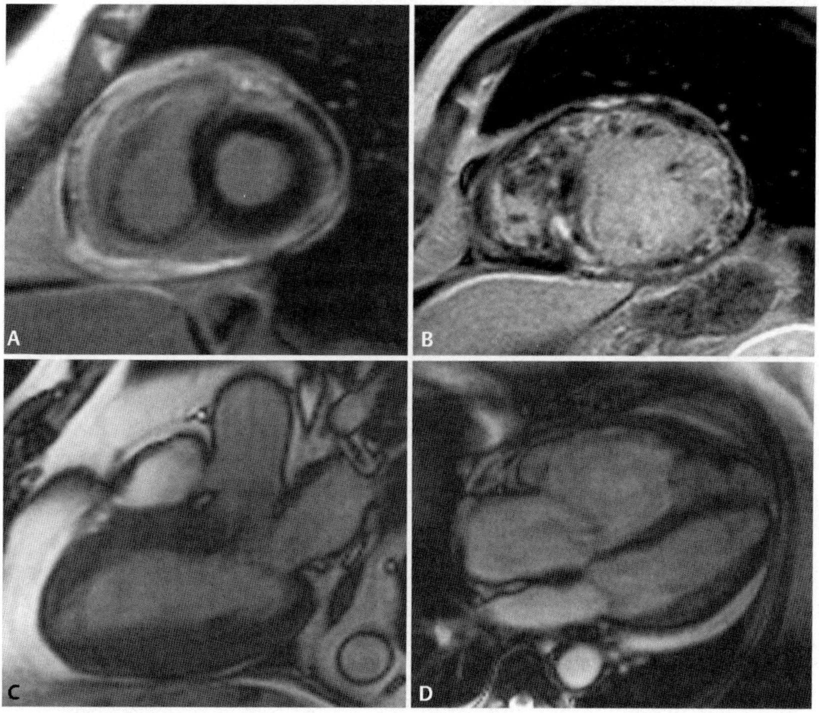

Fig. 57.1 (A–D)

show marked hypertrophy of the left ventricular myocardium involving the interventricular septum and significantly constricting the outflow of blood from the left ventricle. This turbulent flow through this narrowed left ventricular outlet manifests as a low SI jet. Septal thickness greater than 1.5 times that of the posterolateral wall is diagnostic. In severe cases, mid-myocardial or subepicardial enhancement may be present in hypertrophic areas indicating fibrosis or ischemic injury. Similar fibrotic or fatty infiltration also occurs in arrhythmogenic right ventricular dysplasia. In this disorder, myocardial high SI fat from the epicardial surface may displace lower SI myocardial fibers within the right ventricle. Pathognomonic for this condition and demonstrated in the four-chamber view cine SSFP sequence in **Fig. 57.1D** are aneurysmatic dilatations within the "dysplastic triangle" consisting of the right ventricle inflow-outflow tracts and its apex. The right ventricle is markedly dilated as well, and a low SI jet is located at its junction with the atria, representing tricuspid valve regurgitation. A final entity warranting mention is myocardial noncompaction of the ventricle—a congenital cardiomyopathy, characterized by a thickness ratio greater than 2.3 at end diastole between noncompacted, trabeculated, endocardial myocardium and compacted, epicardial myocardium.

58 Ischemic Heart Disease

Although currently limited to a primarily adjunctive role, MRI evaluation of cardiac ischemia demonstrates the wide versatility of the modality. Typically, cine images are obtained to evaluate general function and morphology, followed by first-pass perfusion studies (under rest and/or stress), then T1W IR sequences to evaluate myocardial viability. MRI stress testing exploits the fact that extravascular, extracellular gadolinium chelates pass through the myocardial interstitium within minutes of bolus injection, allowing detection of perfusion differences. Within 10 minutes, washout occurs, and a stress-inducing agent and additional contrast may be given. Stress-inducing agents include dobutamine, dipyridamole, or adenosine. The latter two are coronary vasodilators that are contraindicated in obstructive lung disease and necessitate aminophylline administration should angina be induced. In the presence of vascular stenosis, normal vessels are dilated by these agents, such dilatation stealing flow from the distribution of the stenotic vessel. Areas lacking normal perfusion (enhancement) are characterized as fixed (present on both acquisitions) or reversible (present on stress only). Reduced subendocardial perfusion may also represent reversible microvascular disease, severe three-vessel disease with poor reserve, or even artifact. The latter is favored by a deficit of inconsistent size and SI, not localized to a coronary arterial distribution or present only on rest images. Dobutamine increases heart rate and contractility allowing MRI evaluation of wall motion with higher spatial resolution, scan quality, and reproducibility than echocardiography. For wall motion evaluations, cine images are obtained and 17 myocardial segments graded before and after dobutamine in terms of normal wall thickening during systole. Grade 1 constitutes normal wall motion, whereas grades 2, 3, and 4 correlate with hypokinesis, akinesis, and dyskinesis, respectively.

The two-chamber viability study in **Fig. 58.1A** was obtained 10 to 15 minutes following contrast bolus with IR (set to attenuate normal myocardial SI) T1WI in a patient with a history suggestive of acute ischemia. Viability studies exploit the fact that extravascular, extracellular gadolinium chelates only enter cells when membrane damage is present, resulting in persistent enhancement of infarcted, nonviable myocardium. Cardiac MRI thus delineates stunned (or hibernating) from truly infarcted myocardium—the former predicting a positive outcome with revascularization. Although contractility, as visualized with cine sequences, is variably impaired with viable, stunned myocardium, such tissue consistently demonstrates normal, early enhancement with brisk washout on viability studies, whereas enhancement of nonviable, infarcted tissue is early and persists. In **Fig. 58.1A**, myocardial enhancement from the mid left ventricle to apex confirms the presence of acute myocardial infarction within the distribution of the left anterior descending artery. No-reflow phenomenon is occasionally present on MRI viability studies, with the characteristic appearance of an area of low SI in the center of brightly enhancing myocardium. No perfusion or subsequent contrast penetration occurs in the low SI region secondary to microvascular occlusions, whereas the larger, enhancing area corresponds to a region of infarction reperfused (and contrast delivered by) a patent larger artery. In contrast to normal myocardium, diminished enhancement within an area of no reflow also exhibits progressive enhancement over time and persists as low SI even as the timing of the IR pulse (usually set to suppress normal myocardial SI) is varied.

Enhancement within a specific arterial territory and subendocardial predominance, as seen in **Fig. 58.1A**, implicates the delayed enhancement of ischemia rather

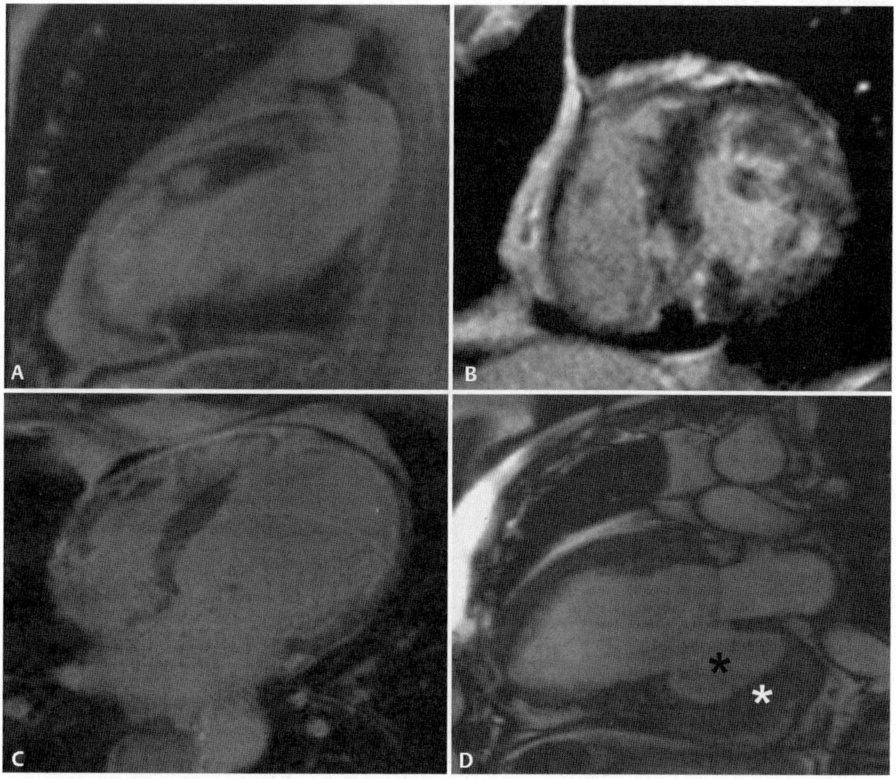

Fig. 58.1 (A–D)

than that of myocarditis. This pattern is not always reliable, as seen in the patchy, less predominant enhancement in the short axis contrast-enhanced IR T1WI image in **Fig. 58.1B**—a case of ischemia secondary to embolic phenomenon in a patient with coronary artery ectasia (a condition associated with coronary aneurysm formation). Delayed enhancement may also occur with myocardial scarring—the end product of myocyte damage—in which contrast is retained within the widened interstitium between collagen fibers. Wall thickness may help distinguish enhancement of infarction from that of fibrosis: a thin enhancing wall—as seen in the left ventricular wall in the four-chamber view of the contrast-enhanced IR T1WI in **Fig. 58.1C**—implies chronic scarring, whereas a thick, enhancing wall signifies acute ischemia. Complications of myocardial infarction are also readily visible on MRI. The two-chamber cine image in **Fig. 58.1D** demonstrates an intraventricular aneurysm with wall dilatation. Although flow is present within portions of the aneurysm (*black asterisk*), low SI clot is also present (*white asterisk*). Unlike regions of scarring or ischemia, clot does not exhibit delayed enhancement on contrast-enhanced IR T1WI. Pericardium surrounding a true aneurysm (**Fig. 58.1D**) is less likely to enhance than that surrounding a false aneurysm. The latter consists of ruptured myocardium, its contents are enclosed by thickened pericardial adhesions.

59 Valvular Heart Disease

The cardiac MRI evaluation of valvular disease is aided by the ability to calculate (typically on short-axis cine images) ejection fraction, end systolic volume, and cardiac output—values typically and less precisely obtained by echocardiogram. Manual (or automatic) outlining of the ventricular endocardial border in a slice allows calculation of intraventricular area. Multiplying this by slice thickness and adding this value for all relevant slices yields the intraventricular volume. The difference in volume between systolic and diastolic cine images represents stroke volume from which ejection fraction and cardiac output may be calculated. Regurgitant flow or valve pressure gradients may be obtained with velocity-encoded MRI. In this sequence, a gradient is applied in the expected direction of blood flow and phase (as well as magnitude) information acquired. Velocity of protons within a given voxel is obtainable based on proportionality between velocity and degree of phase change. Flow volume may be calculated by multiplying velocity by the cross-sectional area (acquired from magnitude information). Integration of flow volume over the cardiac cycle yields the total ejection volume. Comparing the ratio of retrograde to anterograde flow over the cardiac cycle yields a regurgitant fraction; pressure gradients may be estimated from peak flow rates across a valve.

The morphology of the typically low SI cardiac valves is not easily assessed on MRI due to their small size, rapidity of movement, and surrounding (low SI) turbulent flow. The normal tricuspid aortic valve—insufficiency of which was shown in **Fig. 57.1D**—normally lacks a significant pressure gradient when open and exhibits a total area of 3 to 4 cm^2. Stenosis is graded by surface area as severe (<1 cm^2), moderate (between 1 and 1.5 cm^2), and mild (>1.5 cm^2 but with a measurable pressure gradient). A pressure gradient resulting from stenosis can be obtained by applying the Bernoulli equation (Δ pressure $= 4 \times$ peak velocity^2) to peak velocity values obtained by velocity-encoded MRI. In **Fig. 59.1A** a low SI jet, correlating with rapidly dephasing protons in this area of turbulent flow, extends across the stenotic left ventricular outlet into the aorta, consistent with aortic stenosis. In this patient with rheumatic valve disease, a similar jet is seen extending across the closed but regurgitant mitral valve into the left atrium. Mitral insufficiency may also be caused by prolapse, perforation, or annular dilatation with myxomatous degeneration constituting the most common underlying etiology. Nonbacterial vegetations of Libman-Sacks endocarditis are occasionally seen. If possible, valve morphology and root size should be assessed. In prolapse, identification of a culprit leaflet is crucial, as a solitary dysfunction is reparable without full surgical replacement. Quantification of regurgitation severity, ejection fraction, and chamber dimensions should be made. In isolated mitral regurgitation, a regurgitant fraction can be calculated by (in addition to previously described methods) computing the difference in ejection fraction between the right ventricle, which is elevated secondary to systolic ejection of the regurgitant volume, and the left ventricle. Mitral stenosis is rare and seen almost exclusively with rheumatic disease in which leaflet scarring limits motion. The area of the mitral valve is typically between 4 to 5 cm^2, and the valve normally lacks a pressure gradient when open. An open, stenotic mitral valve is shown in the diastolic three-chamber cine images of **Fig. 59.1B**. Significantly increased pressures across the valve may be transmitted retrograde, resulting in dilation of the left atrium, as also seen in the figure. Aortic insufficiency is concurrently present, the regurgitation correlating with a low SI diastolic jet crossing the left ventricle

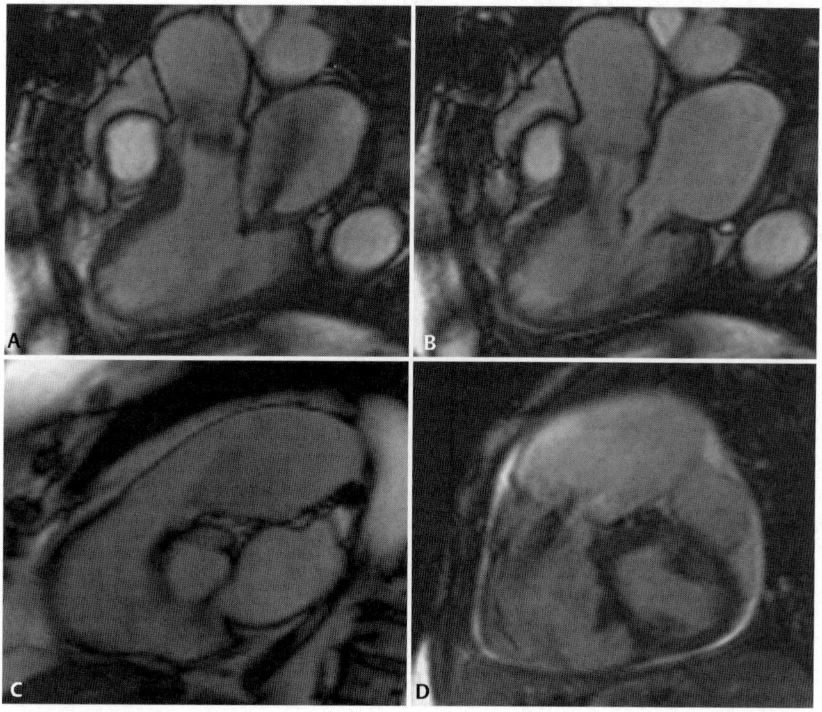

Fig. 59.1 (A–D)

into the aorta. Possible etiologies include endocarditis, rheumatic disease, congenital valve defects, and Marfan syndrome. Quantitative flow calculations should not be performed too close to the aortic valve, as retrograde flow filling the coronary arteries naturally occurs during diastole. An ejection fraction less than 45% or left ventricular end systolic diameter greater than 55 mm warrant surgical intervention. Pulmonic valve stenosis is often congenital, as in the tetralogy of Fallot (see Chapter 60). Moderate and severe disease are defined by valve pressures greater than 50 and 75 mm Hg, respectively. The cine right-ventricular outflow systolic view of **Fig. 59.1C** demonstrates a stenotic right ventricular outlet with marked dilatation of the trunk and turbulent low SI flow present therein. Although some degree of pulmonary regurgitation is considered normal on echocardiogram, hemodynamically significant lesions may occur secondary to pulmonary hypertension or as a result of a prior valvotomy to correct pulmonary stenosis. Clearly regurgitant flow across an insufficient pulmonary valve is visible as a low SI jet on the diastolic cine image of **Fig. 59.1D** with marked accompanying dilatation of the pulmonary trunk. When regurgitation is suspected to have resulted from postoperative valvotomy, MRI evaluation is often useful.

60 Congenital Heart Disease

MRI evaluation of congenital heart disease is a minimally invasive alternative to cardiac angiography, although sedation of uncooperative pediatric patients may be required. The most common congenital disorder of the heart is a bicuspid aortic valve of which aortic stenosis is the most frequent complication (see Chapter 59). Ventricular septal defects (VSD) are the second most common, their significance depending upon the size of and flow through the defect. Absent other shunting, comparison of pulmonary artery and aortic outflow (with velocity-encoded MRI) or left and right ventricular volumes (the right is normally larger with a VSD) allow quantification of shunt volume with MRI. The four-chamber cine image of **Fig. 60.1A** demonstrates a VSD of the muscular septum—as opposed to the more common membranous defect—and resulting right ventricular hypertrophy. A low SI jet into the left ventricle identifies the reversal of normal left to right flow across the defect, corresponding with an Eisenmenger-type physiology. Atrial septal defects (ASDs) are classified as secundum, arising from a defect in the fossa ovale, and less common primum types, arising from sinus venosus defects. ASD in association with a cleft of the anterior mitral leaflet occurs in a partial or complete arteriovenous canal.

Defects in the thin atrial septum are best visualized in four-chamber view cine images. Resulting dilatation of the right atrium and ventricle may occur, and septal configuration progressively loses concavity to the right (best seen in short axis cine views) as pressures therein increase. Quantitative measurements may be made with techniques similar to those above. A patent ductus arteriosus is best visualized on contrast-enhanced MRA and once detected warrants further scrutiny for other congenital disorders (such as tetralogy). Velocity-encoded MRI must be obtained to evaluate flow across the ductus with other quantitative measurements performed as above. Aortic coarctation also frequently presents with other congenital abnormalities. A high-grade coarctation is demonstrated on the volume-rendered thoracic contrast-enhanced MRA in **Fig. 60.1B** with prominent collateralization of the thoracic vasculature. ECG (and possibly respiratory) gated cine images of the heart and arch allow a detailed evaluation of cardiac function and aortic morphology to the level of the renal arteries. Velocity-encoded MRI of the ascending and descending aorta allow assessment of the lesion's hemodynamic significance; black blood images may aid detection of both focal areas of stenosis and lesions within the descending or abdominal aorta. Vascular rings are particularly well seen with contrast administration, allowing assessment of arterial impingement on the low SI trachea.

The major cyanotic congenital disorders include transposition of the great arteries and tetralogy of Fallot. In transposition, the left ventricle is connected to the pulmonary arteries and the right to the aorta. The dextro type of transposition relies on anatomic shunting to maintain oxygenation as deoxygenated blood is pumped through the aorta by the right ventricle and oxygenated blood through the pulmonary arteries via the left ventricle. Surgical interventions include atrial—whereby a baffle directs blood from the vena cava to left ventricle and pulmonary arteries, while pulmonary venous return is directed into the aorta via the right ventricle—and arterial switches—whereby the pulmonary arteries and aorta are reattached to their normal ventricles. MRI evaluation of postoperative atrial switches requires assessment of the baffle for leaks and of the right ventricle for hypertrophy and dysfunction. Outflow tract obstructions, valvular regurgitation, and associated shunts may be quantitatively

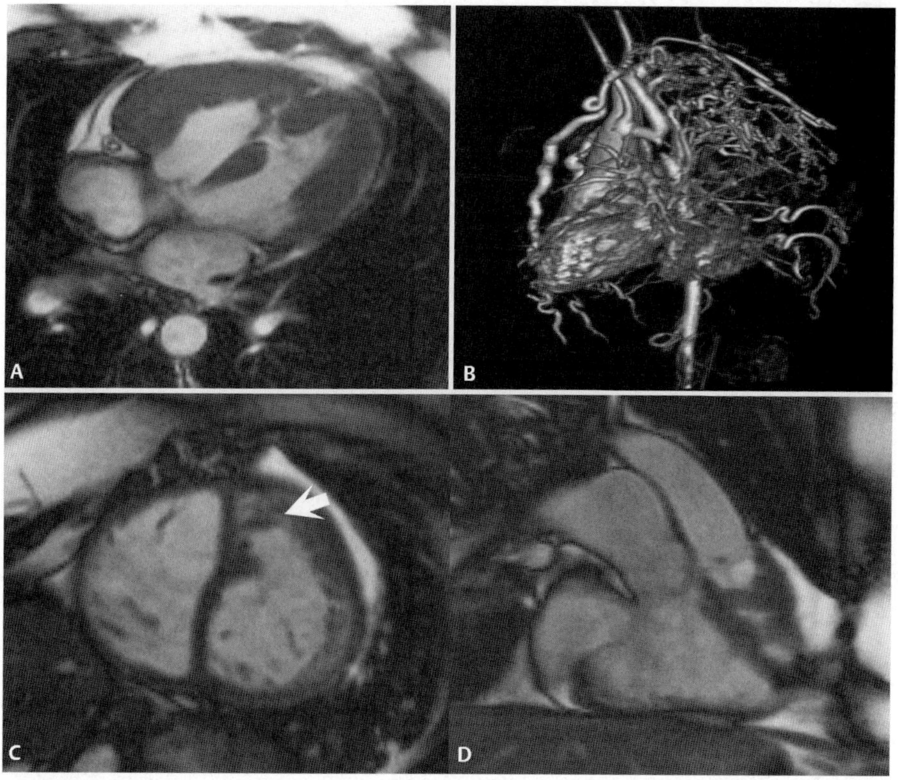

Fig. 60.1 (A–D)

analyzed. With arterial switch procedures, additional attention should be paid to any pulmonary artery stenosis or aortic root dilatation. Levo transposition consists of atrioventricular and ventriculoarterial discordance, whereby the systemic blood flow returns to the right-sided but morphologically left ventricle, which empties into the pulmonary arteries; pulmonary venous blood enters the left-sided but morphologically right ventricle which empties into the aorta. This appearance is demonstrated on the short-axis cine images of **Fig. 60.1C**. Here the identity of the posterior, although morphologically right ventricle is established by the moderator band (white arrow). Additional cine images adapted to focus on the large vessels show the essentially parallel course of the ascending arteries (**Fig. 60.1D**). Tetralogy of Fallot is the most common cyanotic congenital disorder, consisting of an overriding aorta, pulmonary stenosis, right ventricular hypertrophy, and a VSD. Preoperatively, cine MRI assesses right ventricular morphology and function, whereas contrast-enhanced MRA delineates aortopulmonary collaterals and determines ductus arteriosus patency. In operative planning, specific coronary artery imaging may be useful, particularly in detecting the relation of the arteries to the right ventricular outflow tract, a portion of which is often resected surgically. Postoperatively, the right ventricle should also be carefully examined for evidence of dysfunction, aneurysm, or recurrent stenoses in the right ventricular outflow tract or the pulmonary arteries.

61 Thoracic Vasculature

In the workup of pulmonary embolism, contrast-enhanced CT is most commonly used; MRI is reserved for patients with iodinated contrast allergies or in whom radiation exposure should be minimized. Nevertheless, MRI remains promising due to its ability to obtain a variety of morphologic and functional information about the lungs, their vasculature, and other relevant structures within a single exam. On SE images the pulmonary vasculature appears as low SI distinct from a high SI intraluminal embolus. Peripherally, less uniform blood flow leads to inconsistent signal voids, rendering this pattern less useful. On cine SSFP sequences embolus appears as low SI against high SI blood. By far the most commonly acquired MRI scan for the assessment of pulmonary embolism is contrast-enhanced 3D MRA. Both pulmonary perfusion studies and high-resolution contrast-enhanced GRE T1WI may be obtained. In the latter, embolus appears as a foci of low SI against the enhancing vasculature. Chronic emboli may demonstrate an alternative appearance as in the contrast-enhanced MIP MRA image of **Fig. 61.1A** where enhancing vasculature is absent in the right middle and inferior lobes and the central pulmonary arteries are dilated. A four-chamber cine image of the same patient demonstrates right ventricular dilatation and hypertrophy (**Fig. 61.1B**). Together these findings suggest pulmonary hypertension and cor pulmonale secondary to chronic pulmonary emboli. In pulmonary hypertension, cine imaging may also demonstrate paradoxic bulging of the intraventricular septum toward the left ventricle in systole and low SI jets of tricuspid regurgitation. Right ventricular ejection fraction may be diminished and pulmonic arterial flow inhomogeneous on velocity-encoded MRI. Pulmonary perfusion MRA involves acquiring contrast-enhanced T1WI in short-succession (<20 seconds). Digital subtraction of images prior to parenchymal enhancement from images with maximal enhancement is performed, allowing for perfusion evaluation. These images may improve detection of subsegmental infarcts as wedge-shaped areas of hypoperfusion and allow monitoring of reperfusion after anticoagulation. Concurrent evaluation with ventilation scans utilizing aerosolized contrast, helium, or alternatively oxygen-enhanced MRI (wherein the T1 shortening effect of molecular oxygen provides contrast) allows the distinction between hypoxic vasoconstriction (without ventilation-perfusion mismatches) and pulmonary embolus. Although not commonly performed, concurrent acquisition of lower extremity magnetic resonance venography (MRV) further highlights the versatility and potential of the modality.

Pulmonary AVMs—associated with hereditary hemorrhagic telangiectasia (i.e., Osler-Weber-Rendu syndrome)—are also well visualized on contrast-enhanced MRA. A MIP from a patient with the latter entity is presented in **Fig. 61.1C**, with large AVMs noted within the right lower lobe. Preoperatively, contrast-enhanced 3D MRA allows identification and evaluation of feeding vessels. Within the thoracic aorta, MRI can be useful in the detection of aneurysms and quantification of their size—dilatation of ascending aortic aneurysms over 5.5 cm necessitates surgical intervention. Aneurysms are divided into saccular (circumferentially localized) and fusiform (circumferentially diffuse) types: false aneurysms (contained by fewer than three layers of vessel wall) tend to be the former, and true aneurysms (contained by the entire wall) the latter. Longitudinal span and the number of aneurysms present as well as involvement of any branching arteries should be evaluated. MRI also effectively depicts concomitant processes, such as internal thrombus formation, compression of adjacent structures by an aneurysm, leakage, and paraaortic hematoma. Dissections of the aorta result from

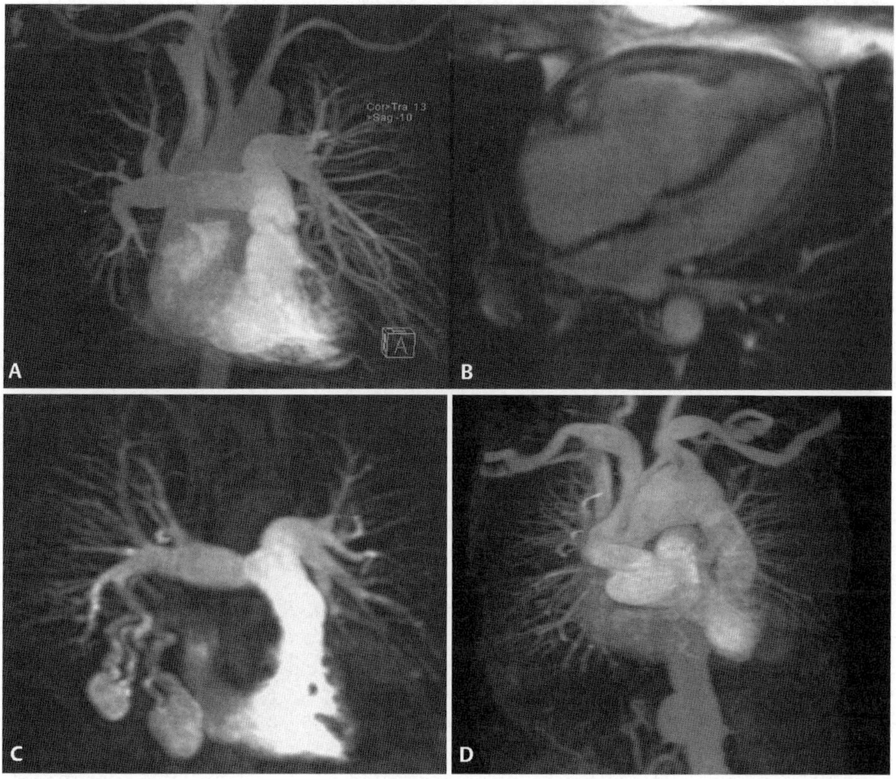

Fig. 61.1 (A–D)

an intimal tear that allows blood to enter the aortic wall, creating a false lumen. Ninety-five percent start in the thoracic aorta: Stanford type A (DeBakey 1 and 2) involve the ascending aorta and type B (DeBakey 3) do not. Type A dissections may involve the aortic valve or coronary arteries, and due to their severity require immediate intervention after detection. In hemodynamically stable patients, MRI is preferred for evaluation. Cine SSFP sequences and contrast-enhanced 3D MRA allow for identification of an intimal flap, detection of thrombus within the false lumen, and the determination of branching vessel origins. The contrast-enhanced MIP MRA image of **Fig. 61.1D** demonstrates a Stanford type A aortic dissection. In this case, the patent false lumen appears to feed the right brachiocephalic artery. In comparison, a thrombosed false lumen will demonstrate a more heterogeneous SI on delayed contrast-enhanced MRA, a lower SI than the true lumen on cine SSFP, and a lack of flow void (higher SI) on SE T1WI. A completely thrombosed false lumen may be difficult to distinguish from an aneurysm with mural thrombus. Characteristics favoring the former include longitudinal extension of the thrombus, a noncircular, compressed false lumen, or a change in the position of the thrombus as a result of the spiral configuration of the dissection membrane.

62 Thoracic Neoplasia

Metastatic tumors are the most common neoplasias involving the heart; primary lipomas and myxomas are rarer. The latter is demonstrated in the axial cine image in **Fig. 62.1A** as a large moderate SI mass attached to the left atrium—the most common site of origin—and extending into the left ventricle. Detection of such an atrial attachment distinguishes a myxoma from intracardiac thrombus. Myxoma SI characteristics vary depending on the amount of blood products and calcification present. Enhancement is also variable. Intracardiac lipomas are distinguished by their high SI (due to the presence of fat) on T1WI. Malignant cardiac tumors (i.e., rhabdomyosarcomas) are rarer still and are suggested by a wide base of attachment or the concomitant presence of a hemorrhagic pericardial effusion.

Unlike those of the heart, lung malignancies are extremely common. Lung MRI presents similar difficulties to that of the heart, typically requiring cardiac or respiratory gating. Other problems include intrinsically low tissue proton density and susceptibility artifact at the interface of air and soft tissue. Although alone the SI characteristics of a pulmonary lesion cannot establish malignancy and CT is generally used for lung cancer staging, MRI may be used in patients with iodinated contrast allergies and in several other scenarios. Given its superior soft tissue contrast, multiplanar capabilities, and lack of bone artifact, thoracic outlet tumors (i.e., Pancoast tumor) are better evaluated by MRI. Mass effect on blood vessels or the brachial plexus may be visualized without contrast administration. The above characteristics also allow clear visualization of chest wall invasion particularly on axial cine images. Irregular margins and infiltrative growth characterize malignancy, whereas lipomas—the most common primary chest wall tumor—demonstrate uniform high SI on T1WI. Surgical contraindications include vascular, brachial plexus, spinal cord, and pericardial involvement—all well seen on MRI. Postoperatively, recurrent tumor is distinguished from fibrosis by its higher SI on T2WI. Mediastinal involvement is likewise better visualized on MRI than on unenhanced CT, as the low SI of blood vessels and the tracheobronchial tree appear distinct from higher SI fat and soft tissue, easily differentiating a small vessel from a pulmonary nodule or lymph node. **Figure 62.1B** depicts a bronchogenic carcinoma, demonstrating moderate SI against the low SI of the air-filled lungs on half-Fourier acquisition single-shot turbo spin-echo (HASTE) T2WI. Invasion of the mediastinum with encasement of the bronchi is evident. Contrast-enhanced MRA may help further evaluate arterial invasion.

In primary mediastinal tumors compartmental localization is particularly important. Anterior mediastinal tumors include lymphoma, teratomas, and tumors of the thymus, thyroid, and parathyroid. Teratomas are identified by the concurrent MRI presence of fatty, calcified, and cystic components. The normal thyroid and parathyroid demonstrate moderate and high SI on T2WI, respectively, and both appear as low SI on T1WI. Conventional MRI and contrast-enhanced imaging may be helpful in presurgical localization of the parathyroid glands. None of the above tumors can be classified as benign or malignant on conventional MRI, rendering its main use that of tumor extent delineation. For example, the thymoma to the left of the pulmonary trunk on the T1WI of **Fig. 62.1C** is clearly situated within the anterior mediastinum and demonstrates moderate SI on T1WI. A right pleural metastasis is also clearly visualized. Although not present here, MRI SI characteristics of pleural fluid content may help elucidate its contents: chylothoraxes demonstrate high SI on T1WI, and diffusion

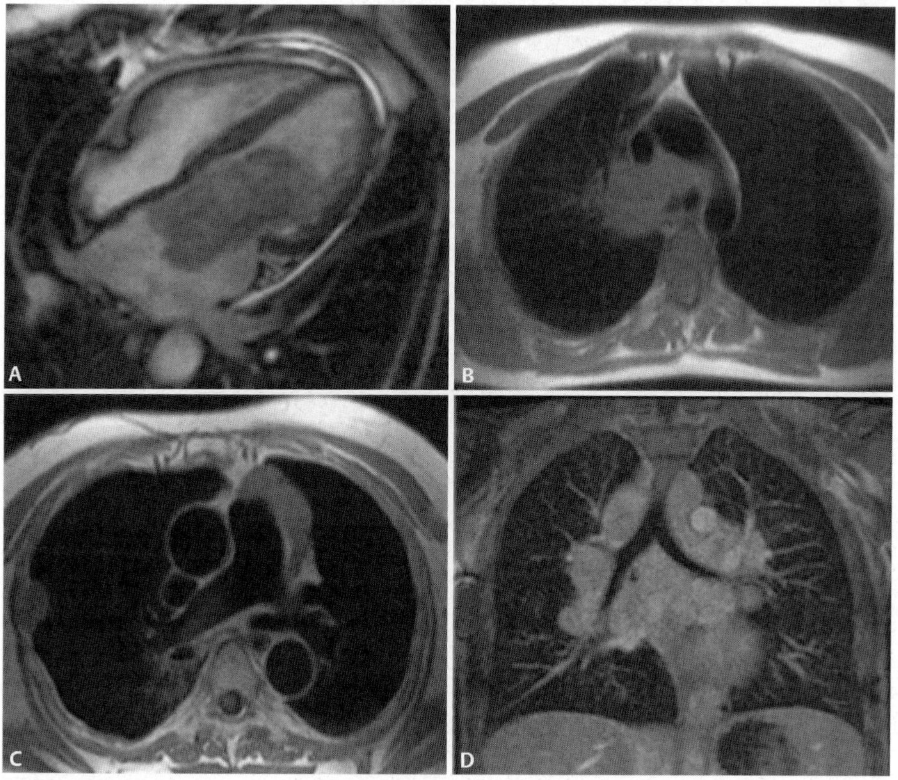

Fig. 62.1 (A–D)

restriction and contrast enhancement typifies exudative fluid. In the middle mediastinum, tracheobronchial and esophageal cysts may occur. Pure fluid within these lesions demonstrates low and high SI on T1WI and T2WI, respectively, whereas greater protein-content increases and decreases these SI, respectively. Lymphoma occurs throughout the mediastinum, appearing as homogeneous lower SI on T2WI, although this appearance is nonspecific. Malignant lymphadenopathy from other causes may also be seen, although the MRI diagnosis may be difficult, in part due to poor visualization of calcification—a marker of benign nodularity and lymphadenopathy. Benign lymph nodes demonstrate a homogeneous SI and fatty (high SI on T1WI) hilum; malignancy is suggested by a short axis diameter exceeding 1 cm and early (within 1.5 minutes) contrast enhancement with rapid washout. Enhancement characteristics of infectious or inflammatory etiologies—other potential causes of mediastinal mass—may be similar. Such characteristics are demonstrated in the case of sarcoidosis illustrated on the coronal contrast-enhanced T1WI in **Fig. 62.1D**, where enlarged, enhancing perihilar and mediastinal lymph nodes are present. Other MRI SI characteristics of infectious and inflammatory lymphadenopathy are nonspecific. Further considerations within the posterior mediastinum include neurogenic neoplasms (see Chapter 39).

63 Breast Neoplasia

Due to its high sensitivity (approaching 100%) breast MRI is indicated for the screening of patients who are genetically positive for breast cancer or certain other predisposing conditions. Alternative indications are a first-degree relative meeting this criteria, prior radiation to the chest between the ages of 10 and 30, or a calculated lifetime risk of 20 to 25% using standard risk models. Imaging protocols for MR mammography have in recent years become more standardized, typically including the acquisition of non-FS T1WI and FS T2WI followed by dynamic postcontrast scans, the latter performed every minute for 5 minutes. Dynamic post-contrast MRI improves upon conventional MRI's relatively low specificity for breast cancer. In dynamic imaging, elimination of fat signal may be achieved by spectral FS or by digital subtraction of pre- from postcontrast T1WI. Inhomogeneity of FS (due to field inhomogeneity) is the major pitfall of the former technique; the latter being limited by patient movement between acquisitions. MIPs, whereby the greatest SI pixels from 3D space are projected to create a 2D image, may be obtained. Slice thickness using 2D Fourier transform techniques should be less than 2 mm (with in-plane resolution of <1 mm); however, 3D imaging is likely superior due to a lack of interslice gaps. In dynamic imaging, a balance must be struck between requirements of high spatial resolution and adequate temporal resolution—a conflict eased by the advent of high field and parallel imaging. Other technical considerations include the performance of breast MRI between days 7 and 14 of the menstrual cycle when background enhancement is minimized.

Figure 63.1 demonstrates a typical appearance for breast carcinoma on MRI. On **(A)** precontrast T1WI, a spiculated area of low SI is noted distinct from the surrounding high SI fat. Dynamic postcontrast imaging at 5.5 minutes **(B)** reveals a persistent (type 1) enhancement pattern. Typically, type 1 enhancement is predictive of a benign lesion ($>$ 90%), whereas a plateau in enhancement (type 2) is moderately associated with malignancy. A pattern of rapid, early enhancement ($>$ 80% of maximum within 2 minutes) and prompt washout (type 3) suggests the presence of leaky vasculature and is strongly predictive ($>$ 85%) of malignancy. Kinetic curves constructed from dynamic measurements are helpful in identification of these patterns. As mentioned, the mass in **Fig. 63.1A** demonstrates a spiculated pattern—a pattern highly suggestive of neoplasia. Masses with irregular margins are likely neoplastic; those with smooth or lobulated borders are more likely benign. The malignancy in **Fig. 63.2** demonstrates a lobulated pattern on T1WI **(A)** and STIR **(B)**, although dynamic postcontrast MIP revealed prompt enhancement at 1.5 minutes **(C)** with subsequent washout. A slight rim-enhancing pattern—a pattern highly predictive of neoplasia ($>$ 70%)—was also present, although not seen here. More benign enhancement patterns include that of nonenhancing septations, which, along with a smooth border and high SI on T2WI, suggest fibroadenoma. The absence of enhancement, although suggestive of benignity, does not fully rule out neoplasia (88–94% negative predictive value). **Figure 63.2** also demonstrates a suspicious, although indeterminate lymph node. In **Fig. 63.3** a small lesion (1 cm in diameter) is clearly seen on the

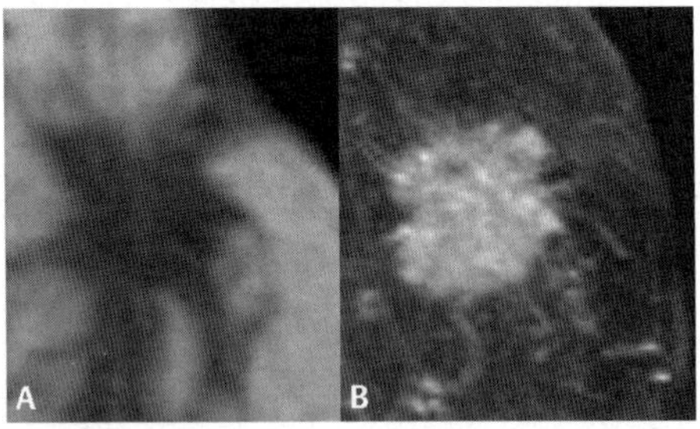

Fig. 63.1 (A,B)

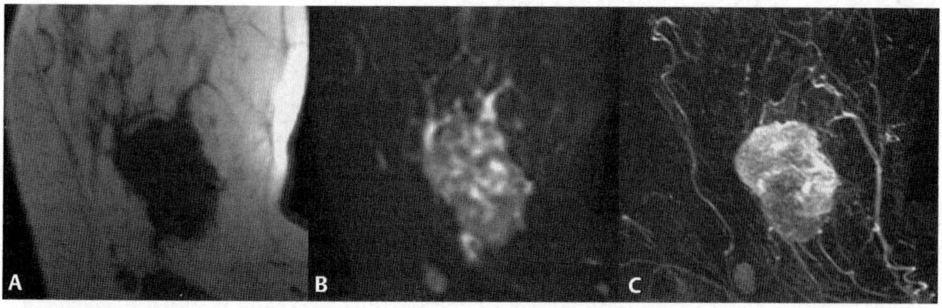

Fig. 63.2 (A–C)

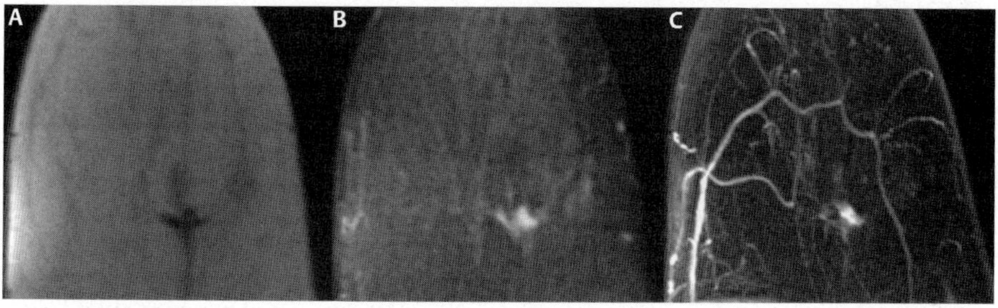

Fig. 63.3 (A–C)

T1WI (**A**), STIR (**B**), and dynamic postcontrast MIP at 4.5 minutes (**C**) with washout kinetics in the latter suggesting neoplasia. Much smaller lesions (<5 mm) may be too small to otherwise characterize and are defined as foci of enhancement. The significance of these lesions varies with the setting in which they occur, their number, and associated findings. A ductal (linear enhancement radiating to the nipple) or segmental pattern (an arrowhead-like focus pointed at the nipple) is suggestive of neoplasia, especially ductal carcinoma in situ (DCIS), as is any pattern of coalesced, focal clusters (clumped enhancement). Biopsy of these lesions by conventional means may be impossible secondary to a lack of visualization on conventional modalities. Likewise, the patient in **Fig. 63.4** was initially found on mammography to have only a solitary mass (confirmed as invasive ductal carcinoma), until breast MRI 10 days later for staging revealed two additional masses, which enhanced briskly on dynamic postcontrast imaging at 1.5 minutes. A targeted, second-look ultrasound may localize such lesions, facilitating biopsy; however, if visualization on mammography or ultrasound is not possible, MRI-guided biopsy is performed.

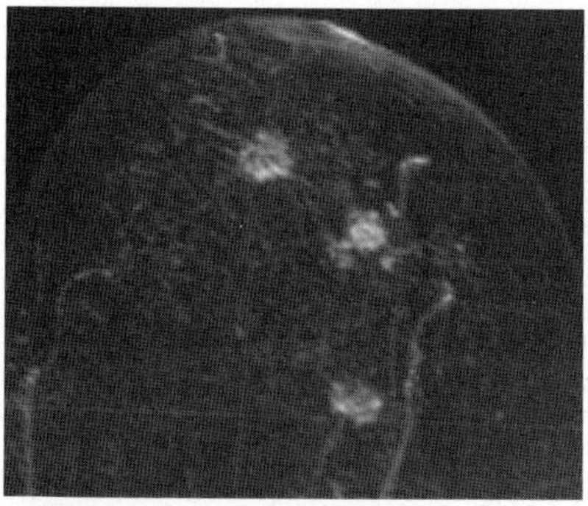

Fig. 63.4

64 Breast Implants

MRI is the most sensitive study for the detection of breast implant rupture and in the detection of cancer in women with implants. Rupture of saline implants usually occurs quickly and completely; thus imaging is rarely performed. Silicone implants are more common. On T2WI the SI of silicone is between that of water and fat. Thus when suspicion of a ruptured implant is high, water and fat suppression are implemented to facilitate visualization. Fat signal suppression is achieved by the addition of an initial inversion pulse (similar to STIR; see Chapter 34). Water signal is suppressed by a spectral technique (similar to that for fat; see Chapter 48). T2WI in **Fig. 64.1** and **Fig. 64.2** show the effect of these measures, where silicone is the only component demonstrating high SI. T1WI are not obtained due to the low SI of silicone. With appropriate suppression, the normal appearance of a single lumen implant includes a high SI silicone core surrounded by a low SI implant shell and outer fibrous capsule. Although the shell can be smooth, more modern implants are typically textured (with the intent of reducing capsular contraction). Folds of this shell may be evident, often with a complex appearance but only encroaching upon the implant lumen peripherally. Implant encapsulation within a rim of reactive collagen and fibrotic tissue is the most frequent complication of breast augmentation, although it is usually a clinical diagnosis. The Baker classification grades degrees of contracture from an encapsulated but normal appearing breast (I)—present in most cases—to one that appears natural but firm (II), to a visibly distorted breast (III), to a hard, painful, and distorted breast (IV) requiring surgical intervention. Rarely visualized on MRI, findings of breast encapsulation include focal, asymmetric folding of the fibrous capsule leading to deformity in the implant's normal oval shape.

Intracapsular rupture refers to breach of the implant shell but containment of leaking silicone within the surrounding fibrous capsule. The MRI appearance of an intracapsular rupture is demonstrated on the axial and sagittal images of **Figs. 64.1A,B**, respectively. The appearance of low SI free strands of silicone envelope within the high SI silicone implant is termed the linguine sign and is the most reliable marker of implant rupture on MRI. Here this sign is present bilaterally, indicating bilateral intracapsular rupture. Often water and fat suppression are not necessary to visualize this, although normal folds of the shell may appear similar and confuse the diagnosis. The keyhole, inverted noose, or tear drop sign refers to the appearance of silicone both inside and outside a radial fold of the implant wall, as seen bilaterally in the axial

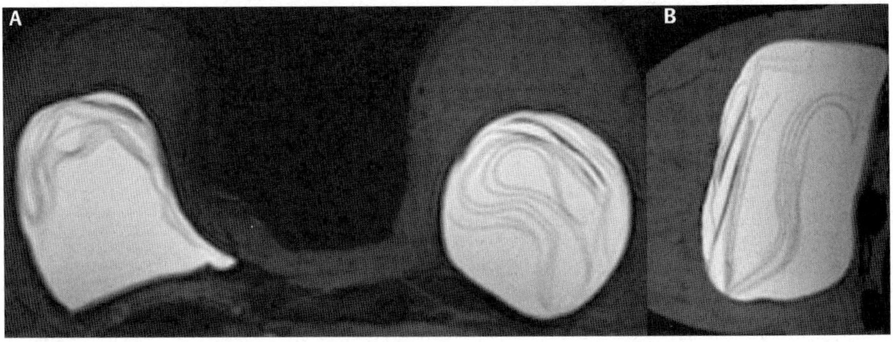

Fig. 64.1 (A,B)

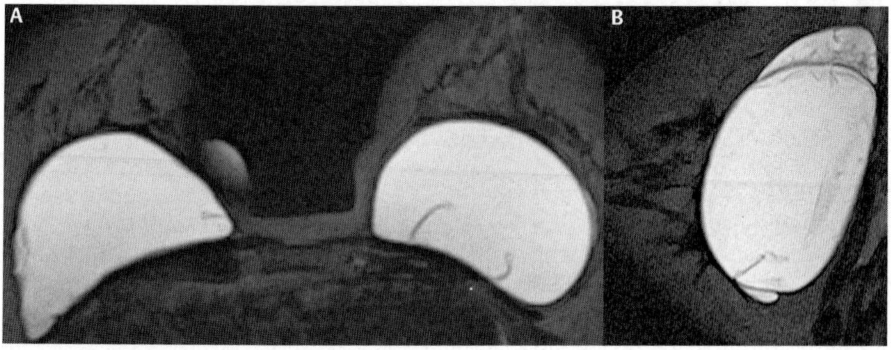

Fig. 64.2 (A,B)

images of **Fig. 64.2A**. The presence of the keyhole sign alone indicates a noncollapsed rupture, but in this case silicone between the shell and fibrous capsule within the left breast, laterally, indicates collapse. **Figure 64.2B** gives the appearance of having two separate lumens both superiorly and inferiorly: the outer wall of the outer lumen is formed by the capsule alone and the inner lumen wall is formed by the collapsed implant envelope. Although **Figs. 64.2A,B** demonstrate bilateral intracapsular rupture, a component of extracapsular rupture in the left breast is noted laterally on axial images **(A)** and superiorly on sagittal images **(B)**. Superior extravasation of silicone is most common, although lateral and inferior are also frequent. The MRI finding most suggestive of extracapsular rupture is simply the presence of high SI silicone within surrounding tissues. Poorly suppressed water SI can mimic this appearance. As in this case, simple gel extravasation can occur, as can extrusion (whereby the extracapsular component is continuous with the implant lumen). Granuloma or cyst formation may occur, and regional lymph nodes may be involved.

An asymptomatic palpable mass in a woman with silicone breast implants is worrisome for neoplasm or implant rupture. Although neoplasm may theoretically be excluded in part by alternatively accentuating and suppressing the SI of silicone, contrast-enhanced examinations are by far more commonly performed (see Chapter 63). Considerations are similar as those in patients without implants, although progressive enhancement of the entire fibrous capsule may occur and is a normal finding. Silicone granulomas may also enhance, but will display SI consistent with silicone on unenhanced MRI.

65 Benign Hepatic Masses

Abdominal MRI examinations typically consist of breath-hold precontrast in and out-of-phase GRE T1WI, volumetric interpolated breath-hold examination (VIBE) 3D T1WI, and HASTE T2WI in addition to STIR and postcontrast T1WI. Dynamic contrast-enhanced examinations (described below) are best performed with agents such as Gd BOPTA (gadobenate dimeglumine; MultiHance, Bracco Diagnostics, Inc., Princeton, NJ) or Gd EOB-DTPA (gadolinium ethoxybenzyl diethylenetriamine pentaacetic acid; Primovist/Eovist, Bayer Healthcare, LLC, Shawnee Mission, KS)—gadolinium chelates partially excreted through the biliary system. Other gadolinium chelates (with sole renal excretion) can be employed, but do not offer the possibility of delayed phase imaging. Hepatic cysts are the most common benign entity involving the liver and appear on T2WI as sharply demarcated, nonseptated, hyperintense lesions (FS T2WI, **Fig. 65.1A**). Simple cysts do not enhance on postcontrast T1WI as seen in **Fig. 65.1B**—a VIBE breath-hold image wherein a solitary, hypointense hepatic cyst is present. Occasionally, hemorrhage into a cyst increases its SI on T1WI, adding mucinous cysts of foregut origin—a lesion usually involving the superficial liver and expanding its margin—to the differential. Mucinous metastases may also appear similar on unenhanced imaging. Echinococcal cysts (*E. granulosis*) are characterized by a hypointense fibrous capsule, which may enhance. Multiple daughter cysts are classically contained within the capsule, with extrinsic cysts termed satellite lesions. Hepatic alveolar echinococcosis (*E. multilocularis*) is more aggressive, demonstrating involvement (and thus enhancement) of the heart, lungs, and their serosa. Biliary hamartomas are benign cystic lesions distinguished by their small size (<1.5 cm) and multiplicity. Thin, peripheral contrast enhancement reflecting nearby compressed hepatic parenchyma may occur, an appearance potentially mimicking that of abscess or metastatic disease. Unlike the latter, progressively central enhancement is not seen and surrounding tissue involvement is sparse. Hemangiomas are the most common neoplastic hepatic lesion. A lobulated giant hemangioma demonstrating typical hyperintensity on HASTE T2WI is illustrated in **Fig. 65.2A**. Hemangiomas are less lobulated when they are smaller in size with all varieties generally exhibiting homogeneously low SI on T1WI. Several enhancement patterns have been described. Type 1 enhancement is intense and uniform in the arterial phase (30 seconds postcontrast) with diminishing enhancement on subsequent images. Hypervascular malignant lesions may appear similar with a lack of surrounding parenchymal enhancement favoring hemangioma,

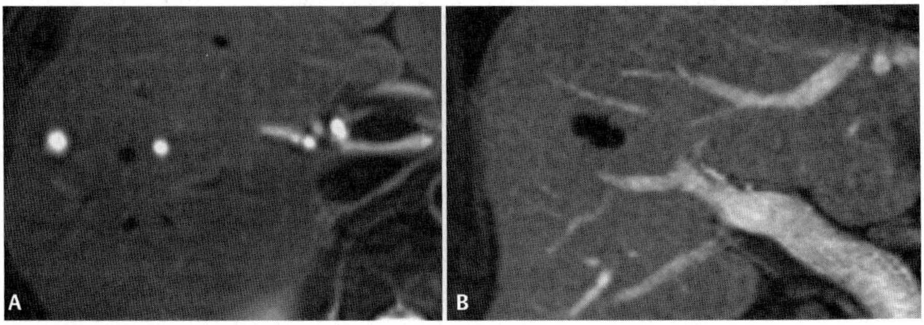

Fig. 65.1 (A,B)

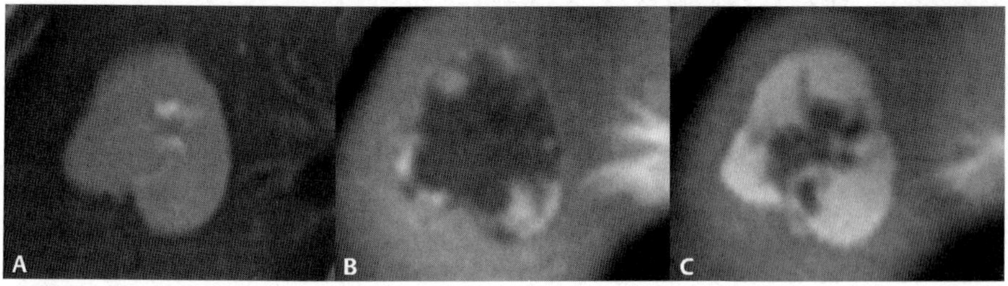

Fig. 65.2 (A–C)

although this finding is unreliable due to enhancing draining veins yielding a similar appearance. Peripheral, nodular, and discontinuous arterial-phase enhancement, characteristic of a type 2 or 3 pattern, is demonstrated in **Fig. 65.2B**—a breath-hold VIBE T1WI obtained one minute following contrast injection. If enhancement progresses centripetally to occur homogeneously throughout the lesion, a type 2 pattern—most common in nongiant (<5 cm) lesions—is present. If an area of central scar is spared, then a type 3 pattern is present. The T1WI (10 minutes postcontrast) in **Fig. 65.2C** demonstrate a type 3 enhancement pattern, the most common seen in giant hemangiomas. Biliary phase enhancement is absent in hemangiomas—a characteristic distinguishing them from focal nodular hyperplasia (FNH). An FNH is illustrated in **Fig. 65.3A**, demonstrating immediate, avid arterial phase (30 seconds postcontrast) enhancement with sparing of its central scar. Enhancement aids in detection of these lesions as they may be essentially isointense to the liver on conventional MRI sequences. Washout of contrast has occurred by the **(B)** venous phase (1 minute postcontrast), with **(C)** 3-hour delayed images using Gd-BOPTA demonstrating biliary retention of contrast—attributable to the malformed biliary ducts within FNH. FNH is also associated with a central hyperintense scar on T2WI, correlating with chronic inflammation and fibrosis. The scar does not typically enhance **(A)** in the arterial phase, but **(B)** enhancement thereafter increases. A similar scar may also be present in hepatic adenomas, the substantial fat content of which leads to characteristic lesion dropout on out-of-phase GRE T1WI. As biliary ducts are absent within hepatic adenomas, delayed enhancement with Gd-BOPTA is absent. Faint uniform arterial phase typically fades after one minute, and a fibrous capsule if present will enhance on interstitial phase images (2 minutes postcontrast).

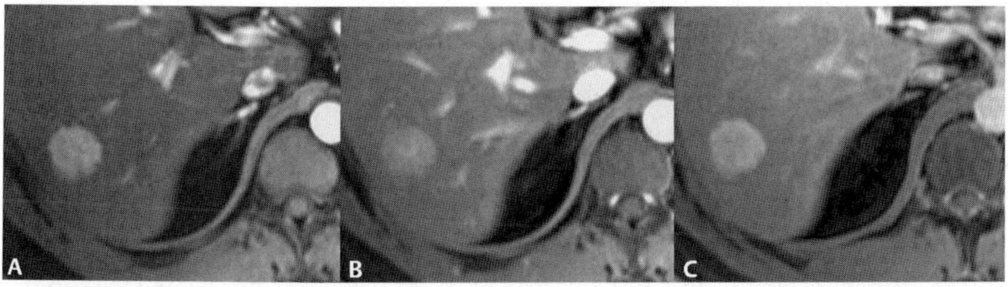

Fig. 65.3 (A–C)

66 Malignant Hepatic Masses

The most common primary hepatic malignancy presenting with arterial phase enhancement (30 seconds postinjection) is hepatocellular carcinoma (HCC), which occurs in a solitary, multifocal, and less-common diffuse pattern. HCC typically appears hypo- and hyperintense to cirrhotic parenchyma on T1WI and T2WI, respectively. Characteristically avid arterial-phase enhancement fades by the interstitial phase (5 to 15 minutes postinjection) except in the case of a late-enhancing pseudocapsule, which is present at least half of the time. In a cirrhotic liver, the major differential for a lesion enhancing in the arterial phase is a regenerative nodule, although these typically remain similar to parenchymal SI on interstitial-phase images, enhance overall more homogeneously, and may demonstrate hemosiderin deposition (low SI on T2WI). Dysplastic nodules, which may be precursors to HCC are larger and may overlap with the latter in appearance. Fibrolamellar carcinoma—a HCC variant found in young patients without cirrhosis—may be confused with focal nodular hyperplasia due to its central scar, which is hyper- and hypointense to hepatic parenchyma on the respective T2 and GRE T1WI of **Figs. 66.1A,B**. This lesion enhances on (**Fig. 66.1C**) arterial-phase contrast-enhanced T1WI with sparing of the scar. With time, overall enhancement of this type of lesion tends to fade. The hypointense capsule surrounding this particular lesion is atypical for FNH, and subsequent biopsy revealed fibrolamellar carcinoma. Gd-BOPTA may be used to distinguish benign and malignant hepatic lesions. HCC demonstrates a target-like appearance on 3-hour postcontrast images due to central necrosis, hemorrhage, and subsequent fibrosis, in the face of preserved, peripheral hepatocytes that take up Gd-BOPTA. Superparamagnetic iron oxide particles, specifically ferumoxides, are phagocytized by reticuloendothelial macrophages (i.e., Kupffer cells), and shorten tissue T2*, resulting in diminished SI on T2WI. Because liver tumors, other than FNH, lack Kupffer cells, they appear hyperintense to parenchyma when imaged 1 to 4 hours postcontrast. Ferumoxides, although rarely utilized, may be useful in the detection of HCC when cirrhotic morphology impairs accurate evaluation with extracellular gadolinium-chelates. Cholangiocarcinoma is another differential consideration for an (late) enhancing hepatic mass, and is further discussed in Chapter 68.

Metastatic disease within the liver may demonstrate avid arterial phase contrast enhancement or more commonly enhance less than the surrounding parenchyma. Unlike HCC, however, such lesions do not possess functioning hepatocytes, and thus uniformly lack delayed enhancement with GD-BOPTA. Mangafodipir (Mn DPDP)—a manganese-based contrast agent no longer available in the United States—is similarly taken up by hepatocytes, allowing differentiation of HCC from metastatic lesions.

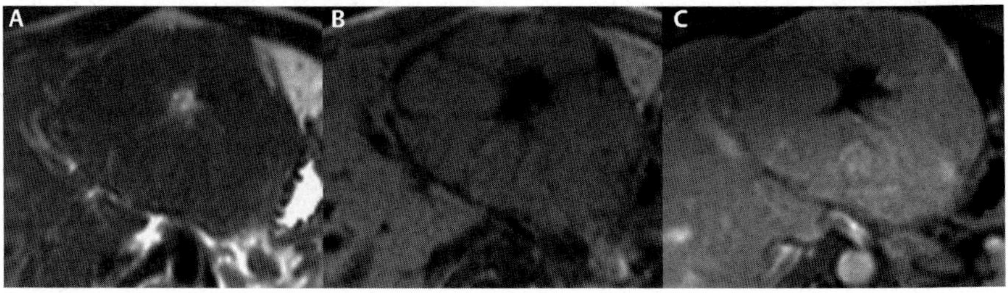

Fig. 66.1 (A–C)

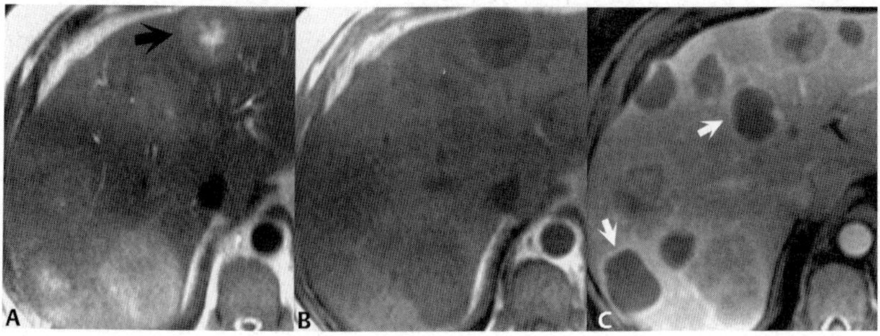

Fig. 66.2 (A–C)

Sources of metastatic disease may be distinguished, in part, by MRI SI and enhancement characteristics. Neuroendocrine tumors appear as very bright lesions on T2WI and demonstrate avid arterial-phase enhancement, thus mimicking a type 1 hemangioma. Lesions of inhomogeneous high SI on T2WI that enhance avidly in the arterial phase include renal cell carcinoma, pheochromocytoma, breast cancer, and melanoma. The latter, along with ovarian cancer and hemorrhagic neoplasias may appear with high SI on T1WI. A fatty liver is often present in metastatic disease, in some instances secondary to chemotherapy; thus lesions with high SI on T1WI may be better detected on out-of-phase imaging. Metastatic colon carcinoma is illustrated on the respective HASTE T2WI, precontrast T1WI, and early venous phase contrast-enhanced FS T1WI of **Figs. 66.2A,B,C**. Multiple, large lesions are evident, one of which demonstrates a characteristic donut sign (**A**, *black arrow*) on T2WI signifying central necrosis, a typical finding in adenocarcinoma. This necrotic area appears as central hyperintensity surrounded by moderate SI tumor. A halo sign may alternatively be present, referring to a high SI rim of viable cells surrounding rims of alternating decreased SI, correlating with mucin, necrosis, or fibrosis, and increased SI, representing liquefactive necrosis. The centrally necrotic area does not enhance on **(C)** FS postcontrast T1WI. Colorectal carcinoma, like most adenocarcinomas, is frequently hypovascular in the arterial phase, demonstrating only a rim of enhancement on arterial and (**C**, *white arrows*) early venous-phase imaging with subsequent washout 5 to 15 minutes postcontrast. Cystic metastases of ovarian cancer may enhance similarly, but with internal septations and of course a cyst-like appearance on unenhanced images. Ill-defined rim enhancement persisting past the venous phase without central contrast uptake, may be seen with a pyogenic or amebic abscess, the latter preferentially involving the right hepatic lobe. Treated metastatic lesions may appear identical although a septated cystic appearance is rarely present, and clinical history should aid in distinction. Lymphoma is also hypovascular in the arterial and portal venous phases, but often iso- rather than hypointense to parenchyma in the interstitial phase. Metastases of leiomyosarcoma and GI stromal tumors may occasionally show delayed, persistent enhancement, as may hemangioendotheliomas or hemangiosarcomas. The latter can be distinguished from benign hemangiomas by its irregular borders and heterogeneous internal appearance secondary to hemorrhage. The fibrous stroma of diffuse HCC may also result in late-phase enhancement.

67 Diffuse Hepatic Pathology

Figures 67.1A through 67.1C illustrate findings characteristic of a fatty liver on FSE T2WI, in-phase, and out-of-phase GRE T1WI, respectively. An area of subtly decreased SI relative to the higher SI fat on **(A)** T2WI represents focal fatty sparing. On **(B)** in-phase T1WI, the liver appears of high SI. **(C)** Out-of-phase images clearly demonstrate signal loss diffusely within the liver with the exception of the spared focus, the SI loss resulting from negation of opposed water and fat signals as described in Chapter 69. FS imaging detects mild fatty infiltration less sensitively than in and out-of-phase imaging, as SI suppression from fat saturation when a small amount of fat is present is approximately half of that obtained in out-of-phase images, which suppress both fat SI and that of water (when present in the same voxel) due to destructive signal interference. Fat-predominant lesions are, however, better detected with FS imaging. The T2WI of **Fig. 67.1D** demonstrates a hypointense lesion (*white arrow*) in fatty liver, as further evident on **(E)** in and **(F)** out-of-phase images. As with neoplasia, no out-of-phase dropout is present, but a lack of abnormal enhancement on **(G)** in-phase contrast-enhanced T1WI implies an area of focal fatty sparing near the gallbladder fossa. Postcontrast out-of-phase imaging results in a paradoxical loss in fatty tissue SI: tissues consisting of mainly fat still contain some amount of water, the SI contribution from which is disproportionately small due to the long T1 of water. Gadolinium chelates shorten the T1 time of water in the extracellular space, resulting in a greater contribution of water protons to SI. With out-of-phase images, this results in more destructive interference with fat, decreasing SI.

Accumulation of intracellular paramagnetic iron products—in distinction to copper (as in Wilson disease)—results in magnetic field inhomogeneities that increase T2* decay and lead to a low SI on GRE T2WI. The patient in **Fig. 67.2** had received multiple blood transfusions, resulting in secondary hemochromatosis with reticuloendothelial iron content leading to diminished SI on **(A)** axial and **(B)** coronal HASTE T2WI within both the liver and bone marrow. Iron deposition in the reticuloendothelial system in

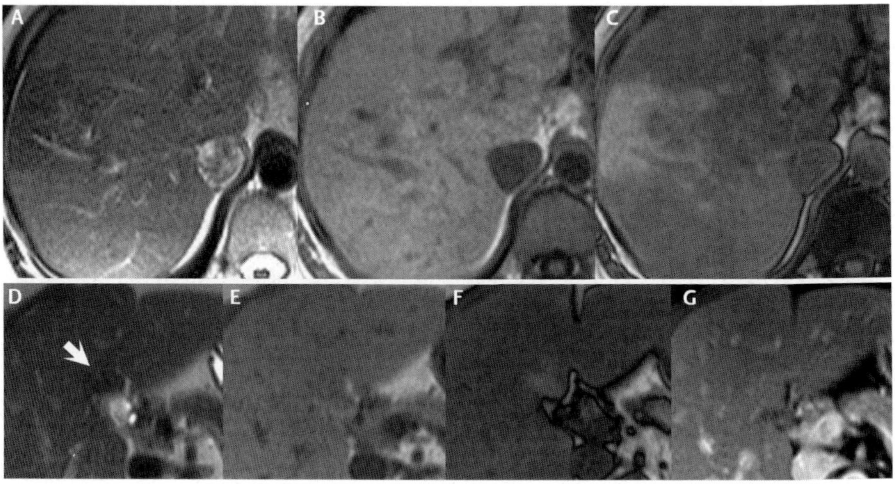

Fig. 67.1 (A–G)

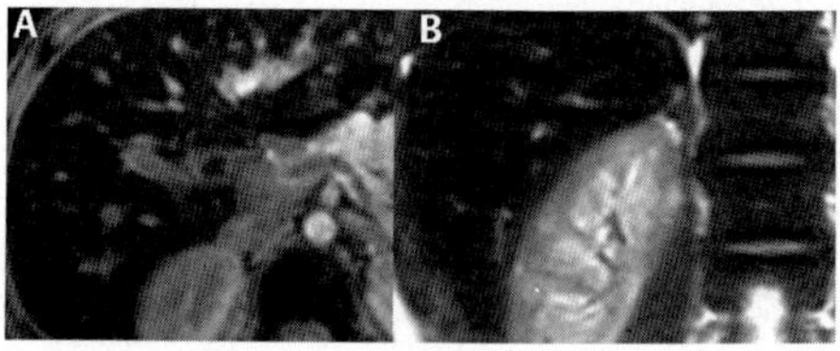

Fig. 67.2 (A,B)

secondary hemochromatosis and hemosiderosis does not directly damage parenchymal cells and spares the pancreas, progressively affecting the liver, spleen, and myocardium. Parenchymal iron deposition occurs directly in primary hemochromatosis, affecting the liver, pancreas, and myocardium but not the spleen. A dysfunctional or saturated reticuloendothelial system in secondary hemochromatosis may blur the latter point of distinction. Resulting hypointensity in the liver on T2* and T2WI provides natural contrast—similar to that obtainable with SPIO contrast agents—to aid in the detection of hepatocellular carcinoma, a condition predisposed by hemochromatosis.

The earliest findings of liver cirrhosis include medial segment atrophy and hilar enlargement with fatty infiltration. Atrophy of the entire right lobe occurs later with left lateral and caudate lobe hypertrophy. Focal or diffuse fibrotic changes may occur, the former illustrated in **Fig. 67.3** where a focus of fibrosis is hyperintense to parenchyma on **(A)** HASTE and **(B)** STIR T2WI. **(C)** Lack of contrast enhancement on T1WI makes hepatocellular carcinoma less likely. Liver contour in **Fig. 67.3** is typically nodular. Dysplastic regenerative hepatic nodules often demonstrate high and low SI on T1WI and T2WI, respectively, and do not enhance, whereas those associated with hepatocellular carcinoma are of moderate to low SI on T1WI and high SI on T2WI and enhance avidly in the arterial phase. Siderotic regenerative nodules, appearing as low SI structures on GRE T2WI, predispose to hepatocellular carcinoma, and may also be seen in the spleen, resulting from hemorrhagic changes secondary to portal hypertension (i.e., Gamna-Gandy bodies). Splenomegaly—present in **Fig. 67.3**—typifies portal hypertension, as does the presence of varices at porto-systemic anastomoses, the latter appearing as prominent flow-voids on T2WI. Portal venous flow may be assessed via MRA, with venous anatomy well depicted on 2D TOF imaging and flow direction confirmed on phase contrast studies. Contrast-enhanced MRA is especially useful if portal vein thrombosis is suspected or if stagnant flow impairs 2D TOF. Areas of avid parenchymal enhancement are seen in portal vein thrombosis due to the increased dependance of the parenchyma on systemic blood supply. The wedge shape of such lesions distinguishes them from the heterogeneous enhancement seen in congestive heart failure due to increased sinusoidal pressure delaying parenchymal arterial flow. Acute hepatitis may be detected as patchy enhancement on arterial-phase postcontrast imaging.

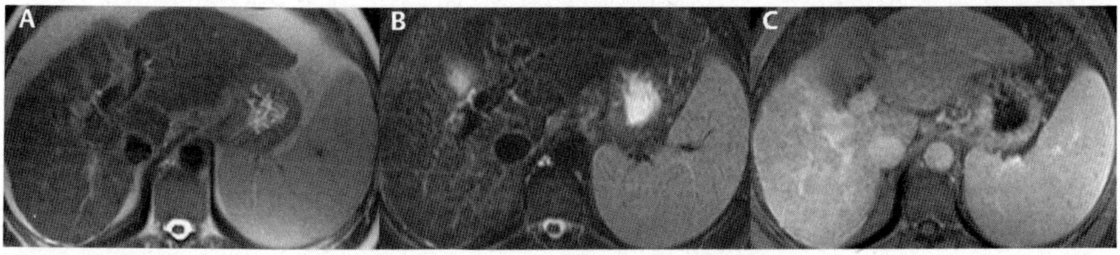

Fig. 67.3 (A–C)

68 Biliary Disease

Magnetic resonance cholangiopancreatography (MRCP) clearly depicts high SI static biliary fluid, which has a long T2 time, against surrounding structures of low SI on images acquired with long echo times. Typically, a series of conventional T1WI and T2WI are acquired in various planes followed by thick slab (4–5 mm), single-shot 2D acquisitions with long echo times. A 3D scan with isotropic spatial resolution—to allow for reconstruction in any desired plane—is then acquired, typically with navigator echoes to avoid motion artifact. MIP images are then constructed. Contrast-enhanced MRCP may also be performed utilizing agents with biliary excretion such as Gd-BOPTA or Gd EOB-DTPA; precontrast T1WI and T2WI allow precise evaluation of surrounding structures. MRCP offers noninvasive imaging comparable to ERCP (endoscopic retrograde cholangiopancreatography) in accuracy without operator dependence or ionizing radiation.

The normal gallbladder wall appears as low SI on T2WI and enhances homogeneously. The SI of bile itself increases with fasting on T1WI due to increasing bile salt concentrations. Cholelithiasis is a common incidental finding on MRI. A gallstone appears hypointense on T1WI and T2WI due to a lack of mobile protons within its internal lattice. Stones with high protein concentration may appear hyperintense on T1WI. Multiple low SI gallstones are present on the thick-slab MRCP image of **Fig. 68.1A**. A gallstone may be distinguished from a polyp by its dependent location and lack of enhancement. Both MRCP and axial T2WI, **Figs. 68.1A,B**, respectively, also demonstrate a solitary common bile duct stone at the level of the ampulla (*white arrows*). Pneumobilia may mimic gallstones, but is nondependent in location. Acute cholecystitis is sensitively detected by wall enhancement and enhancement of reactive adjacent hepatic parenchyma. Gallbladder wall thickening and pericholecystic fluid are well detected on T2WI. A shrunken gallbladder with only mild, homogeneous enhancement of a thickened wall typifies chronic cholecystitis, whereas wall calcification—hypointense on T2WI has been classically associated with an increased risk of gallbladder carcinoma. Carcinoma appears as a heterogeneously enhancing gallbladder lumen mass often with associated wall thickening, local invasion, and lymphadenopathy. In distinction, adenomyomatosis demonstrates high SI cystic spaces (which do not enhance postcontrast) within a thickened gall bladder wall on T2WI. Intrahepatic (peripheral) cholangiocarcinomas may be confused

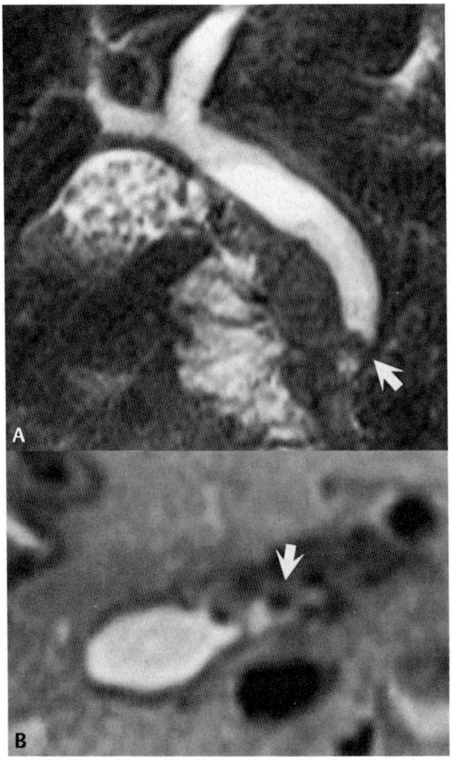

Fig. 68.1 (A,B)

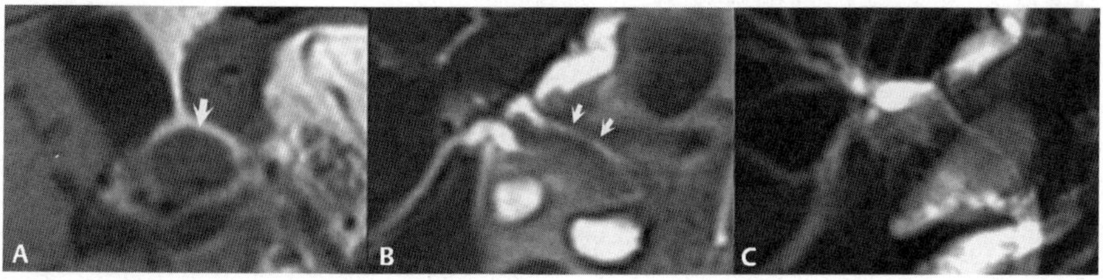

Fig. 68.2 (A–C)

with HCC, but demonstrate low SI on T1WI and T2WI and delayed enhancement due to their fibrous composition. Concurrent cirrhosis and vascular involvement favor HCC. The extrahepatic cholangiocarcinoma (*white arrow*) in **Fig. 68.2A** demonstrates a typically moderate to low SI appearance on GRE T1WI. The coronal T2WI in **Fig. 68.2B** localizes this lesion near the common bile duct (*white arrows*). **(C)** Thick-slab MRCP images, which suppress the mass's SI due to the long TE, allow better biliary visualization, specifically of the shoulder sign, a finding characterized by abrupt narrowing of the otherwise dilated common bile duct at the level of tumor. Ductal wall thickening (>5 mm) also suggests cholangiocarcinoma, with wall irregularity signifying infiltration. So-called Klatskin tumors occur at the confluence of the hepatic ducts. Primary sclerosing cholangitis, illustrated in **Figs. 68.3A,B**, is an important predisposing condition to cholangiocarcinoma. **(A)** Thick-slab MRCP images demonstrate multifocal areas of stricture and dilatation within the intrahepatic biliary system. Fibrosis of peripheral ducts lends a pruned appearance to the intrahepatic biliary tree. Characteristic periportal inflammation and edema appear as high SI on T2WI (**Fig. 68.3B**), whereas thickened, enhancing ductal walls may be seen on contrast-enhanced T1WI. Focal wedge-shaped regions of hepatic parenchymal hyperintensity may arise secondary to edema and inflammation. Similar involvement exclusive to the intrahepatic biliary system suggests primary biliary cirrhosis with hepatic cirrhosis mimicking both diagnoses. Parenchymal and wall findings are similar with infectious cholangitis but biliary dilatation is more diffuse with abscesses often present.

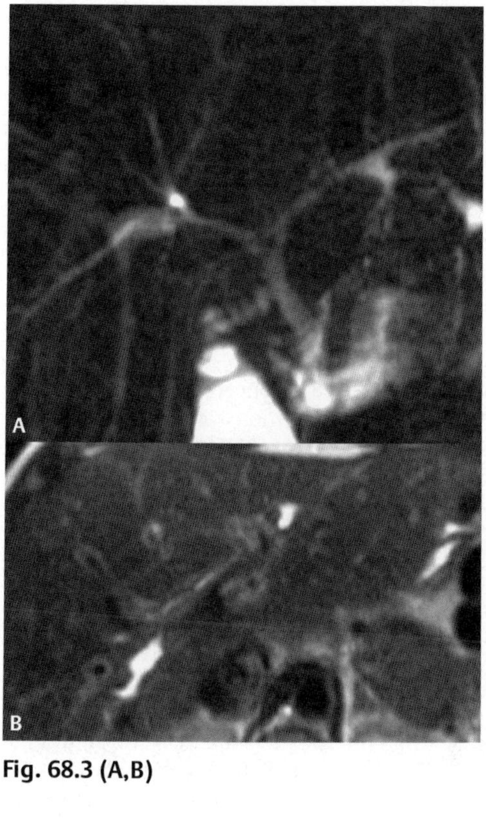

Fig. 68.3 (A,B)

69 Adrenal Disease

MRI is useful in localizing and characterizing masses of the adrenal gland due to its ability to detect fat content of a lesion. Like spectral fat suppression techniques, in- and out-of-phase GRE T1WI sequences exploit differential resonance frequencies of fat and water protons. Within a given voxel immediately following an initial RF excitation pulse (i.e., the factor enabling T1 and T2 relaxation) both lipid and water protons are in phase. Due to their differing resonance frequencies, however, the relative phases of water and fat protons begin to immediately change. TE can thus be selected such that water and fat protons are completely in- or out-of-phase with each other. In the latter case, SI from such protons cancel, manifesting as low SI on out-of-phase images. Voxels solely possessing water or fat protons, however, appear relatively unchanged on out-of-phase images. In practice, in- and out-of-phase images are typically obtained as part of a double-echo sequence, an approach for which clinical utility rests on the selection of a relatively short TE for out-of-phase images: GRE is sensitive to T2* effects, which will be more pronounced at longer TEs. Thus, losses in SI from T2* decay may masquerade as SI dropout from fat on out-of-phase images obtained with a long TE.

Figures 69.1A and 69.1B illustrate a homogeneous left adrenal lesion on in- and out-of-phase GRE T1WI, respectively. On the former, the lesion is isointense to the liver. Lesion SI decreases significantly on **(B)** out-of-phase GRE T1WI owing to SI dropout—due to the presence of fat and water within the same voxel as described above. These features are characteristic of a benign adrenal adenoma. Out-of-phase images are identifiable by the prominent outlining of masses or organs at their interface with fat by a thin artificial low signal intensity line ("etching" artifact). This is appreciable in the out-of-phase GRE T1WI of **Fig. 69.1B** at the medial edge of the liver. On FSE T2WI fatty adrenal adenomas may appear hyper- or isointense to the liver; enhancement is less prominent than that of more ominous lesions, often washing out rapidly on dynamic contrast-enhanced imaging. Nonfatty adenomas represent a diagnostic conundrum, the solution to which may be provided by delayed enhanced CT or confirmation of stability on follow-up imaging. Adrenal myelolipomas are slow-growing, benign masses characteristically possessing macroscopic fat, the presence of which is better detected by SI dropout on FS T1WI than on out-of-phase imaging. This is illustrated in the T1 and FS T1WI of **Figs. 69.2A,B**, respectively, with focal areas of fat suppressed within the adrenal lesion in the latter sequence.

Lesions lacking SI dropout on out-of-phase images are concerning for malignancy. A characteristic-appearing adrenocortical carcinoma is demonstrated in **Fig. 69.3**: a large, heterogeneous, partially hypointense mass is seen on **(A)** T1WI. Opposed phase images (not shown) showed no significant SI dropout. **(B)** Contrast-enhanced FS T1WI demonstrates diffuse, heterogeneous enhancement, consistent with malignant degeneration. The tumor illustrated in **Fig. 69.3** also exhibited delayed contrast washout—another characteristic of adrenal carcinoma. MRI accurately detects the spread of adrenal carcinoma to the inferior vena cava, demonstrating loss in the normal flow voids of that structure on FSE imaging. The adrenal gland is overall the fourth most common

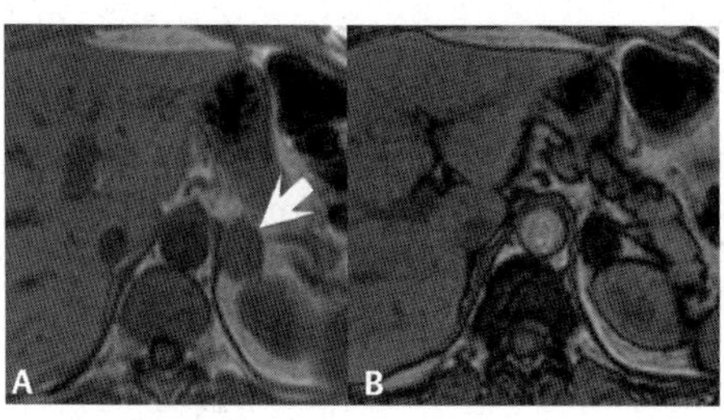

Fig. 69.1 (A,B)

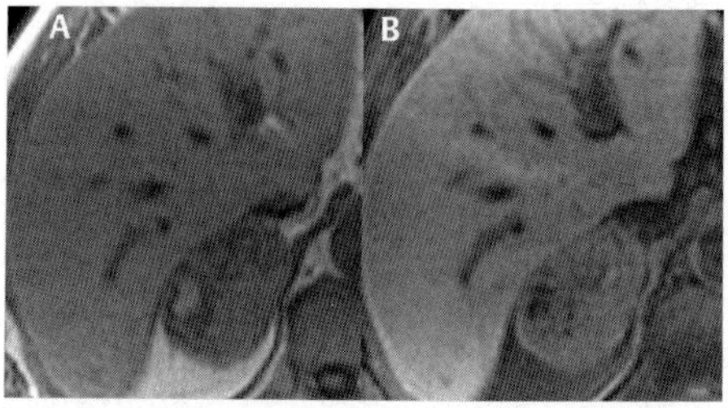

Fig. 69.2 (A,B)

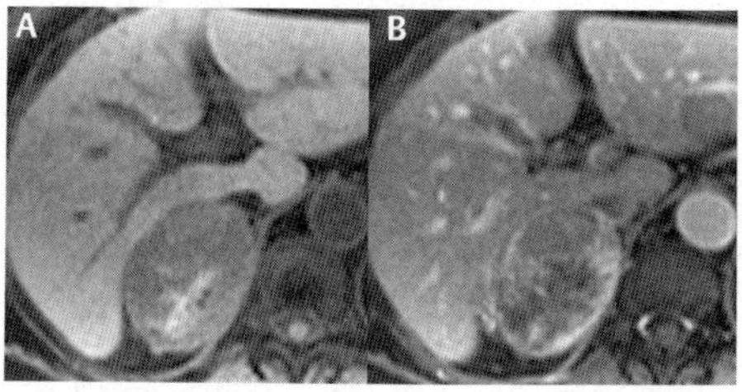

Fig. 69.3 (A,B)

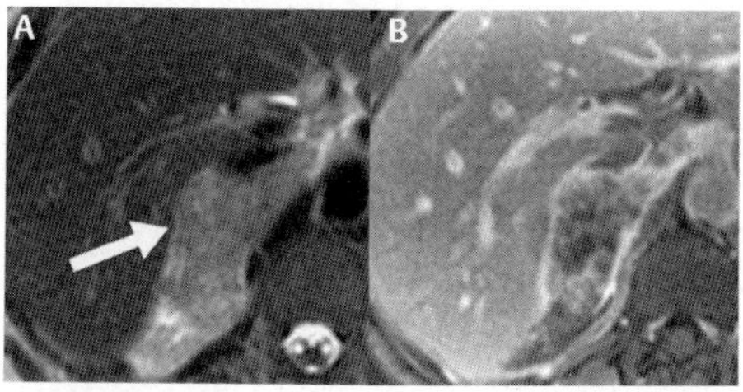

Fig. 69.4 (A,B)

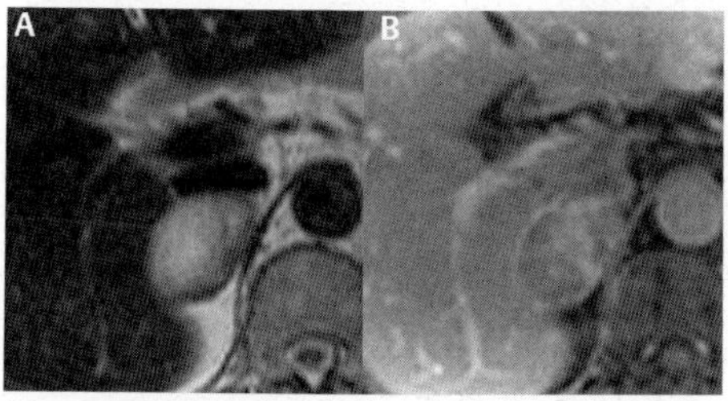

Fig. 69.5 (A,B)

site of metastatic disease. Other than those of clear cell renal carcinoma, adrenal metastases are typified by a lack of SI dropout on out-of-phase GRE T1WI. **Figure 69.4** demonstrates the typical appearance of a metastasis, revealing a large, heterogeneous adrenal mass (*white arrow*) on **(A)** T2WI. **(B)** Contrast-enhanced FS T1WI show heterogeneous lesion enhancement with irregular, enhancing margins. Pheochromocytomas are potentially malignant tumors for which MRI is both sensitive and relatively specific for diagnosis. These medullary tumors are devoid of fat, exhibiting classically, due to high water content, marked hyperintensity on T2WI. This is shown in the T2WI of **Fig. 69.5A**. Simple adrenal cysts may demonstrate higher SI than pheochromocytomas on T2WI, the distinction lying in the early, bright CE with delayed washout seen in the latter. The enhancement of the lesion illustrated in the FS T1WI of **Fig. 69.5B** is less typical, being heterogeneous in nature. Ten percent of pheochromocytomas are bilateral and the same percentage calcify—the latter feature better detected with CT. Tuberculosis, also often bilateral, is a further differential concern, along with histiocytosis, both of which may appear as cystic or rim-enhancing masses. Adrenal hemorrhage demonstrates SI characteristics varying with the stage of the hemorrhagic blood products. GRE images are especially sensitive to the detection of hemorrhage. A large adrenal hematoma may present as a mass-like lesion, although hematomas will usually resolve over time, not enhance, and possibly develop into a pseudocyst over time. Considerations for an adrenal mass in a pediatric patient are described in Chapter 72.

70 Renal Masses

MRI of the normal kidneys clearly differentiates between the cortex and medulla, the latter exhibiting fluid-like SI due to the presence of urine. Cortical enhancement occurs at 20 to 30 seconds following contrast injection with uniform medullary and cortical enhancement at 80 seconds—the time at which masses are most sensitively detected. Simple renal cysts are the most common lesions in adults. A case of adult polycystic kidney disease is illustrated in **Figs. 70.1A,B**. Cysts of varying complexity are present, but the lesion denoted by the *black arrow* appears simple with typical low and high SI on **(A)** T1 and **(B)** T2WI, respectively, and no clearly identifiable wall or septation. The lesion denoted by the *asterisk* demonstrates SI compatible with a hemorrhagic cyst—high SI on **(A)** T1 and low SI on **(B)** T2WI—specifically the SI characteristics of intracellular methemoglobin. The vertebral body SI in the above figures is abnormal as these sequences were not acquired with fat saturation. The low SI correlates with the patient's diagnosis of hemosiderosis (see Chapter 67). Simple cysts do not exhibit enhancement with contrast administration and are classified as Bosniak type I lesions. A Bosniak 2 cyst is illustrated in the **(A)** axial T2 and **(B)** contrast-enhanced T1WI of **Figs. 70.2A,B,** respectively. The **(A)** T2WI demonstrates a single, thin low SI septation that enhances minimally on **(B)** contrast-enhanced images. Bosniak 2F cysts have multiple, thin septae or smooth, minimal wall thickening and require follow-up. The septum of the lesion in **Figs. 70.2C,D**—a Bosniak 3 lesion—is thickened and somewhat irregular on **(C)** precontrast T1WI, findings confirmed on **(D)** parenchymal-phase contrast-enhanced T1WI. Irregularly thickened, enhancing walls also constitute Bosniak 3 lesions, which are by definition not characterizable as benign or malignant on MRI. Bosniak 4 lesions are cystic renal cell carcinomas. Such a lesion is illustrated in **Figs. 70.2E,F**, the cystic component appearing as low SI on **(E)** T1WI. **(F)** Three minutes following contrast administration, the thickened irregular rim of this cyst avidly enhances along with a nodule in the adjacent kidney. A solid renal cell carcinoma is illustrated in **Fig. 70.3**. Here **(A)** a coronal T2WI illustrates dilatation of the superior renal collecting system by a moderate to low SI mass arising from the lower renal pole. The mass demonstrates heterogeneous enhancement on **(B)** 5-minute postcontrast FS T1WI. This particular lesion extended to invade the renal vein and inferior vena cava, establishing a Robson stage of 3A. Other stage 3 lesions may involve regional lymph

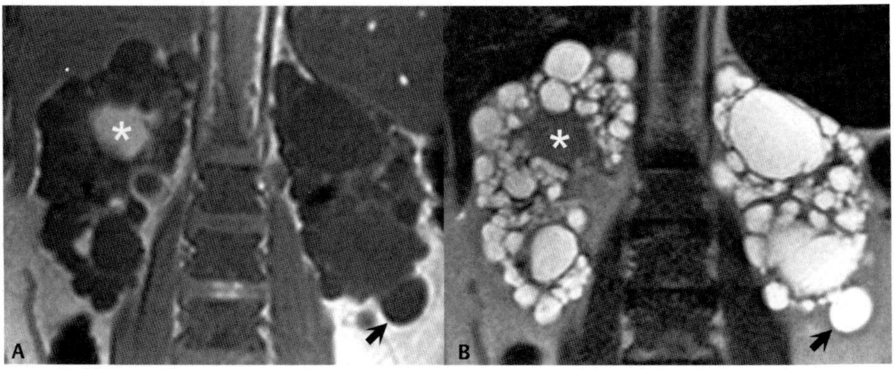

Fig. 70.1 (A,B)

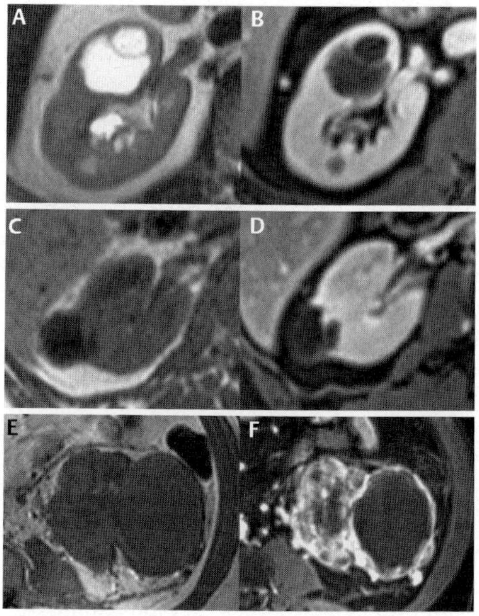

Fig. 70.2 (A–F)

nodes (stage 3B) or both the aforementioned venous structures and lymph nodes (stage 3C). Lesions not extending beyond the renal capsule or Gerota fascia are classified as stage 1 and 2 lesions, respectively. Local visceral invasion (with the exception of ipsilateral adrenal invasion) or distant metastases constitute a stage 4 lesion. The presence of a pseudocapsule, appearing as a hypointense linear band surrounding tumor on both T1WI and T2WI, signifies a lack of perinephric fat invasion. Benign renal oncocytoma may be confused with renal cell carcinoma; the two are not readily distinguishable on imaging. Oncocytomas are better defined and enhance more homogeneously, often with a central nonenhancing stellate scar. If an oncocytoma is favored in the differential diagnosis, nephron-sparing surgery may be performed. Renal angiomyolipomas, illustrated in **Fig. 70.4** are commonly encountered benign renal masses. **(A)** Coronal T2WI demonstrates a hyperintense mass near the inferior pole of the right kidney. Linear areas of low SI likely correlate with flow voids from contained vascular structures. On **(B)** axial T1WI the lesion demonstrates SI similar to that of perinephric fat, with loss of SI on **(C)** axial FS T2WI. **(D)** Contrast-enhanced FS T1WI demonstrate the lesion to remain low SI, with only linear, likely vascular enhancement. Clear and papillary cell renal carcinoma may also contain small amounts of fat, complicating the diagnosis.

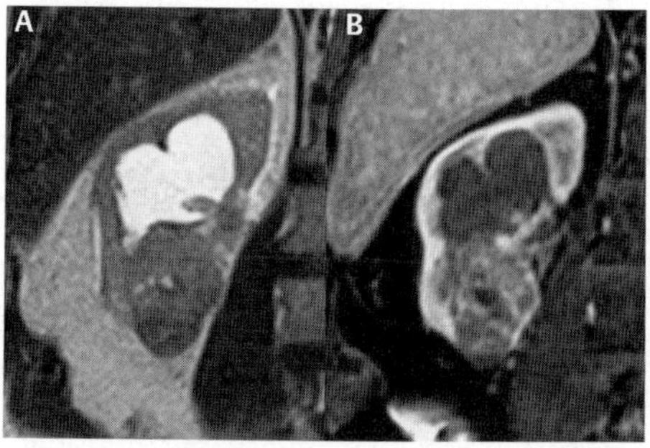

Fig. 70.3 (A,B)

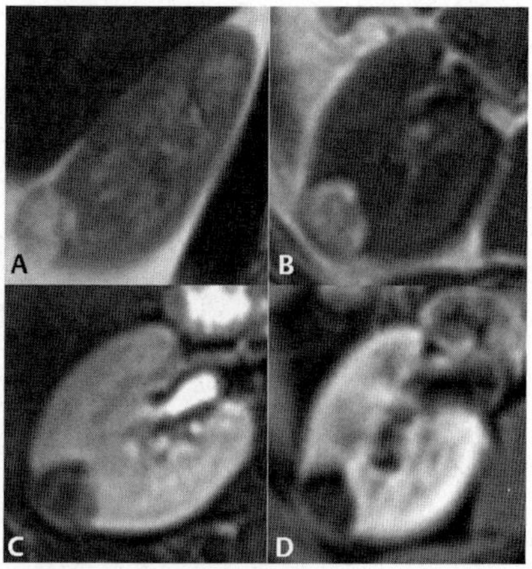

Fig. 70.4 (A–D)

71 Pancreatic Disease

Fat saturation is important to improve the differentiation between pancreatic parenchyma and peripancreatic fat, both of which demonstrate high SI on conventional T1WI, the former due to aqueous proteins within acinar cells. Contrast-enhanced T1WI is also performed with FS, the normal pancreas exhibiting enhancement peaking in the arterial phase and fading thereafter. Pancreatic adenocarcinoma is hypointense to parenchyma on such images. Carcinomas with prominent fibrous components, however, will demonstrate progressive enhancement, appearing hyperintense to parenchyma on delayed imaging. The pancreatic head mass (*white arrow*) in the region of the ampulla illustrated in the axial images of **Figs. 71.1A,B** demonstrates moderate to low SI on both **(A)** T2WI and **(B)** T1WI. This mass obstructs the confluence of the common bile and pancreatic ducts, resulting in dilatation of both structures—the so-called double-duct sign—best seen in the thick-slab MRCP image of **Fig. 71.1C**. Pancreatic adenocarcinoma and focal, chronic pancreatitis may appear similar. Chronic pancreatitis is less well defined, enhances in the early hepatic venous phase relative to the parenchyma, and is more hyperintense on T2WI due to prominent edema. Pancreatic carcinoma is favored by the presence of lymphadenopathy, distant metastases, or vascular encasement. Optimal sequences for detection of lymphadenopathy vary based on nodal location. Interstitial-phase contrast-enhanced FS T1WI are generally helpful, but porta hepatis nodes are better seen against the background liver on T2WI. Mesenteric and retroperitoneal nodes are well detected against abundant surrounding fat on T1WI. Pancreatic carcinoma metastatic to the liver exhibits an MRI appearance similar to that of colorectal metastases and other adenocarcinomas (See Chapter 66).

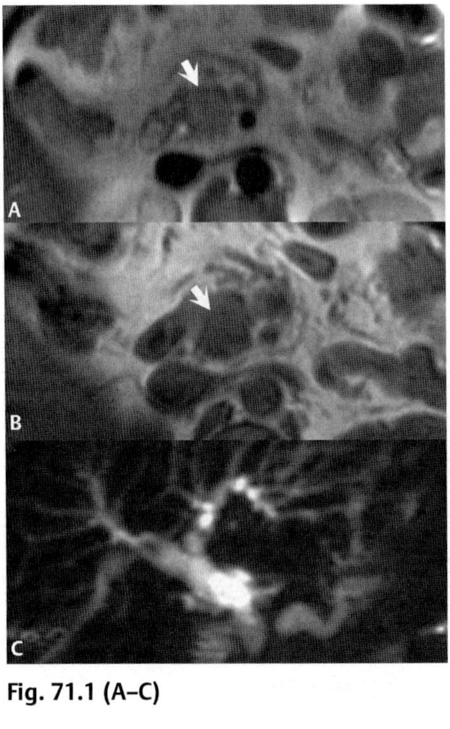

Fig. 71.1 (A–C)

Rarer endocrine neoplasms (i.e., gastrinoma, insulinoma, carcinoid) demonstrate moderately high and low SI on T2 and T1WI, respectively, with homogeneous arterial-phase enhancement on contrast-enhanced T1WI. Ductal and vascular involvement is rare. Cystic neoplasms are of benign serous and malignant mucinous types. Serous cystadenomas exhibit multiple fluid-like SI cysts on T2WI. Occasional low SI septations often demonstrate mild enhancement. These characteristics are also seen in mucinous cystadenomas and cystadenocarcinomas—essentially indistinguishable by MRI—which typically involve the pancreatic body and tail. Larger cysts and high SI on both T1WI—due to mucinous content—and T2WI favor these lesions over typically benign serous tumors. Mucinous metastases avidly enhance on arterial-phase imaging. Intraductal papillary mucinous neoplasms may involve the main pancreatic duct or its branches and appear similar to other cystic tumors except for their communication with the pancreatic duct. Ductal dilatation may be seen secondary to copious mucin production.

Inflammatory pancreatic disease and peripancreatic fluid collections are best visualized on FS or STIR T2WI as high SI edema stands out against suppressed peripancreatic fat on such images. The peripancreatic fluid collection (*white arrows*) anterior to the pancreatic head in **Fig. 71.2A** demonstrates low SI on axial **(A)** T1WI. Peripancreatic fat stranding is also present. High SI areas on **(B)** T2WI correspond to the fluid collection although hyperintensity also involves the pancreatic head. The peripancreatic fluid collection shown here lacks a definable, progressively enhancing wall on **(C)** contrast-enhanced T1WI and is thus not likely to represent a true pseudocyst. Heterogeneous pancreatic enhancement on contrast-enhanced images is characteristic of pancreatitis as shown on the illustrated **(C)** early venous-phase contrast-enhanced T1WI. Contrast-enhanced imaging may be useful in the detection of necrotic areas, which do not enhance on such images. Hemorrhagic pancreatitis, another potential complication, appears as high SI on FS T1WI. The characteristic MRI appearance of chronic pancreatitis relates to the pathophysiology of the condition: chronic, progressive pancreatic inflammation results in acinar atrophy, leading to diminished overall gland size and a reduction in SI on T1WI due to the reduced presence of aqueous proteins within the acini. Associated chronic fibrosis leads to a pattern of gradual enhancement that peaks in the venous phase. The typical appearance of chronic pancreatitis on T1WI is illustrated in **Fig. 71.2D** wherein pancreatic SI is distinctly lower than that in **Fig. 71.2A**. Atrophy is present, manifested in part by the markedly dilated pancreatic duct (*white arrows*). On the T2 and thick slab MRCP images of **Figs. 71.2E,F**, respectively, a dilated pancreatic duct is again present, demonstrating numerous tiny outpouchings on the latter image. Findings of chronic pancreatitis on MRCP are graded via the Cambridge criteria: a normal appearance is Cambridge 1, whereas dilatation in fewer than three side branches is equivocal for pancreatitis (Cambridge 2). Mild chronic pancreatitis (Cambridge 3) consists of dilatation or obstruction in more than three side branches, moderate pancreatitis (Cambridge 4) of main pancreatic duct dilatation and stenosis, and severe pancreatitis (Cambridge 5) of main duct stenosis with concurrent cysts and ductal calculi. Secretin-enhanced MRI—leading to increased ductal dilatation—may aid in assessment of such criteria.

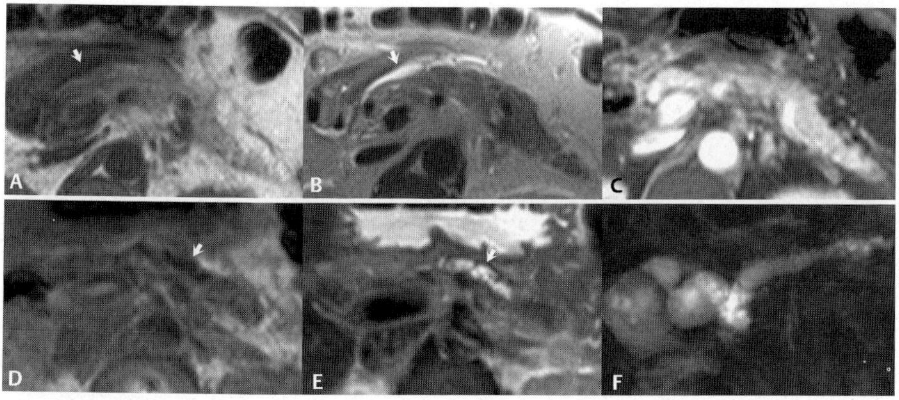

Fig. 71.2 (A–F)

72 Pediatric Abdominal Disease

MRI of the pediatric abdomen poses several challenges: in younger patients (<6 years old), it is difficult to appropriately minimize voluntary patient motion. As such, conscious sedation may be necessary. Persistent physiologic motion due to respiration and bowel peristalsis may be minimized by utilization of sequences with short acquisition times, possibly to the detriment of image quality, or employing motion robust imaging techniques such as PROPELLER (periodically rotated overlapping parallel lines with enhanced reconstruction). Pediatric abdominal masses most commonly involve the kidney with nephroblastoma (Wilms tumor) being the most common, often appearing as a large heterogeneously hyperintense and hypointense mass on T2WI and T1WI, respectively. Inhomogeneity on T2WI may result from hemorrhagic, cystic, or necrotic foci, the latter identifiable by a lack of contrast enhancement. **Figure 72.1A** illustrates contrast-enhanced FS T1WI of a large, somewhat homogeneously enhancing nephroblastoma. Because normal retroperitoneal lymph nodes are not commonly visible in children, the presence of such nodes, which often enhance and demonstrate increased SI on T2WI, is suspicious for metastases. Infiltration of the perirenal fat or renal veins is an important determination, the latter manifesting as loss of normal vascular flow voids on FSE imaging or as luminal hypointensity on GRE images. MRV may further delineate such spread if invasion is questioned, as this finding may alter the surgical approach. The true origin of a retroperitoneal mass in a child may be difficult to delineate: a neuroblastoma arising from the adrenal medulla or paraspinal sympathetic chain may appear similar. A neuroblastoma is shown on the T2WI of **Fig. 72.1B**. Unlike nephroblastomas, neuroblastomas are less well defined, encase the retroperitoneal vascular structures, extend posteriorly to the aorta, and calcify more frequently—a finding not well detected on MRI. Localization of lesion origin to the adrenal may be aided by the multiplanar capabilities of MRI. Extension to the midline is an important staging factor. More than half of neuroblastomas metastasize to bone—a more difficult finding to appreciate given the normal low marrow SI on T1WI in infants. Progressively more benign neurogenic tumors—ganglioneuroblastoma then ganglioneuromas—occur with advancing age, the former lesion illustrated in the coronal contrast-enhanced FS T1WI of **Fig. 72.2A** (*asterisk*). Such lesions do not encase vasculature like a neuroblastoma. The left kidney in **Fig. 72.2B** (contrast-enhanced FS T1WI) is affected by a mesoblastic nephroma (i.e., fetal renal hamartoma)—the most common solid renal tumor

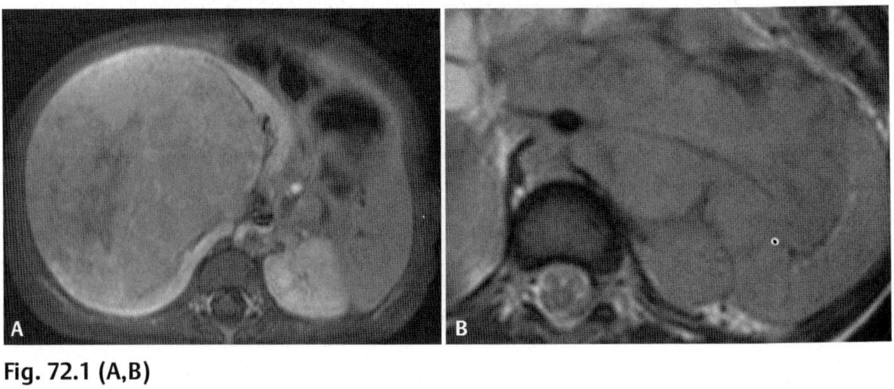

Fig. 72.1 (A,B)

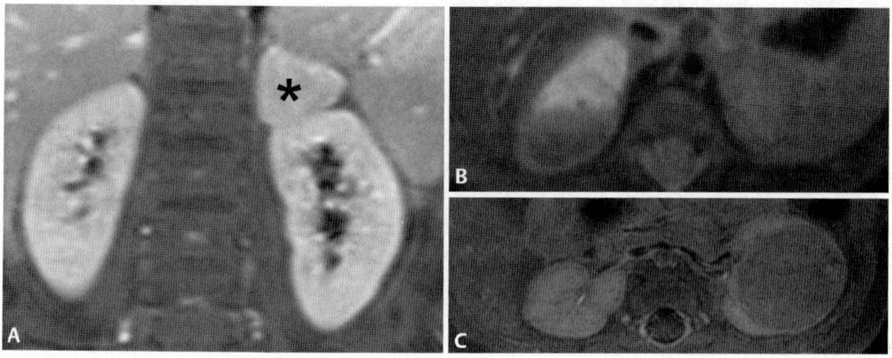

Fig. 72.2 (A–C)

in patients less than 6 months old. This lesion is benign with an MRI appearance essentially indistinguishable from that of a nephroblastoma. Such lesions may be hyperintense on T2WI despite their typically fibrous content and enhance variably. Metastases from lymphoma and leukemia may also involve the kidney. Nephroblastomatosis is the rare persistence of the fetal renal blastema that predisposes to nephroblastoma development, a lesion more likely to develop from central rather than peripheral (perilobar) lesions. These lesions often manifest as bilateral, oval-shaped entities with irregular hypointense foci on T1WI and contrast-enhanced T1WI and high SI on T2WI. Hemorrhage into the adrenal glands, often from birth trauma, may occasionally mimic a retroperitoneal neoplasm. In distinction to neoplasia, adrenal hemorrhages often preserve the triangular shape of the gland. SI characteristics of such hemorrhages vary depending on the stage of their contained blood products: the axial STIR T2WI image in **Fig. 72.2C** demonstrates hyperintensity consistent with the hemorrhage's subacute timeframe.

Hepatoblastomas and hepatocellular carcinoma, both malignant, constitute the major pediatric liver masses. The former—associated with Beckwith-Wiedemann, fetal alcohol, and Gardner syndromes—affects a younger population (~1 year old), whereas hepatocellular carcinoma typically affects children between 5 to 15 years old with hepatitis or congenital liver disease. These two entities appear similar on MRI, both preferentially involving the right hepatic lobe and occurring commonly as a solitary mass. The hepatoblastoma in the contrast-enhanced T1WI of **Fig. 72.3** exhibits this appearance. Early heterogeneous enhancement is typical and reflective of the contained fibrous structures that are more prominent in hepatoblastomas than in hepatocellular carcinoma. Assessment involvement of both nearby vascular structures and portal lymph nodes should be made. Prominent flow-voids are present in the hepatoblastoma of **Fig. 72.3**, a feature complicating its distinction from a hemangioendothelioma (infantile cavernous hemangioma). Enhancement patterns similar to those of adult hemangiomas typify the latter (see Chapter 65).

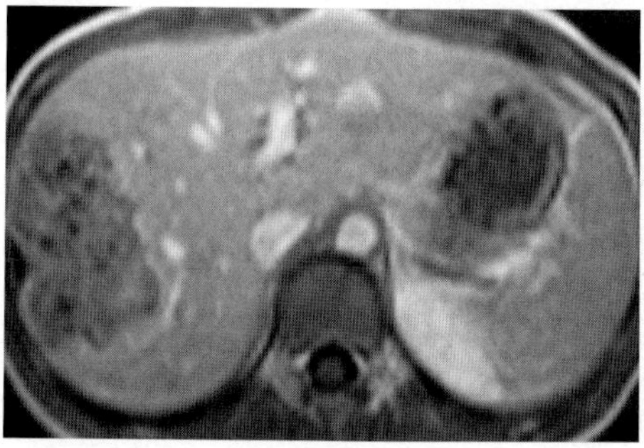

Fig. 72.3

73 Urinary Bladder and Male Pelvis

Urinary bladder carcinoma, a case of which is illustrated in **Fig. 73.1**, is best locally staged with MRI. **(A)** Sagittal FSE T2WI illustrate high SI urine, moderate SI bladder mucosa, low SI bladder musculature, and high SI perivesicular fat, the latter useful for delineating the bladder wall. A thickened wall (>5 mm) is a nonspecific finding seen in an underfilled bladder, acute cystitis, fibrosis, and infiltrative cancer. On **(B)** axial GRE T1WI low SI urine is surrounded by the moderate SI wall. T1WI readily detect superficial mucosal lesions as well as enlarged, low SI lymph nodes contained in perivesicular fat. Use of GRE T1WI, in addition to short acquisition times and adaptability to 3D acquisitions, allows distinction of nodes from high SI vascular structures. In **Fig. 73.1A**, an intermediate SI mass-like lesion interrupts the low SI of the muscular layer (*white arrow*); **(B)** T1WI demonstrates a moderate SI lesion involving the right bladder wall without infiltration of the surrounding fat. Carcinoma enhances earlier and more avidly than the normal wall. Delayed (>2 minutes) postcontrast image acquisition limits evaluation of the bladder wall due to urinary excretion of the administered gadolinium chelate. Cystitis enhances similarly, as opposed to the late enhancement seen with wall fibrosis. Bladder carcinoma is staged by the TNM (tumor, node, metastasis) system based on whether the tumor is superficial to the muscular layer (T1), invades the layer superficially (T2) or deeply (T2b), invades the perivesicular fat micro- (T3a) or macroscopically (T3b), or extends to adjacent organs (T4). An intact low SI muscular layer signifies a T1–T2 lesion on MRI, whereas T2b and T3a lesions (see **Fig. 73.1**) cannot be readily distinguished on MRI. Nodal evaluation by MRI is guided by size with accuracy comparable to CT, and staging based on whether a solitary lymph node measuring less than 2 cm in dimension is involved (N1), a single node between 2 to 5 cm or multiple nodes less than 5 cm are involved (N2), or nodal metastases greater than 5 cm are present (N3). Detection of distant metastases to bone (M1) is best identified, due to the high SI of the metastasis, on FS or STIR T2WI. The seminal vesicles are posterosuperior to the prostate, exhibiting loss of their normal hyperintense fluid SI on T2WI if involved with cancer. Seminal vesicle cysts, associated with urogenital abnormalities, are the most common congenital abnormality of the seminal vesicles.

MRI plays an evolving role in preoperative staging of prostate cancer and in assessing therapeutic response. At 1.5 T high resolution, imaging necessitates transrectal coil use, although improved SNR at 3 T may allow use of an overlying pelvic coil.

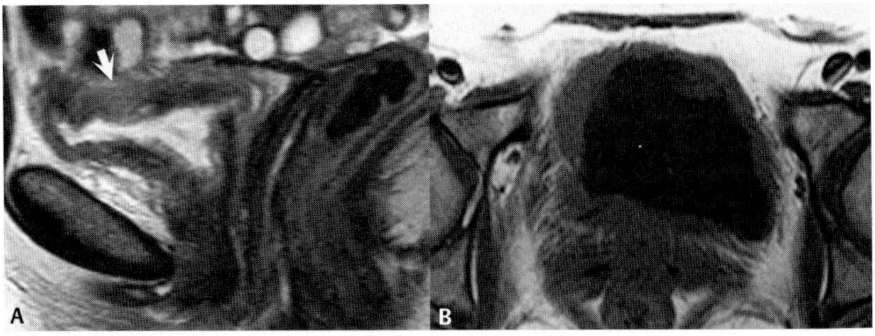

Fig. 73.1 (A,B)

The normal prostate appears homogeneous on T1WI, the majority of the gland (i.e., the peripheral 60%) appearing hyperintense on T2WI. Hyperintensity on T2WI correlates with predominance of fluid-filled acinar elements peripherally as opposed to smooth muscle elements in transitional and periurethral regions. **Figures 73.2A and 73.2B** illustrate a case of benign prostate hypertrophy, showing a symmetrically enlarged prostate on **(A)** axial T2WI with nodular enlargement of the central gland. On **(B)** contrast-enhanced T1WI such regions are hypointense to the otherwise heterogeneously enhancing gland. In distinction, prostate carcinoma may manifest as a hypointense lesion in the gland's periphery on T2WI, although this guideline is less reliable for the detection of higher SI mucinous tumors. The finding of capsular invasion is important for staging purposes. **Figure 73.2** illustrates on **(C)** FS T2WI and **(D)** contrast-enhanced FS T1WI a case of prostate carcinoma clearly invading the capsule (*white arrow*) and extending to the right pelvic side wall. A useful finding denoting extracapsular extension, illustrated in this case, is loss of the normal recto prostate angle—a normal angle denoted by the *asterisk* in **Fig. 73.2A**. Other suggestive findings on T2WI include irregular bulge of tissue beyond the low SI capsule, smooth capsular bulges, and neurovascular bundle asymmetry. Periurethral or transitional zone neoplasms are difficult to identify on T2WI. Furthermore, the classic finding of peripheral cancer on conventional MRI—a hypointense peripheral lesion—is nonspecific for prostate cancer occurring in hemorrhage, prostatitis, and prostate atrophy or fibrosis. Several MRI techniques may be combined to more accurately identify prostate cancer. DWI is useful both in initial detection of neoplasm and in assessing tumor recurrence postoperatively. Increased cellularity of prostatic neoplasia restricts the extent of Brownian water (proton) motion in the extracellular space, a condition manifest as high SI and low ADC values on DWI. Whole body DWI may eventually play a role in

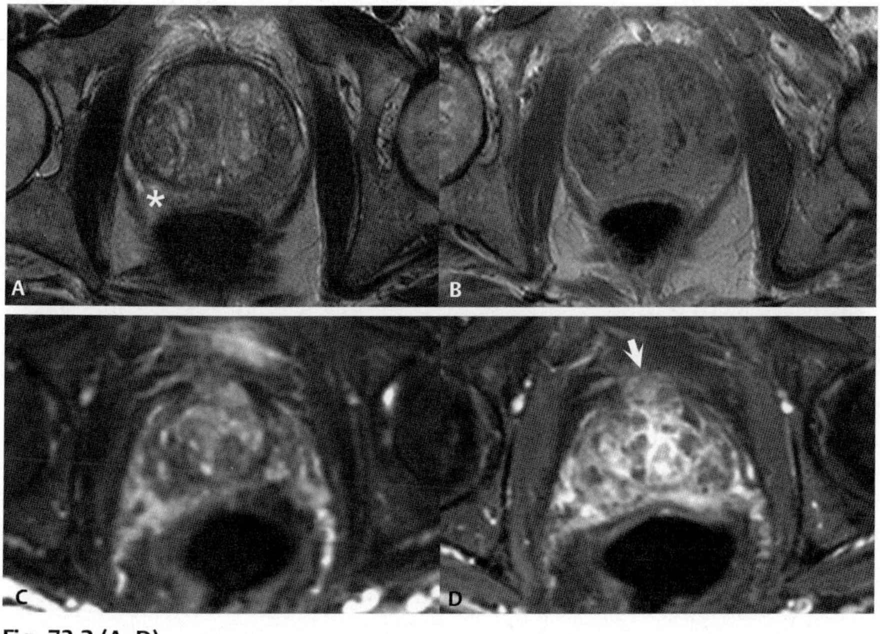

Fig. 73.2 (A–D)

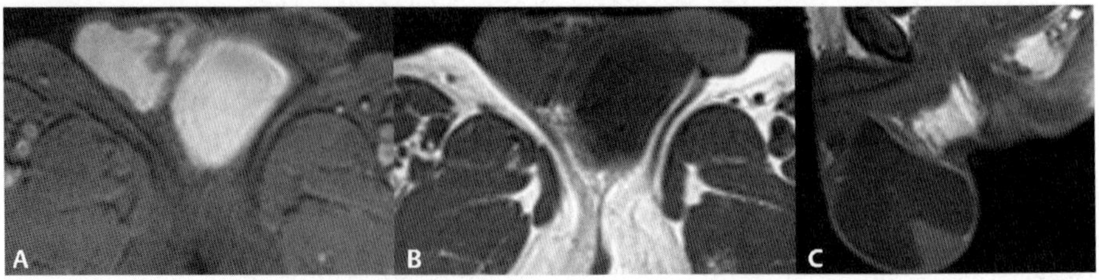

Fig. 73.3 (A–C)

detecting prostatic metastases. MRS findings of prostate cancer include increased choline + creatine to citrate ratios, although such alterations may also be seen with prostatitis or focal atrophy. Dynamic contrast-enhanced MRI—commonly used in breast imaging (see Chapter 63)—can be utilized to construct pharmacokinetic models of tissue gadolinium concentration, although semiquantitative approaches have been shown to be equally effective in identifying prostate malignancy. Enhancement patterns consistent with neoplasia include early enhancement onset, short time to peak, high levels of peak enhancement, and early washout of enhancement. The most discriminating parameter is derived from subtraction of peak enhancement values in the region of concern from that of adjacent peripheral or central glandular tissue, termed relative peak enhancement. A high relative peak enhancement is characteristic of prostate carcinoma.

Scrotal abnormalities are not uncommonly evaluated on MRI, with positioning important when using a surface coil to assure that side-to-side differences involving the testicles reflect pathology, not simply distance from the coil. The normal testes are intermediate SI between fluid and fat SI on T1WI, slightly hypointense to fluid on T2WI, and covered by a hypointense layer of fibrous tissue—the tunica albuginea. Bilateral hydroceles are illustrated in the **(A)** axial T2WI, **(B)** T1WI, and **(C)** sagittal T1WI of **Fig. 73.3**. The testes in these images are not clearly seen, but the hydroceles demonstrate the expected SI of **(A)** hyperintensity on T2WI and **(B,C)** hypointensity on T1WI. Testicular cysts are a commonly identified, fluid-like SI lesion on MRI. MRI characteristics of neoplastic testicular masses are dependent on tumor pathology with seminomas exhibiting homogeneous hypointensity on T2WI possibly with low SI fibrous bands, which enhance more than the remainder of the tumor. Nonseminomatous tumors are more heterogeneous both pre- and postcontrast. Acute testicular infarctions, as seen in the setting of torsion, likewise manifest as edema-like SI, with more chronic lesions appearing as low SI scar.

74 Benign Lesions of the Female Pelvis

Respiratory and bowel motion are minimal in pelvic imaging, but can degrade image quality if unaccounted for. Fasting should commence 4 to 6 hours prior to pelvic MRI. Administration of intramuscular glucagon may be helpful. Utilization of a compression band to restrict motion may decrease motion-induced artifact, as may respiratory gating, triggering, and utilization of navigator echoes. The bladder should be only moderately distended, in part to minimize truncation artifacts on T2WI. Positive or negative oral contrast is not routinely utilized in MRI in the United States. T2WI but not T1WI illustrate uterine junctional anatomy, distinguishing among the endometrium—high SI due to glandular tissue—junctional zone—hypointense muscular structures—and the myometrium—a moderate SI structure on T2WI during the proliferative phase but hyperintense during the secretory phase due to increased edema and vascular flow.

Embryologically, two Müllerian ducts fuse to form the upper vagina, cervix, uterus, and fallopian tubes. Cysts arising from this fusion are similar in MRI appearance and are named by location: nabothian cysts in the cervix; Bartholin gland cysts in the posterolateral vulvovaginal vestibular glands inferior to the pelvic diaphragm; and Gartner cysts, associated with congenital genitourinary abnormalities, above the diaphragm in the anterolateral vagina. **Figure 74.1** demonstrates the characteristic appearance of a Bartholin cyst—that is, low SI on **(A)** axial T1WI and high SI on **(B)** axial and **(C)** coronal FS T2WI. Cyst SI varies depending on content, and walls of noninfected cysts do not enhance. Congenital defects in Müllerian duct fusion are reliably characterized on MRI. Class 1 lesions consist of Müllerian hypoplasia or agenesis. The uterus, if present, appears as a low SI structure on T2WI. A unicornuate uterus (class 2) results from unilateral Müllerian duct hypoplasia, the formed uterus appearing as a low volume, off-midline structure. The contralateral horn, if not aplastic, is either cavitary—with approximate preservation of junctional anatomy—or noncavitary—with asymmetric low SI thickening on T2WI. The (**A**) axial T2WI of **Fig. 74.2** illustrates uterus didelphys (class 3)—a fusion abnormality resulting in two normal-sized uteri and cervices with a myometrial septum at the upper vagina. Junctional anatomy, as in **Fig. 74.2A**, is typically preserved. In this particular case, the uterine fundi lie opposite one another; an endometrioma (*asterisk*) is incidentally present within the left ovary. A bicornate uterus (class 4)—with preserved junctional anatomy and partially duplicated uterine fundi that merge eventually more caudally—is illustrated in axial T2WI of **Fig. 74.2B**. A septate uterus (class 5) represents failure of resorption of the fibrous septum between otherwise fused Müllerian ducts. An arcuate uterus (class 6) may represent an anatomic variant and is illustrated in the **(A)** sagittal and **(B)** axial T2WI

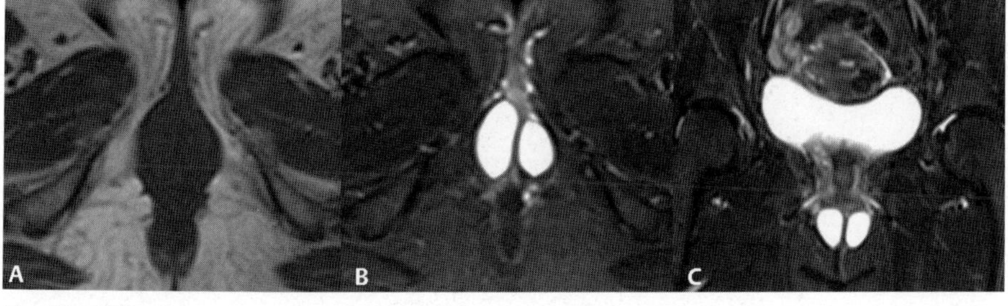

Fig. 74.1 (A–C)

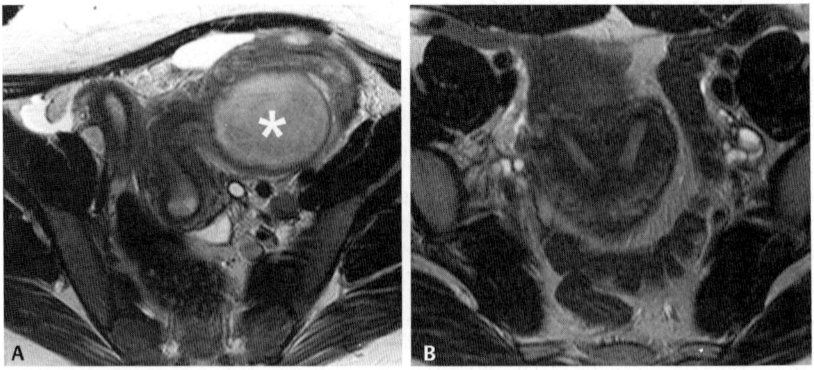

Fig. 74.2 (A,B)

of **Fig. 74.3**. Here, no low SI fibrous component is present, only midline thickening of the fundal endometrium with indentation into the fundal cavity in a uterus with otherwise normal contour. T-shaped uteri from in utero exposure to diethylstilbestrol constitute class 7 abnormalities.

Leiomyomas are optimally evaluated on T2WI, as in **Fig. 74.4A** where multiple heterogeneous lesions are present. The fundal lesion (*white arrow*) is characteristic in appearance—a well-defined, mass hypointense to myometrium on T2WI. Hypointensity correlates with predominant smooth muscle and fibrous content. The lesion is distinct due to its surrounding pseudocapsule of compressed myometrium. On **(B)** contrast-enhanced T1WI, the leiomyomas all appear well-demarcated but with diminished enhancement compared with the normal uterus. Leiomyoma enhancement does vary, with hypervascularity correlating to favorable outcomes with uterine artery embolization. Foci of hyperintensity on T2WI, evident in the largest leiomyoma in **Fig. 74.4** (*asterisk*), are nonspecific correlating with hyaline, fatty, cystic, hemorrhagic, mucinous, and myxomatous degeneration. Hemorrhagic degeneration is, however, reliably identified by hyperintensity on T1WI and a lack of contrast enhancement—characteristics foretelling a poor outcome with uterine artery embolization. Cellular leiomyomas may also appear hyperintense on T2WI, and exhibit avid contrast enhancement. Differential

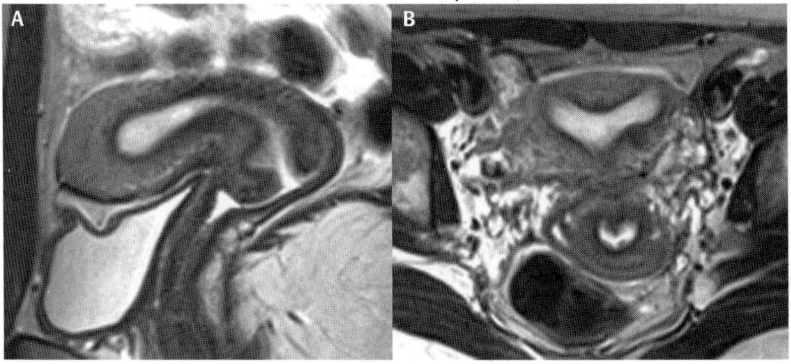

Fig. 74.3 (A,B)

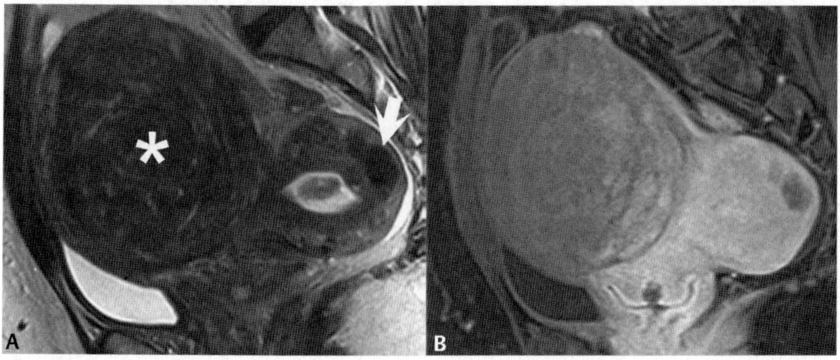

Fig. 74.4 (A,B)

considerations for leiomyomas vary by lesion location: subserosal lesions may be confused with ovarian fibroids, both lesions being benign; myometrial contractions may also appear as myometrial hypointensity presumably due to decreased perfusion within contracting tissue. Such contractions deform the endometrium, sparing the uterine contour. Transience is their most characteristic feature. Rare leiomyosarcomas are not reliably distinguished from benign leiomyomas but have less-distinct borders, their distinguishing feature being sudden enlargement on serial imaging. Focal adenomyosis is the major differential consideration for an intramural leiomyoma. **Figure 74.5** illustrates a typical appearance of an adenomyoma on **(A)** sagittal and **(B)** axial FS T2WI. The lesion (*white arrows*) appears as ill-defined thickening (> 8 mm) of the junctional zone on both images, the hypointensity correlating with smooth muscle hyperplasia. The lack of endometrial mass effect and **(B)** hyperintense foci and striations—potentially representing hemorrhage or ectopic endometrium—leading from the endo to the myometrium are also characteristic. Adenomyosis may also appear as interspersed foci of hyperintensity corresponding to ectopic endometrium. Foci of hemorrhage may appear bright on T1WI. On contrast-enhanced T1WI, an adenomyoma may enhance less rapidly than the normal myometrium and take-on a so-called Swiss cheese appearance due to the lack of enhancement of ectopic endometrial glands.

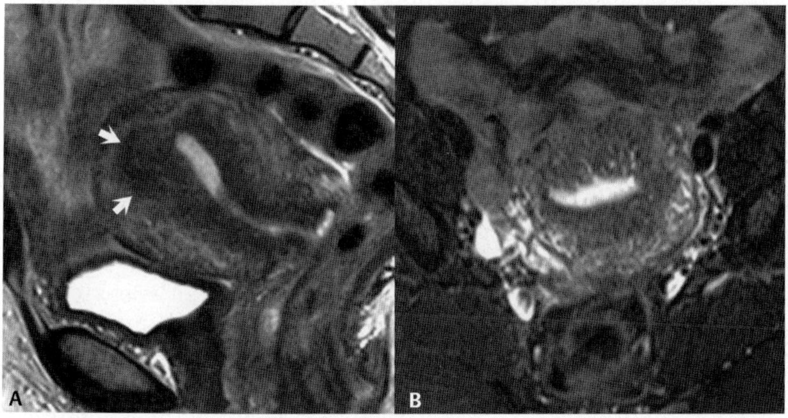

Fig. 74.5 (A,B)

75 Uterine and Cervical Cancer

Endometrial carcinoma is predisposed by the development of endometrial hyperplasia and polyps, MRI being of little utility in distinguishing benign and malignant varieties of the latter. Both benign and malignant polyps are of variable SI, the latter identifiable only by myometrial invasion. Submucosal fibroids may appear similar but arise from the myometrium and display uniformly low SI unless degenerative. MRI may be performed if ultrasonographic evaluation of endometrial hyperplasia is not possible. Normal myometrial thickness is less than 5 mm in postmenopausal women and 8 mm in the proliferative (16 mm secretory) phase of premenopausal women. Cystically dilated high SI glandular structures on T2WI are often present in hyperplastic endometrium and do not typically enhance. Findings of endometrial hyperplasia are indistinguishable from those of endometrial carcinoma on MRI with only myometrial invasion proving the latter—the most common invasive carcinoma of the female genital tract. Treatment is guided by grade, but early staging is performed with MRI due to accurate depiction of zonal anatomy on T2WI. Stage 1A lesions, as in **Fig. 75.1**, are manifest as endometrial thickening without junctional zone disruption. On **(A)** coronal T2WI, a low SI lesion (*white arrow*) involves the right side of the endometrium. A hypointense lesion is present on **(B)** axial T1WI without depiction of the zonal anatomy. The junctional zone, disrupted in 1B lesions, in the **(A)** T2WI is clearly intact, thus establishing the stage as 1A. If distinction between the junctional zone and myometrium is poor, as in adenomyosis or postmenopausal patients, contrast-enhanced T1WI aids in diagnosis by depicting areas of absent early-phase myometrial enhancement, corresponding with endome-trial carcinoma. Axial contrast-enhanced T1WI in **Fig. 75.1C** exhibits intact hyperintense myometrium with the hypointense carcinoma (*black arrow*) confined to the endometrium. On delayed images, such tumors appear hyperintense to myometrium, similar to fibroids. The distinction between stage 1B and 1C disease is crucial, the latter correlating with a high probability of extrauterine and lymphatic disease. MRI reliably identifies stage 1C lesions, confined to but involving greater than one half of the myometrium, by their complete disruption of the junctional zone. MRI similarly depicts involvement of the endocervical canal (2A) or cervical stroma (2B). The former manifests as endocervical canal widening, whereas the low SI of the normal stromal ring is interrupted in the latter. On contrast-enhanced T1WI stage 2B lesions manifest as a hypointense lesion in the stroma. True invasion of the endocervical canal rather than mere extent of a polypoid lesion must be demonstrated. Invasion of the parametrial fat constitutes a stage

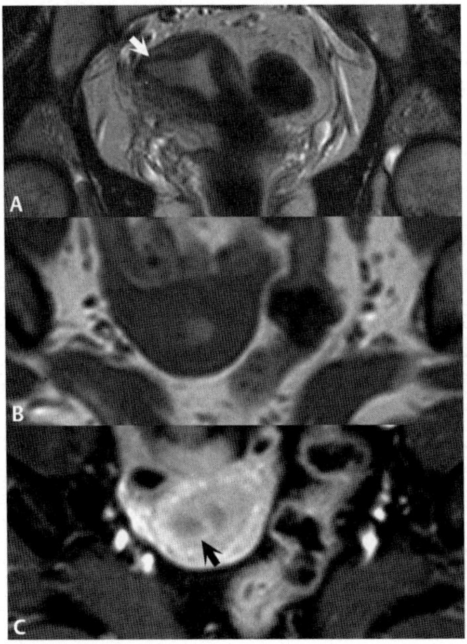

Fig. 75.1 (A–C)

2B lesion or higher. In the absence of rectal mucosal or bladder wall involvement stage 3 lesions involve the uterus, adnexa, or peritoneum (3A), the vagina (3B), or paraaortic or pelvic lymph nodes (3C). Urinary bladder wall and rectal mucosal invasion constitute stage 4A lesions; distant metastases or involvement of other lymph nodes indicate 4B disease. Nodal involvement is best detected on precontrast T1WI as lymph nodes measuring greater than 1 cm in short axis diameter.

MRI is preferred for the staging of cervical carcinoma. Stage 0 or carcinoma in situ is not reliably detected, whereas stage 1A lesions, seen on T2WI as hyperintensity against the low SI cervical stroma, are well seen as microinvasive lesions confined to the cervix. Stage 1B lesions, as in **Fig. 75.2A**, are greater than 5 mm in depth or 7 mm in transverse extent. (**A**) Sagittal T2WI illustrate the intact, low SI stroma of the anterior cervical labium interrupted only by a high SI Gardner cyst. The low SI of the posterior labium is replaced by hyperintense mass without containing low SI stromal capsule. The carcinoma in **Fig. 75.2B** is a stage 2A lesion, involving the upper two-thirds but not the lower third (i.e., stage 3A) of the ventral vaginal wall (*white arrow*). Parametrial invasion, reflected by hyperintensity on T2WI constitutes a stage 2B lesion, whereas pelvic sidewall invasion signifies a stage 3B lesion. Postradio chemotherapeutic edema can masquerade as tumor involvement of these structures in its hyperintensity on T2WI. Distant metastases or involvement of the rectal or bladder mucosa constitute stage 4 lesions. The latter case is illustrated in the sagittal T2WI of **Fig. 75.2C** with heterogeneously hyperintense cervical tumor infiltrating the upper third of the vagina and interrupting the low SI bladder wall (*white arrow*). A similar appearance is present on the axial contrast-enhanced T1WI of **Fig. 75.2D,** where the irregularly enhancing tumor protrudes into the bladder wall. Contrast enhancement of cervical cancer is variable, but contrast-enhanced T1WI may greatly aid in evaluating the extent of an invasive cervical carcinoma.

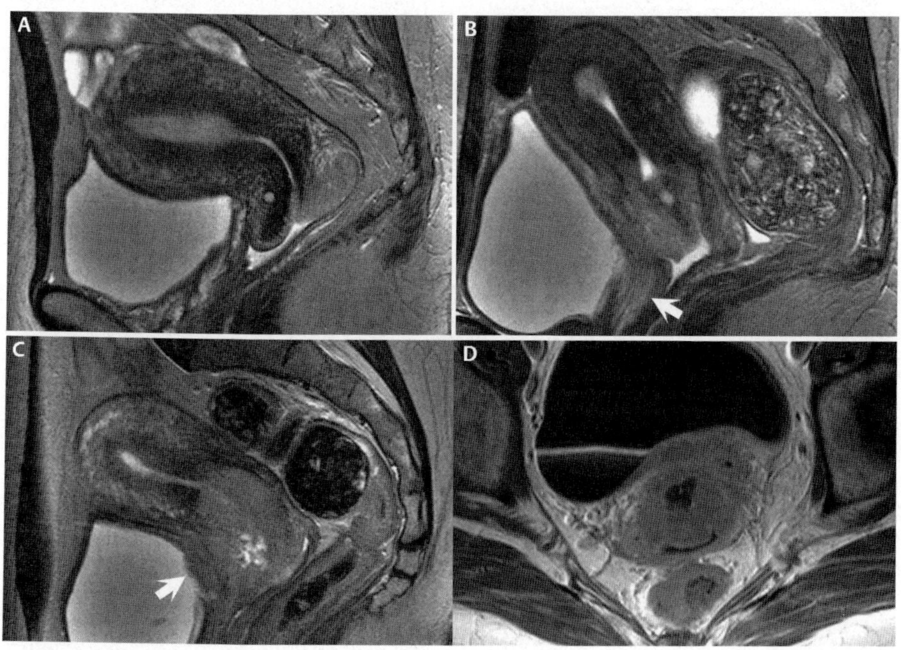

Fig. 75.2 (A–D)

76 Ovarian Pathology

Functional follicular ovarian cysts are common, benign entities, typically appearing as unilocular, thin-walled lesions with fluid-like SI (**Fig. 76.1**, axial T2WI). Nonfunctional cystic lesions are differential considerations, but because cystic neoplasia may appear similar, a newly diagnosed follicular cyst should be reassessed by ultrasound in 6 weeks. Walls of corpus luteum cysts are typically thicker, as illustrated in the coronal T2WI of **Fig. 76.2A** (*white arrow*), with the **(B)** contrast-enhanced T1WI demonstrating avid wall enhancement. Hemorrhagic corpus luteum cysts are common and are illustrated in **Figs. 76.2C,D** as high and low SI on axial (**C**, *white arrow*) T1 and **(D)** T2WI, respectively. Multiple bilateral cysts are seen in polycystic ovarian syndrome and ovarian hyperstimulation syndrome. Such cysts are small, peripheral, and subcapsular adjacent to prominent low SI central stroma. Accompanying ascites and pleural effusions are often seen in hyperstimulation syndrome. Teratomas may possess a cystic component. A dermoid (i.e., mature cystic teratoma) often contains prominent ectoderm, which secretes fatty sebaceous material. A solid nonenhancing protuberance (i.e., the Rokitansky or dermoid plug) containing fat, hair, bone, or teeth is often present. **(A)** T1WI in **Fig. 76.3** illustrate a heterogeneously appearing cystic mass with prominent high SI components. Such hyperintensity is seen in hemorrhagic cysts and endometriomas, but SI loss on (**B**) spectrally fat-suppressed T2WI confirms the presence of a dermoid. Fat suppression with STIR is nonspecific (i.e., all protons with short T1 are suppressed) and cannot make the above distinction. Microscopic fat content may be undetectable with spectral saturation and be better identified by SI dropout on out-of-phase GRE T1WI. Enhancing, solid components favor a malignant, immature teratoma. Dermoid cysts predispose to ovarian torsion, initially manifest as edema-like stromal SI but varying in appearance with time due to necrosis and hemorrhage. Nonenhancement on contrast-enhanced T1WI is specific for ovarian infarction, but not sensitive for torsion given the dual ovarian blood supply. Other findings include ipsilateral uterine deviation, ascites, and engorged ovarian vasculature. Endometriomas, hyperintense on T1WI, are present bilaterally in the axial T1WI of **Fig. 76.4A**. The more specific appearance is that of the **(B)** left-sided lesion in the T2WI, illustrating the "shading sign," seen as either complete loss of signal intensity or as in this case dependent laying. Endometrial plaque—low SI on T2WI—in characteristic locations (i.e., the cul-de-sac or uterosacral ligaments) also suggests endometriosis. The low SI of fibroma-spectrum neoplasms (fibroma, thecoma, and fibrothecoma) is specific for benignity. Such lesions may be associated with ascites and pleural effusions in Meigs syndrome.

Mucinous and serous cystadenomas are frequently confused for metastatic lesions on MRI. Mucinous cystadenomas are large, more likely to be benign, commonly multiloculated, and demonstrate a high and low SI appearance on T1 and T2WI, respectively. Fluid-like SI is more typical of serous lesions, as illustrated in **Fig. 76.5**. Portions of this lesion's wall and septa are, however, thickened (>3 mm) on **(A)** sagittal T2WI—findings concerning for malignant ovarian neoplasm. **(B)** Sagittal T1WI illustrates a hyperintense focus of hemorrhage within this cystic malignancy. Further suggestive characteristics include an enhancing solid component—as opposed to nonenhancing debris or

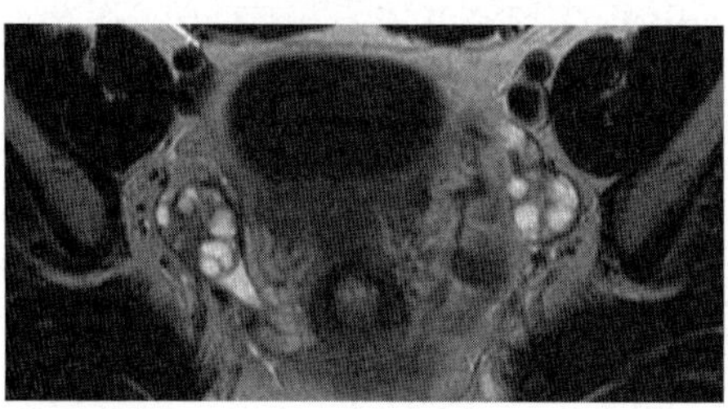

Fig. 76.1

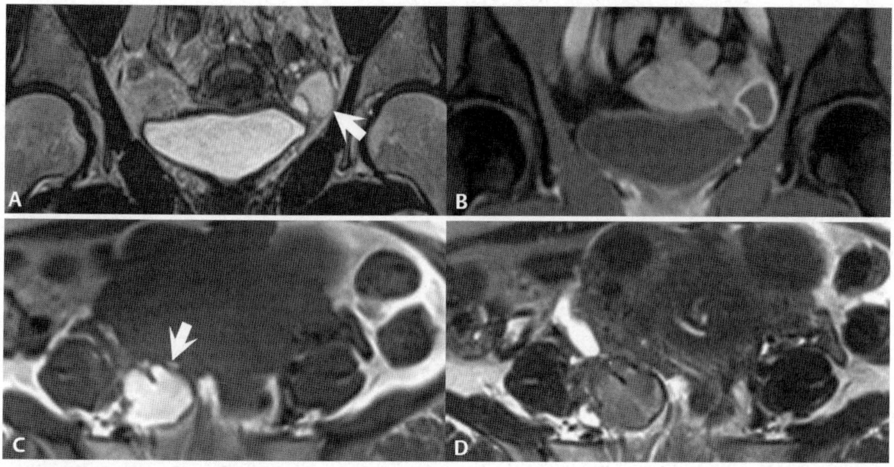

Fig. 76.2 (A–D)

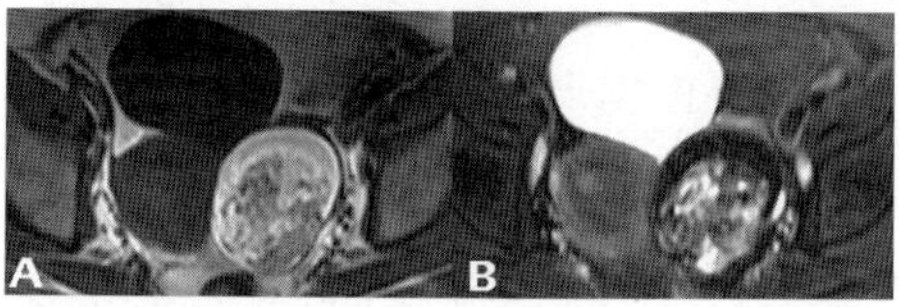

Fig. 76.3 (A,B)

clot—or papillary projections. Necrosis, appearing as a nonenhancing focus on contrast-enhanced T1WI, is concerning as is ascites. Ovarian cancer is staged based upon whether disease is contained to the ovaries (stage 1) or the pelvis (stage 2) or whether there are retro- or extrapelvic intraperitoneal (stage 3) or

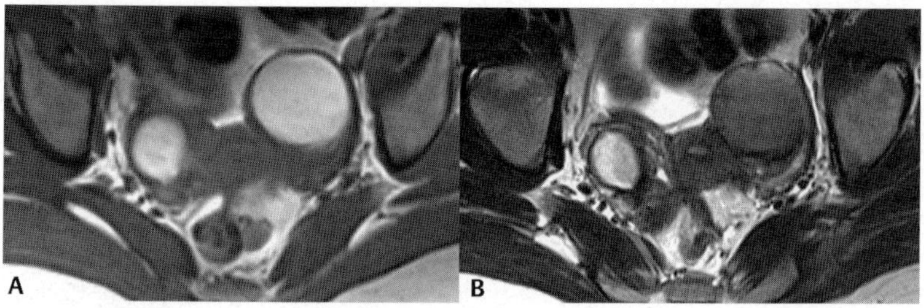

Fig. 76.4 (A,B)

distant (stage 4) metastases. Ovarian carcinoma commonly metastasizes by peritoneal implantation—lesions (if > 1 cm) readily identified on contrast-enhanced T1WI. Direct lymphatic spread to the retroperitoneal space and renal hilum is also common. Metastatic lesions enhance and are heterogeneous on T2WI, whereas bilateral lesions and those of lower SI on T2WI are more suggestive of metastatic gastrointestinal cancer (i.e., Krukenberg tumor).

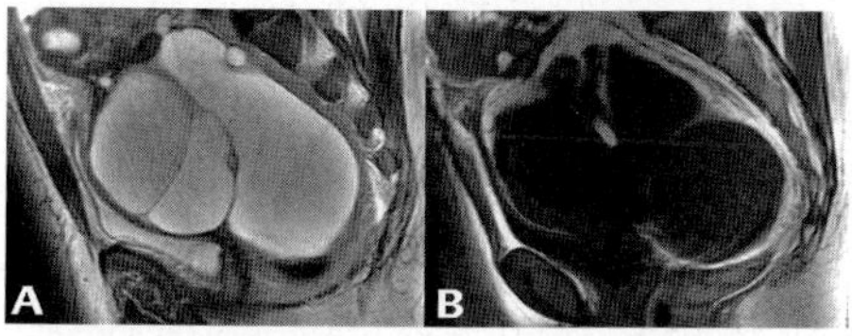

Fig. 76.5 (A,B)

77 Meniscal Tears I

Musculoskeletal MRI has long been hampered by low SNR. The advent of high-field imaging and joint-specific surface coils, however, has obviated this problem to a large extent, establishing the modality at the forefront of musculoskeletal imaging. Striking an optimal balance between SNR and adequate spatial resolution—in particular for small structures such as the carpal tunnel and menisci—however remains difficult given the fact that increased spatial resolution results in fewer recruited hydrogen nuclei per voxel and thus lower SNR. Additional approaches such as sampling at a lower bandwidth frequency (which, depending upon how this is done, may increase image blurring) and increasing the number of scan averages can help improve SNR. Maintaining a reasonable acquisition time is a concern with the latter approach. An additional way to increase image SNR is to acquire fluid-sensitive proton density-weighted images (PDWI). These images are obtained with a long TR and short TE that respectively minimize the effects of tissue T1 and T2 relaxation rates on SI. Tissue contrast in PDWI is based predominately on the number of available protons. PDWI are frequently obtained with spectral fat saturation to improve visualization of high SI pathologies, particularly against the fatty marrow of bone. The choice of fat suppression technique is important in musculoskeletal MRI as areas of inhomogeneous suppression can mimic pathology. This is a problem particularly with spectral fat suppression in which a presaturation pulse is applied at the resonance frequency of fat to suppress SI. Because the resonance frequency of fat varies directly with field strength, field inhomogeneity results in some fat molecules resonating above or below the frequency of the presaturation pulse leading to nonuniform suppression. Presaturation pulse inhomogeneity has similar effects. For high-field imaging—wherein separation of fat and water proton resonance frequencies is increased—with homogeneous magnetic fields (i.e., adequate shimming, no ferromagnetic surgical hardware, a small field of view), spectral saturation is preferred to STIR due to shorter acquisition times and improved SNR. Nonspecific suppression of tissues with T1 values similar to fat is an additional drawback of STIR, although combined sensitivity to entities with long T1 and T2 with the technique increases sensitivity to fluid SI. As fat protons provide signal, suppression techniques, in general, reduce SNR, potentially impairing visualization of small structures. Although fatty marrow is typically dark on conventional T2 SE images, FSE techniques with fat suppression—in which some associated blurring is seen due to use of FSE—are still preferred due to markedly shorter acquisition times. Acquisition times with GRE are shorter still, although these scans are prone to susceptibility artifact. Despite this, these scans may allow for improved visualization of the glenoid and acetabular labrum in the absence of arthrography.

Knee imaging is typically obtained with a dedicated coil with the knee traditionally in 15 degrees of external rotation to align the anterior cruciate ligament (ACL) with the sagittal plane. Similar results are achieved on modern MRI systems by angling the sagittal scan series. Such rotation is less important when slices thinner than 3 mm are acquired, as is possible with GRE and FSE on newer systems. FS FSE PDWI are typically obtained in the axial, sagittal, and coronal planes with T1WI recommended in at least one plane to improve specificity for detection of marrow abnormalities. GRE may detect meniscal lesions missed on FS FSE PDWI due to blurring originating secondary to the multiple echoes sampled in FSE imaging; however, these may not be clinically significant lesions. Decreasing the echo train and sampling at higher bandwidth reduces the time available for T2 decay after a given excitation, decreasing blurring.

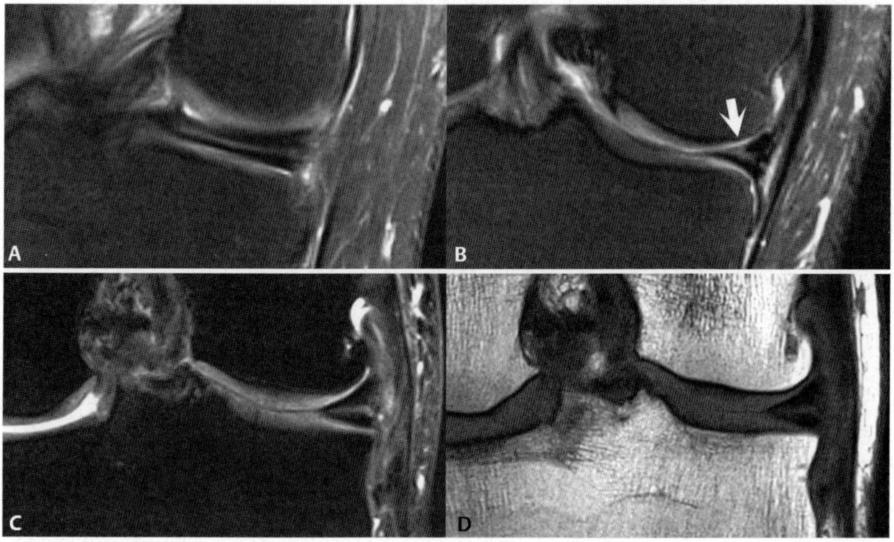

Fig. 77.1 (A–D)

Newer systems with improved slew rates and shorter echo spacing allow for FSE imaging with higher echo train lengths and less blurring.

Meniscal pathology is typically well evaluated on coronal or sagittal images. The medial meniscus is attached to the medial capsule at its periphery; the lateral meniscus is separated from its capsule by the popliteus sleeve. The lateral meniscus is more mobile than its medial counterpart and is thus less frequently torn. Posterior horn tears of the medial meniscus are more common than tears of the anterior horn, although the lateral meniscus demonstrates no such predilection. The normal meniscus typically consists of type 1 collagen: the slowly rotating water molecules within which drastically shorten T2—effects resulting in a low SI appearance on T1WI, T2WI, and PDWI. With edematous change, T2 relaxation is prolonged sufficiently that hyperintensity will be visualized even on images acquired with a short TE (T1WI and PDWI). Not all abnormal SI within the meniscus is representative of tear. Meniscal SI is graded as follows: grade 0 consists of no abnormal intrameniscal signal, grade 1 lesions of a single round or punctate high SI focus present within the meniscal substance, and grade 2 lesions of a linear high SI focus within the meniscus not extending to the articular surface. Grade 3A lesions involve increased SI within a region of meniscal fiber separation, while grade 3B lesions consist of hyperintensity extending to at least one articular surface. Of these SI gradations, only grade 3 lesions represent true meniscal tears. **Figures 77.1A and 77.1B** demonstrate a grade 3B lesion of the body and posterior horn of the medial meniscus on FS PDWI in the coronal plane. In the first image, an area of hyperintensity transversely spans the low SI medial meniscus from its inner free edge, more peripherally. The **(B)** second image clearly shows extension of the tear vertically to the articular surface (*white arrow*), a pattern suggestive of a nondisplaced flap-type of tear (see Chapter 78). A more purely horizontal, cleavage-type of lateral meniscal tear does not extend to the articular surface on the coronal FS PDWI and T1WI of **Figs. 77.1C,D**. This lesion is clearly delineated from the low SI meniscus on (**C**) FS PDWI, but is not as visible on the **(D)** T1WI.

78 Meniscal Tears II

Vertical meniscal tears are oriented perpendicular to the meniscus on coronal images. An example of such a tear within the lateral meniscus is seen in the coronal FS T2WI of **Fig. 78.1A**. This hyperintense tear (*white arrow*) extends to both superior and inferior articular surfaces, establishing it as a grade 3B lesion. In this image, there is also hyperintensity within the lateral femoral condyle and to a lesser extent within the lateral tibial plateau, reflecting edema from bone contusion. Due to the possibility of homogeneous fat suppression, T1WI are superior to FS T2WI for the detection of marrow pathology. Note the relative graininess of the FS T2WI in **Fig. 78.1A** compared with the FS PDWI in **Fig. 78.1B**, owing to the FS T2WI being obtained at a lower field strength (1.5 T vs 3 T) and the intrinsically lower SNR of this sequence compared with PDWI.

Tears may also be grouped based on surface pattern into radial, longitudinal, and flap types. These tears all extend to the superior or inferior articular surface, in contrast to a pure horizontally oriented (cleave) tear (see **Fig. 77.1C,D**). Nonpure horizontal (see **Fig. 77.1A,B**) tears may extend to the surface as flap or longitudinal tears, but only vertical (as viewed in the coronal plane) tears extend as radial tears. In the axial plane, longitudinal tears follow the meniscal long axis. A combination of longitudinal and radial hyperintensity defines a flap tear. In coronal images, the orientation of a flap tear is often, although not uniformly, oblique. Radial tears are oriented perpendicular to the meniscal long axis and occur more frequently in the lateral meniscus. These tears may be associated with additional horizontal and flap tears commonly located in the lateral and medial menisci, respectively. A radial meniscal root tear may be associated with the ghost meniscus sign in which the posterior horn of the structure appears absent sagittally near the intercondylar notch. Root tears are more common in the posterior horn of the medial meniscus and are associated with concurrent ACL tears. Complex tears exhibit a combination of the above types of lesion. Such a lesion is illustrated in **Fig. 78.1B**—a large, complex tear involving the body and posterior horn of the medial meniscus.

A displaced longitudinal tear of the meniscus is termed a bucket handle tear. These most commonly involve the medial meniscus, beginning posteriorly and extending anteriorly. This appearance is demonstrated in **Fig. 78.2A** on coronal FS PDWI where the displaced fragment of the medial meniscus is seen within the intracondylar notch (*white arrow*). If the displaced fragment appears adjacent to the origin of the posterior cruciate ligament (PCL), this appearance is termed the double-PCL sign. A similar appearance is seen in the coronal FS PDWI in **Fig. 78.2B** with the inner heads of the medial meniscus (*white arrow*) being displaced into the intracondylar notch. The remainder of the visualized meniscus also demonstrates a shortened, truncated appearance. A degenerative displaced fragment is less likely to heal, as are tears through the relatively avascular, central "white zone" as opposed to those within the peripheral, vascularized "red zone." Bucket handle tears most often occur in the setting of acute trauma—an etiology often suggested by the presence of joint effusion or osseous contusion. **Figure 78.2C** demonstrates an example of the latter involving the femoral condyle on coronal FS PDWI. Without fat suppression,

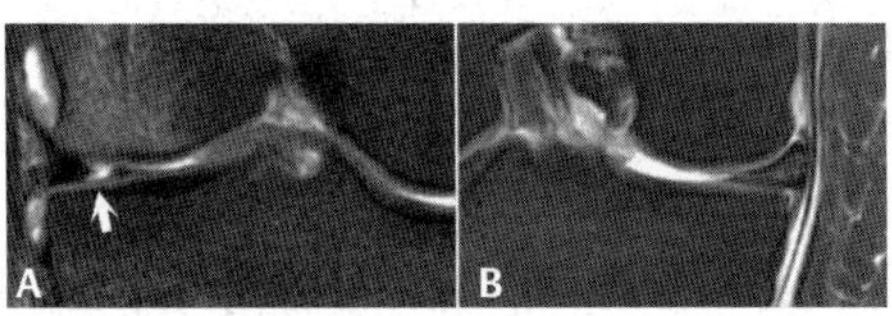

Fig. 78.1 (A,B)

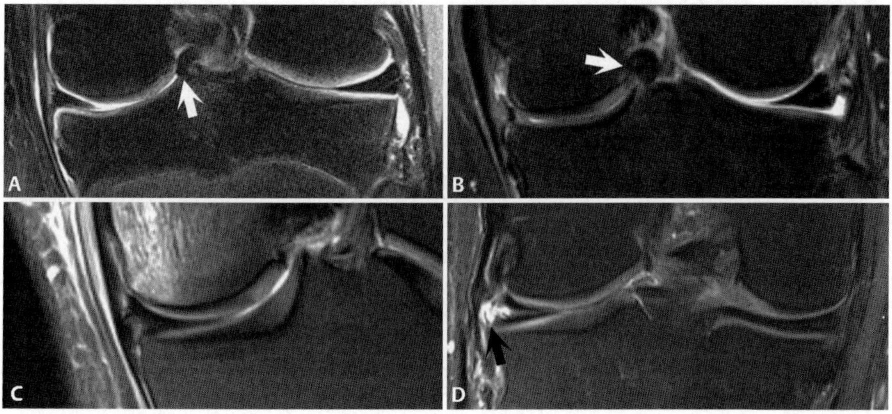

Fig. 78.2 (A–D)

this lesion would not be clearly visible on PDWI. A complex tear involving the posterior horn of the medial meniscus is also present. When synovial fluid extrudes through a meniscal tear, a synovial cyst may form. These typically appear as well-defined areas of fluid-like SI adjacent to a meniscal tear on MRI. The typical appearance of such a cyst is demonstrated in the FS PDWI of **Fig. 78.2D**. In this case there is also a clearly visible horizontal tear of the lateral meniscus. The lateral hyperintense extrameniscal fluid collection (*black arrow*) represents extruded synovial fluid confined within a small meniscal cyst.

Not all abnormal MRI SI within the meniscus is indicative of a tear. Abnormal SI within grade 1 and 2 lesions may represent intrasubstance myxoid degeneration, and abnormal meniscal SI less than 3A in grade does not predispose to tear. SI of meniscal contusions may masquerade as a tear, appearing as globular hyperintensity throughout the menisci without definite evidence of tear. Normal pediatric vasculature may give the appearance of linear hyperintensity. High SI truncation artifacts, which occur at the border of tissues with very high and low SI, may mimic meniscal tears but typically parallel the meniscal surface and are encountered only in a single plane. Higher resolution imaging may decrease this artifact. Partial volume averaging with nearby fat may also mimic meniscal pathology, findings clarified by examination in additional planes. Partial volume averaging with nearby fat may also mimic meniscal pathology, findings clarified by examination in additional planes. Due to restrictions in water motion within tendon collagenous structures, the so-called magic-angle phenomenon may occur in the upsloping portion of the posterior horn of the lateral meniscus when it is angled at 55 degrees to the main magnetic field, resulting in tendinous hyperintensity. The posterior portion of the meniscofemoral ligament—the ligament of Wrisberg (or Humphrey if anterior to the PCL)—may, in an externally rotated knee, at its insertion to the posterior horn mimic the appearance of a hyperintense vertical meniscal tear. Triplanar images may help determine whether abnormal SI extends to the articular surface in a given case. A lesion in which SI fades near the articular surface likely represents a grade 2 closed meniscal tear. Postoperatively, hyperintensity may persist within normally healing menisci, and as such MR arthrography may aid in the diagnosis of postoperative tears.

79 Cruciate Ligaments

Knee MRI identifies tears of the ACL with sensitivity of 95% and specificity approaching 100%. The normal ACL—arising from the posterior inner surface of the lateral femoral condyle and attaching anterolateral to the anterior tibial spine—is seen in **Fig. 79.1A**. The smooth, continuous fibers of this ligament demonstrate low SI on T1WI and T2WI due to its composition of type I collagen, the rigid architecture of which limits motion of free water, accentuating dipole–dipole interactions between nearby molecules. This increases T2 relaxation and thus decreases SI on T2WI. Linear hyperintensity proximally within the ligament on T2WI is normal and results from volume averaging with intercondylar fat which is bright on FSE T2WI. Acquisition of sagittal images with the knee externally rotated 15 degrees may be preferred so as to angle sagittal slices parallel to the ACL, with selection of appropriately angled imaging planes achieving the same result. Optimal PCL evaluation is similarly obtained, its normal appearance seen on the T2WI of **Fig. 79.1B**. The low SI fibers of the PCL span from the medial condyle of the femur to the posterior intercondylar area of the tibia. Any degree of hyperintensity is abnormal within the PCL.

ACL tears typically occur in the midportion or at its attachments. Loss of the ligament's parallel course with the Blumensaat line is best evaluated on sagittal PDWI. A fluid-filled gap within the ligament, appearing as high SI on T2WI and PDWI, is the most sensitive sign of ACL tear. If not completely visualized sagittally, additional T2WI or PDWI in the coronal plane may aid in the detection of abnormal ligamentous SI. The T2WI of **Fig. 79.1C** demonstrates an undulating appearing ACL with high SI throughout correlating with edema. Such undulation signifies ligamentous lengthening typical of a partial (grade 2) ACL tear. Lesions with abnormal ligamentous hyperintensity but no thickening are classified as grade 1. With time the tear in **Fig. 79.1C** progressed to **(D)** complete ligamentous disruption—a grade 3 lesion. The absence of low SI fibers within the lateral portion intercondylar notch is a reliable indicator of a grade 3 lesion. The posterior horn of the lateral meniscus may be uncovered in ACL tears, and concurrent injury to other ligaments, particularly the medial cruciate, frequently occur. Additional acute findings include joint effusions and bone contusions, both of which manifest as edema-like SI. Contusions occur in pivot-shift injuries from external femoral rotation with anterior tibial subluxation, involving the lateral femoral condyle and posterolateral tibia. Such injuries may angulate the PCL leading to a squared appearance, as illustrated. Segond fractures are associated with ACL tears and result from lateral capsular avulsion, seen as edema-like SI involving the location of capsular insertion on the lateral proximal tibia. The tibial tuberosity may also avulse, especially in children. Absence of joint effusion or bone contusion suggests a chronic lesion with the injured ACL adopting a horizontal orientation over time, potentially adhering to the PCL. Scarring or resorption may also occur, the latter signified by the presence of fat on T1WI often at the ligament's insertion. Chronic hyperintensity on T1WI reflects mucoid degeneration. Ganglion cysts within the tendon or intercondylar notch may mimic an ACL tear, demonstrating edema-like SI. MR arthrography is rarely required for the diagnosis of cruciate ligament tears, but the presence of gadolinium within the triangular space between the ACL and PCL or within the ACL itself is suggestive. Surgical ACL reconstruction is performed via tendinous grafts from the patella or hamstrings, which often demonstrate a generally more oblique orientation and within the first year thickening and abnormal hyperintensity on T2WI. Successful reconstruction is contingent upon femoral tunnel placement at the intersection of the posterior

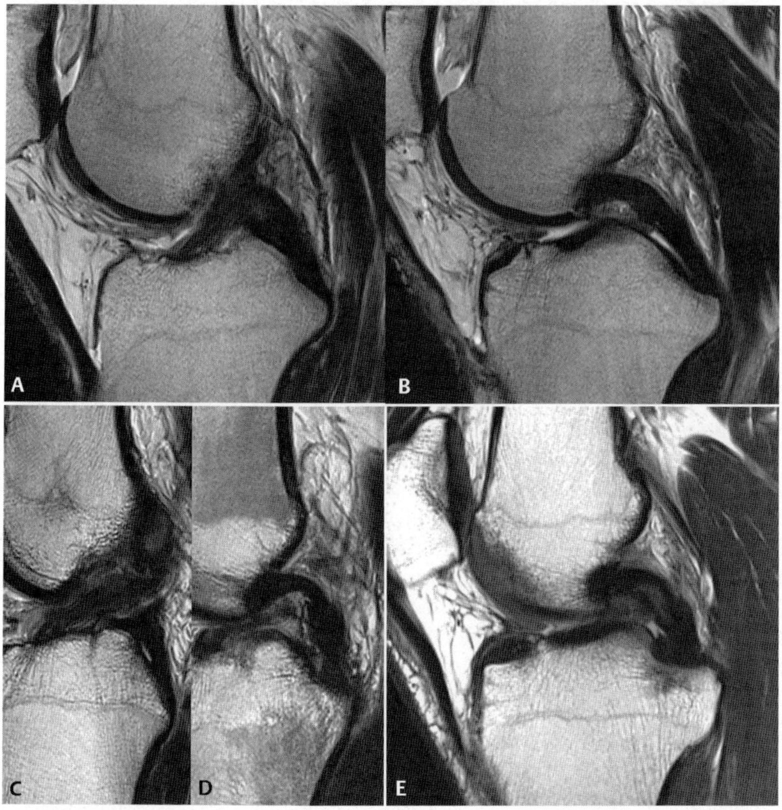

Fig. 79.1 (A–E)

femoral cortex and the posterior portion of the femoral physeal scar. Prior preference of GRE T2WI for the detection of ACL tears has been supplanted by T2 FSE sequences, especially in the postoperative setting to minimize susceptibility artifact. Principles for imaging the PCL are similar for those of the ACL. PCL tears are similarly diagnosed by disruption along the ligament's course or by areas of high SI on T2WI correlating with edema. **Figure 79.1E** demonstrates this appearance with high SI edema involving the midportion of the otherwise low SI PCL on sagittal images. Partial, midsubstance tears, as seen here, are typical in PCL injury. Associated avulsion at the insertion of tibial component of the medial collateral ligament (MCL) from off the medial tibial plateau is known as a medial or reversed Segond fracture. The arcuate sign—avulsion of the superior fibular styloid—is associated with posterolateral corner injuries and cruciate tears, especially the PCL.

80 Collateral Ligaments, Knee

Like other ligaments, type 1 collagen lends the collateral knee ligaments of the knee a hypointense appearance on common pulse sequences. The superficial portion of the MCL arises from the medial femoral condyle and inserts below the joint line, merging with low SI cortical bone posterior to the pes anserinus muscles. The course of this ligament is illustrated on the coronal FS and non-FS PDWI of **Figs. 80.1A,B**, respectively. The superficial MCL fibers are separated from the deep fibers by the Voshell bursa. The pes anserinus bursa lies distal to this, anterior to the tendons of the sartorius, semitendinosus, and gracilis. The deep MCL is best seen in the PDWI of **Fig. 80.1A**, merging with the joint capsule and medial meniscus medial to the superficial portion. Grade 1 lesions (i.e., sprain) demonstrate edema and/or hemorrhagic SI in the tissues superficial to the MCL with the ligament itself remaining normal in SI and thickness. Grade 2 lesions are partial tears marked by displacement from adjacent bone with intraligamentous hyperintensity on STIR and FS PDWI often present. A grade 3 lesion is a complete tear and is illustrated on the coronal FS T2 and PDWI in **Figs. 80.1C,D**. Here, particularly on the **(C)** FS T2WI, thickening and high SI edema within the MCL with full-thickness disruption (*black arrow*) of the proximal fibers of the superficial and deep ligamentous components are visualized. These features are not as clearly demonstrated on the **(D)** PDWI without fat saturation, although compared with a normal MCL (**Fig. 80.1B**), the ligament is clearly less distinct. Tears of the ligamentous substance, as in this lesion, tend to be associated with concurrent ACL injury, whereas peripheral tears often occur in isolation. Simple joint effusions are seen as fluid SI tracking around and along nearby ligaments; subacute hemorrhagic effusions demonstrate hyperintensity on T1WI and T2WI. A hypointense, free body indicates an avulsed bone fragment.

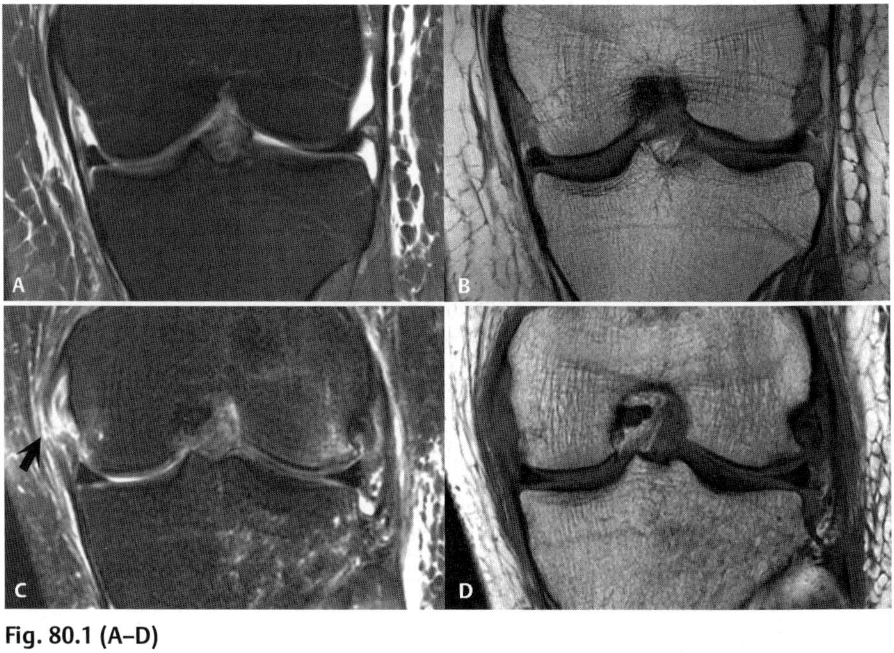

Fig. 80.1 (A–D)

Pellegrini-Stieda disease—a form of heterotopic (calcification or ossification) at the proximal MCL attachment—may occur chronically. Such mineralization is initially seen as hypointensity, but with time the presence of fatty marrow increases the SI on T1 and PDWI. GRE T2WI are most sensitive for the detection of mineralization. Associated bursitis may appear as abnormal edema-like SI within the pes anserinus or Voshell bursa. Due to the proximity of the MCL, inflammation within the latter may be confused with tear.

The posterolateral complex consists of the lateral collateral ligament—spanning from the lateral condyle of the femur to the lateral fibular head—and the biceps femoris, together known as the conjoint tendon, as well as the popliteus muscle and tendon, and the arcuate ligament complex. The latter consists of the popliteofibular, fabellofibular, arcuate, and coronary ligaments; posterolateral joint capsule; and the posterior horn of the lateral meniscus. The popliteus arises from the lateral femoral condyle, running obliquely along the posterior knee to insert in the posterior tibia under the condyles. Its tendon runs medial to the LCL. The popliteofibular ligament extends from the fibular styloid superiorly to the popliteus tendon, which courses medially to the LCL. The arcuate ligament, which may be absent with a prominent fabellofibular ligament, arises from a condensation of fibers at the fibular head, crosses the popliteus, and inserts on the posterior capsule. The LCL itself is best visualized on coronal images. A tear of the conjoint tendon's fibular insertion is seen in the FS PDWI of **Figs. 80.2A,B,C**. The MRI gradation of LCL tears is similar to those of the MCL. In this image there is overlying soft tissue edema with clear (**A**, *white arrow*) hyperintensity at the conjoint tendon's fibular insertion and superior displacement of portions of the ligament. This structure, however, maintains continuity here and **(B)** throughout its course including at **(C)** its insertion at the lateral femoral condyle, consistent with a grade 2 tear. SI changes in LCL injuries generally are of more moderate SI on MRI than those of the MCL as the former is more distinct from the capsule and does not elicit as much joint fluid when torn. Popliteus tendon tears, a case of which is partially visualized in **Fig. 80.2A** as a focus of hyperintensity at the musculotendinous junction, may occur concurrently with other associated injuries including tears of the biceps femoris and iliotibial band. Lateral meniscal and cruciate ligament tears are common with LCL disruption as are fibular head and Segond fractures—an avulsion of the capsular insertion on the lateral tibial plateau.

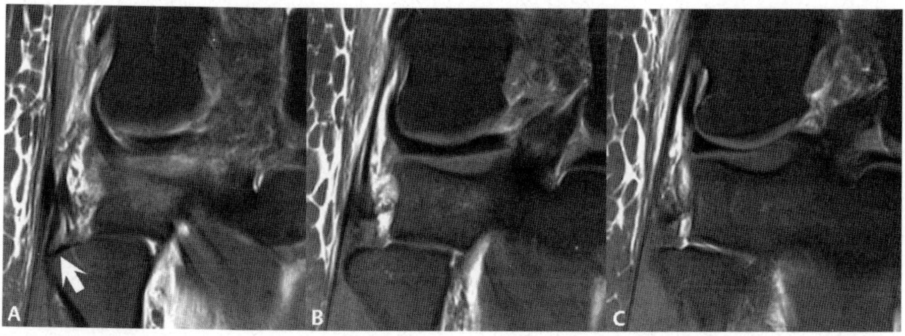

Fig. 80.2 (A–C)

81 Osteochondral Lesions, Knee

Normal articular cartilage consists of three separate zones, variably visualized as distinct layers on MRI depending on spatial resolution. At lower resolutions, truncation artifact, which occurs at interfaces of high tissue contrast, may mimic this trilaminar appearance. Protons within highly organized collagen fibers at the articular surface and superficial zone exhibit accelerated T2 decay, resulting in a decreased SI on T2WI. Fibers within the deeper transitional zone are less organized exhibiting hyperintensity on T2WI. The deep radial zone collagen fibers are also well-organized, correlating again with a decreased SI on T2WI. On T1WI there is little intrinsic tissue contrast between synovial fluid and articular cartilage, therefore FSE T2WI or PDWI, which give an arthrographic effect (partially aided by magnetization transfer), are preferred for visualization of articular cartilage defects. Choice of longer echo times, however, may impair delineation of cartilage from subchondral bone. Other disadvantages with FSE T2WI include the image blur and chemical shift artifacts that may be corrected, respectively, by reducing echo-train length and obtaining FS images. The thinness of articular cartilage renders 3D GRE T1WI a reasonable sequence by which to obtain high spatial resolution scans without interslice gaps. The trilaminar structure of articular cartilage is reliably demonstrated with this technique, although at the cost of longer acquisition times, greater sensitivity to susceptibility artifact, and poorer visualization of nearby other soft tissue structures. Postoperative evaluation is optimally performed with FSE imaging. Low-field MRI has been shown inferior for the detection of cartilaginous lesions due to problems in implementing the above sequences. Direct MR arthrography confirms an unstable fracture when contrast extends underneath the fragment, although the invasiveness of the technique, especially in the serial MRI evaluations that are often performed, impairs its utility.

Cartilaginous injury is graded from 1 to 4: grade 1 injuries correlate with softened cartilage, demonstrating increased SI on MRI without surface extent or clear tear. The increased SI seen in cartilaginous tears reflects the increased and decreased water and proteoglycan content therein, respectively, as well as increasing cartilaginous disorganization. Irregular cartilaginous fibrillation or fissures consuming less than or greater than half of cartilaginous thickness constitute grade 2 and 3 lesions, respectively. Complete absence of cartilaginous SI or exposed subchondral bone constitutes a grade 4 lesion. The FSE FS PDWI of **Fig. 81.1A** demonstrates a 5-mm full-thickness (grade 4) defect at the central aspect of the medial femoral condyle. Adjacent marrow edema—demonstrating high SI on FS T2WI—suggests a recent traumatic etiology or subarticular stress reaction related to altered mechanics from the defect. In the same patient, at a more posterior section an internal (button or stud) osteophyte is seen in the subchondral region of the medial femoral condyle (**Fig. 81.1B**). This term refers to an osteophyte occurring along the articular surface, with bone marrow often filling the entire thickness of the cartilage defect as opposed to typical osteophytes that occur at the joint margin. A large osteochondral lesion is illustrated in **Figs. 81.2A,B** on sagittal PDWI and coronal FS PDWI, respectively. This lesion involves the lateral femoral condyle and demonstrates subchondral degenerative changes, most prominent on the **(A)** sagittal PDWI. Disruption of the overlying articular cartilage is present anteriorly; fluid-like SI is seen undercutting the lesion in **Fig. 81.2B**. The presence of this finding indicates instability, which may lead to lesion dissociation and formation of a free intraarticular joint body. The medial femoral condyle is the most common site of osteochondritis dissecans—an idiopathic osteochondrosis of children and

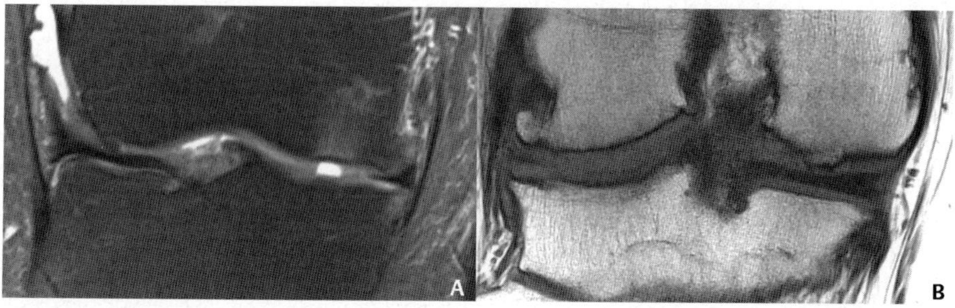

Fig. 81.1 (A,B)

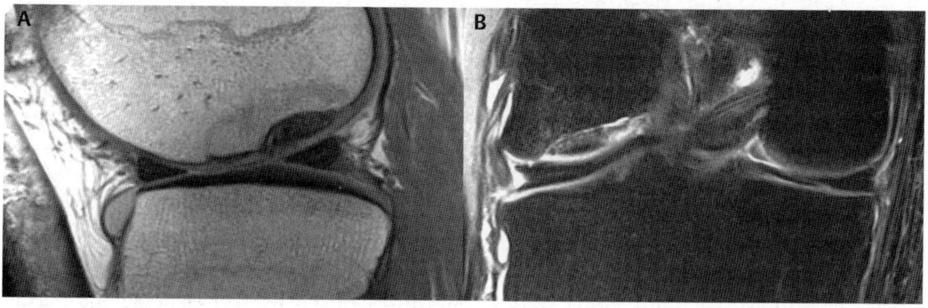

Fig. 81.2 (A,B)

adolescents—typically involving the lateral margin. The first MRI finding with this disease is the development of subchondral edema demonstrating typical fluid-like SI. A fracture line later develops demonstrating low SI on T1WI and high SI T2WI, respectively, eventually disrupting the articular surface. Instability of such lesions is indicated by fluid-like SI on T2WI involving the peripheral fracture rim, entering the defect from articular cartilage disruptions, or the formation of peripheral subchondral cysts. Due to its avascularity, cartilage has a low potential for independent repair and operative intervention is frequently required. A microfracture repair-type is based on the release of stem cells from underlying marrow when microfractures are induced. This undifferentiated cell population responds by producing fibrocartilage. On MRI, such newly formed cartilage is initially hyperintense, and subjacent marrow edema is present due to the utilized surgical technique. With time, the marrow edema should regress with the in-growing fibrocartilage demonstrating hypointense signal. However, if osteoblastic differentiation occurs, reactive bone overgrowth will fill the defect instead of cartilage. Autologous grafts, often from the intercondylar notch, are utilized for osteochondral transplantation and demonstrate early subchondral edema postoperatively. Persistence of this SI beyond 6 months, continued high SI at the implant interface, or graft collapse signify rejection. Low SI at the plug periphery may reflect condensation of trabecula if press-fit or osseous integration techniques were utilized. Autologous chondrocyte implantation involves the injection of chondrocytes derived from autologous tissue culture under harvested periosteum. These are held in place over the defect by glue or fibrin. Initial hyperintense transplanted cartilage is seen with subchondral bone edema, findings that diminish thereafter.

82 Rotator Cuff Tears

A shoulder MRI may require initial acquisition of thin-section (≤3 mm) axial images with the shoulder in neutral or slight external rotation to properly position parasagittal and paracoronal slices parallel to the surface of the glenoid cavity and supraspinatus tendon, respectively. A dedicated extremity coil allows maximization of SNR and spatial resolution. Evaluation of the long head biceps tendon, neurovascular bundles, and the relationship between the humeral head and glenoid labrum is best performed in the axial plane, whereas the paracoronal slices (**Figs. 82.1A,B,C,D**) better demonstrate the rotator cuff muscles, tendons, and associated bursae. FSE T2WI (with or without fat suppression) must be acquired in all imaging planes for accurate characterization of pathology. Axial GRE T2WI and MR arthrography are useful for evaluation of the glenoid labrum. Hyaline cartilage lining the articular surfaces of the humeral head and glenoid cavity normally demonstrates moderate SI on T1WI and T2WI, whereas fibrocartilage, which lacks free mobile protons, composes the glenoid labrum and articular surface of the acromioclavicular (AC) joint and appears of low SI on conventional pulse sequences. Fibrous rotator cuff tendons similarly demonstrate low SI, impairing their differentiation from adjacent low SI cortical bone.

Tendinosis, partial tears, and small full-thickness tears of the rotator cuff represent a continuum of disease and may be difficult to distinguish. Tendinosis demonstrates increased SI on T1WI or PDWI. SI on FS T2WI is less than that of fluid, as illustrated in the case of supraspinatus tendinosis in **Fig. 82.1A**. Here, associated tendinous thickening is present along with subacromiodeltoid fluid, the latter indicating reactive bursitis. Brighter SI within the supraspinatus tendon is present in the FS T2WI of **Fig. 82.1B**, a case of a partial supraspinatus tear. Here, hyperintensity is limited to the more commonly involved articular surface (i.e., a partial articular or inferior surface tear). Reactive bursitis is again present. Partial tears may also demonstrate fluid SI extending to the bursal surface and are classified as low-grade (less than 50% of tendon thickness) or high-grade lesions (>50%). Interstitial partial tears demonstrate high fluid-like SI on T2WI, but do not extend to the tendon's surface. Tendon thickness and partial articular surface tears are also well evaluated by MR arthrography. Contrast infiltrates into the latter, but does not extend into the bursa as with complete tears. Full-thickness tears consist of hyperintensity pervading the entire tendon thickness from its articular to bursal surface (T2WI of **Fig. 82.1C**, *arrow*). Complete tears are classified based on size as small (<1 cm), medium (<3 cm), large (3–5 cm), and massive (>5 cm) lesions. Intraarticular fluid (and gadolinium chelate, in arthrography) typically extends into the subacromiodeltoid bursa. The tendon may retract in severe cases such as in **Fig. 82.1D** (a T2WI), in which the muscle body, although not visualized completely, is correspondingly atrophic. Fatty infiltration often accompanies atrophy, appearing as intramuscular hyperintensity on T1WI. In this case, fluid SI is prominent within the subacromiodeltoid space. Chronically, scar or granulation tissue may infiltrate the area of a tear, AC joint cysts may form, and the acromiohumeral distance may narrow. With supraspinatus tears, stress is progressively propagated to the infraspinatus and biceps tendon, whereas larger or anterior tears may involve the subscapularis. Chronically, the humeral head migrates superiorly, resulting in greater tuberosity sclerosis or hypertrophy, manifesting as low SI on T1WI.

Shoulder impingement syndrome often underlies rotator cuff tears due to the chronic trapping of the supraspinatus or long head of the biceps tendon between the

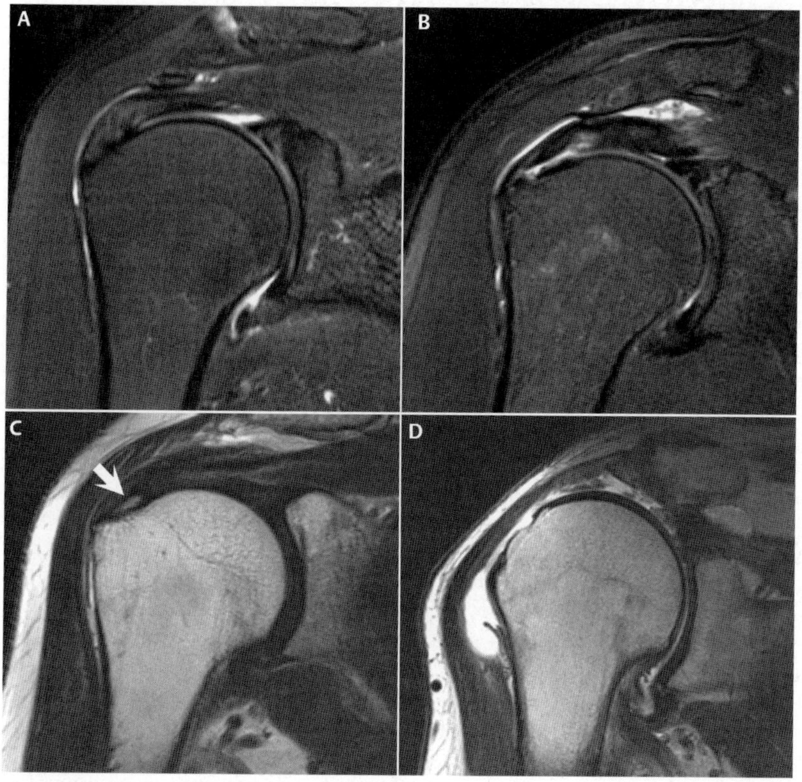

Fig. 82.1 (A–D)

humeral head and anterior acromion, AC joint, or coracoacromial ligament. This is secondary to chronic rotator cuff fatigue and is associated with the inability to maintain a concentrically located glenohumeral joint during the wide range of motion that the shoulder exhibits. Subacromial bone proliferation, osteophytosis, and capsular hypertrophy at the inferior AC joint typify such primary impingement. Small osteophytes consist of cortical bone and thus demonstrate low SI on conventional sequences, potentially leading to confusion with normal insertion points of the coracoacromial ligament or deltoid. Larger, marrow-containing osteophytes demonstrate central, fat-like SI. AC joint hypertrophy and callus formation appear as intermediate SI around the joint on all sequences. An anterolaterally angulated or type 3 (type 1 straight, type 2 curved, type 3 hooked) acromion predisposes to impingement, as does an anteriorly (best seen on sagittal images) or laterally (best seen on coronal images) downsloping acromion. "Secondary" impingement results from joint instability, occurring in athletes who throw overhead and may lack the typical associated coracoacromial abnormalities. Failure of anterior acromial apophyseal fusion (os acromiale) may also contribute, with surrounding high SI correlating to instability or degenerative changes within.

83 Glenohumeral Instability I

The glenohumeral joint is the most mobile joint in the body. Instability may result from traumatic dislocation that can cause tearing of the joint capsule and glenoid labrum. The ovoid glenoid labrum attaches to the osseous glenoid rim, providing attachment for the glenohumeral ligaments. The labrum is uniformly hypointense on MRI. Capsular joint structures are best evaluated with MR arthrography, performed with the intraarticular injection of ~12 mL of dilute (0.1 mL of gadolinium chelate in 20 mL saline) gadolinium chelate. Direct arthrography need not be performed in the presence of a joint effusion in which case thin-section GRE T2WI best evaluate the joint structures. In arthrography, FS T1WI are obtained immediately following contrast injection often with the shoulder abducted and externally rotated. Indirect (IV) arthrography may be performed with joint fluid enhancement improved by postinjection exercise of the shoulder. Indirect techniques do not afford the joint distention associated with direct arthrography. Instability may be considered atraumatic or traumatic. AMBRI refers to atraumatic, multidirectional, often bilateral instability, for which rehabilitation is the first-line therapy followed by capsular shift surgery. This is often manifest as recurrent subluxations or dislocations of the humeral head. Anterior glenohumeral instability is the most common posttraumatic instability and arises following anterior dislocations. The anterior portion of the inferior glenohumeral ligament constitutes the major resistance to anterior dislocation, forming portions of the anterior glenoid labrum. This site of attachment represents the most common site of ligamentous failure—a condition termed a Bankart lesion (actually a spectrum of lesions occurring in this location). Failure at the ligament's midsubstance is the next most common; tears at the ligament's other attachment—the humeral neck—are least common (i.e., humeral avulsion of the glenohumeral ligament [HAGL]). In a typically anteriorly dislocated shoulder with failure of the anterior band of the inferior glenohumeral ligament, the humeral head is displaced anteroinferiorly, contacting the anteroinferior glenoid rim, and resulting in a posterolateral humeral head osteochondral impaction fracture—a Hill-Sachs lesion. Such a lesion is illustrated on the FS T1WI images from an MR arthrogram in **Fig. 83.1A**. This large Hill-Sachs lesion consists of a prominent impaction deformity of the posterolateral humeral head. Extensive marrow edema at this site was better visualized on the FS T2WI (not shown). The bare area of the posterior humeral head should not be confused with a Hill-Sachs defect, which typically occurs at the level above the coracoid process rather than below it. This patient also had a Bankart lesion (**Fig. 83.1B**) consisting of avulsion of the anteroinferior labrum, which remains attached to the anterior glenohumeral ligament. Periosteal disruption off the anterior scapula surface is also present in this softtissue Bankart lesion. Complete labral avulsion is not essential for a Bankart lesion, as any contrast extending between the labrum and glenoid cartilage constitutes a labral tear. In so-called double lesions, avulsion of the labrum from the scapular rim and of the glenohumeral ligament from the avulsed labrum is present. The addition of scapular periosteal disruption to a double lesion is termed a triple lesion. An osseous Bankart (i.e., Bankart fracture) may also occur as illustrated in the MR arthrogram image (FS T1WI) of **Fig. 83.1C**. Here the hypointensity of the anterior labrum is interrupted by a large, linear focus of high SI, correlating to contrast within this tear (with the avulsed component including both labrum and underlying bone). Chronic osseous Bankart lesions tend to heal with osseous hypertrophy resulting in inferiorly convex glenoid curvature. Acute Bankart lesions are more characteristically associated with hyperintensity within the underlying glenoid on fluid-sensitive images. Operative repair of Bankart lesion consists of reattachment of the

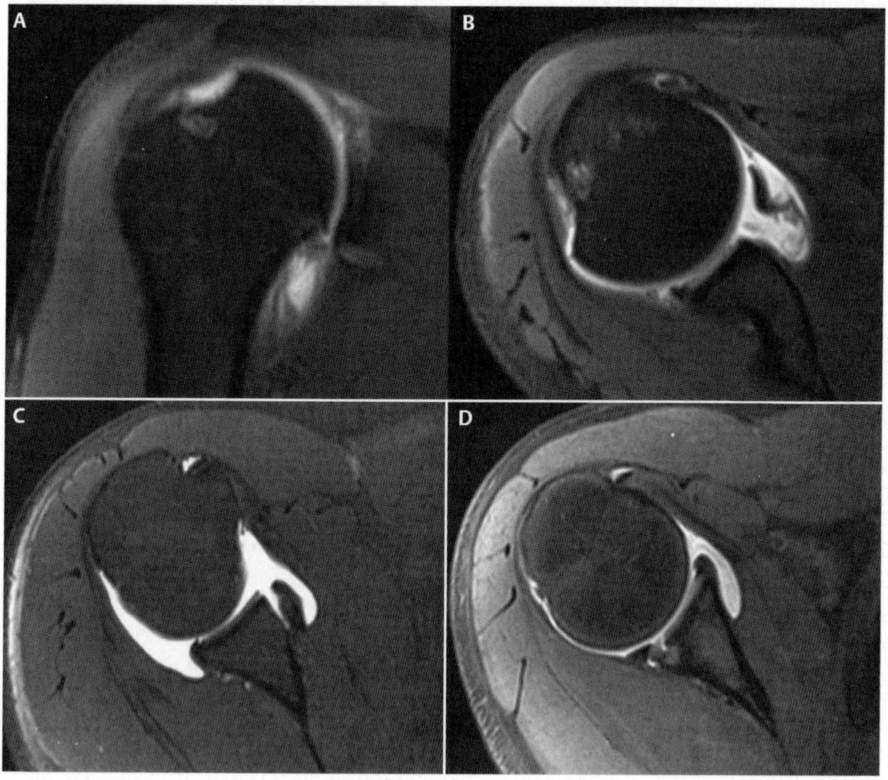

Fig. 83.1 (A–D)

labrum to the glenoid rim with poorer outcome resulting from hypertrophic glenoid convexity as described above. Identification of suture anchors and tacks, which may demonstrate susceptibility artifact, is aided with MRI as is the detection of recurrent Bankart tears. Because normal postoperative findings after Bankart repair include hyperintensity on T2WI, correlating with granulation tissue (often appearing near sutures), evaluation for recurrent tears with direct MR arthrography is preferred.

Posterior instability of the shoulder is less common and is associated with glenoid dysplasia. The relevant anatomy and pathology in posterior instability and dislocations is analogous to that of anterior instability described above: the posterior band of the inferior glenohumeral ligament prevents posterior humeral dislocation, whereas dislocations result in wedge-type impaction deformities on the anteromedial humeral head (i.e., a reverse Hill-Sachs lesion) as well as posterior labral tears (i.e., reverse Bankart) with possible osseous involvement. **Figure 83.1D** demonstrates on an FS T1WI following intraarticular contrast administration, a fracture extending through the articular cartilage of the posterior glenoid and exiting the posterior glenoid cortex, consistent with a reverse Bankart. Contrast is also seen undermining the posterior labrum in this region along with a paralabral cyst. Posterior labral tears are frequently associated with Bennett lesions—an entity commonly found in baseball pitchers and resulting from the posterior portion of the inferior glenohumeral ligament exerting stress traction outside the glenohumeral joint just adjacent to the posterior glenoid.

84 Glenohumeral Instability II, Labrum

Additional causes of anterior glenohumeral stability include Bankart variants of which the Perthes lesion is an example. This lesion occurs when the scapular periosteum remains intact but is stripped medially, while the anterior labrum is avulsed from the glenoid but remains partially attached to the scapula by the intact periosteum. The labrum may assume a normal position and thus a Perthes lesion is difficult to diagnose without imaging the shoulder in abduction and external rotation. A Perthes lesion is illustrated in the MR arthrogram image (FS T1WI) of **Fig. 84.1**. Here, contrast undermines the anterior labrum with stripping of the glenoid periosteum. There is not significant displacement of the former structure, and in distinction to the Bankart lesion (see **Fig. 83.1B**), the attachment of the labrum to the periosteum remains intact. Disruption of the scapular periosteal attachment is also characteristic of anterior labral ligamentous periosteal sleeve avulsion injury (ALPSA), which is essentially a Bankart lesion in which the torn fragment of the anterior labrum is displaced medially and rotated inferiorly (a "medialized" Bankart). Similar lesions may be seen with the posterior labrum and may be referred to as POLPSA (posterior periosteal sleeve avulsion). Avulsions of the anterior band of the inferior glenohumeral ligament may occur at its humeral attachment (HAGL), although midportion tears are more common. On conventional MRI, these lesions are difficult to detect in the absence of a joint effusion but may appear as foci of hyperintensity on T2WI, the T1WI typically demonstrating a thickened, irregular ligament. Arthrographic findings include extravasation of contrast material within the ligament at its humeral attachment. The inferior displacement of the ligament characteristically results in a J shape. Posterior HAGL lesions (PHAGL) are less common and consist of avulsions of the posterior band of the inferior glenohumeral ligament at its humeral attachment. Associated marrow edema or humeral bone avulsions may occur with both of these lesions and are sometimes referred to as BHAGL.

Superior labral tears are also common, although these lesions do not result in instability. The detection of anterosuperior lesions may be difficult given the frequent presence of normal variants in this region, including the sublabral foramen (common) and Buford complex (uncommon). A sublabral foramen is a normal variant in which the anterosuperior labrum is not well attached to the glenoid above the superior epiphyseal line of the glenoid. A sublabral foramen is often confused with a superior tear. Features suggesting tear over this anatomic variant include an irregular labral margin, abnormal labral hyperintensity, and separation between the glenoid and labrum. In the Buford complex, the anterosuperior labrum is absent and there is a thick, cord-like medial glenohumeral ligament attaching to the superior labrum directly. True tears of the superior labrum are best detected in the coronal plane, with arm placement in external rotation during scanning potentially aiding in detection. Tears involving the superior labrum, extending anteriorly and posteriorly are termed SLAP (superior labrum anterior posterior) lesions, 10 types of which are described. The typical appearance is seen on the direct arthrographic MRIs

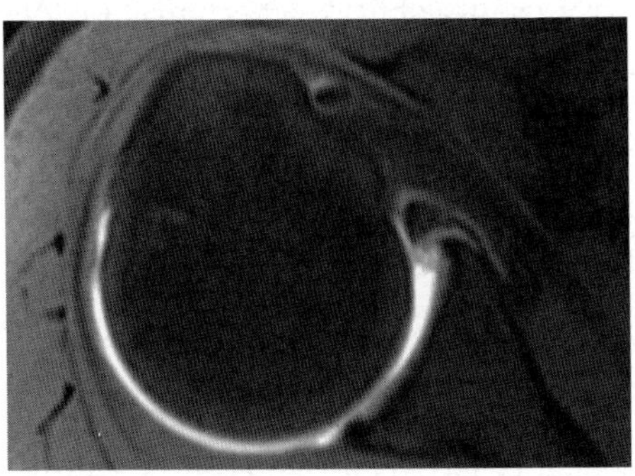

Fig. 84.1

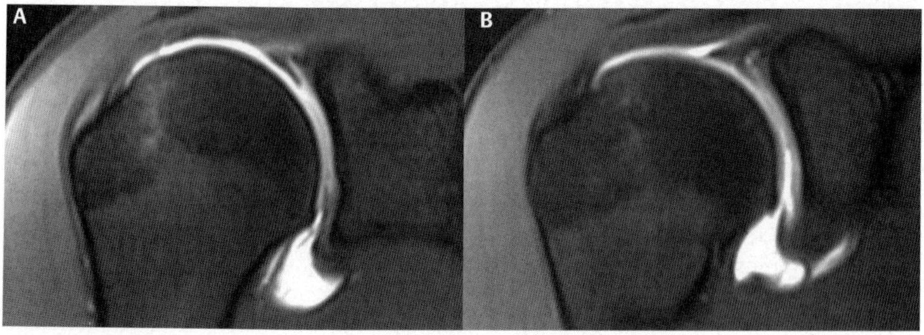

Fig. 84.2 (A,B)

(FS T1WI) of **Figs. 84.2A,B** in which intraarticular gadolinium chelate undermines portions of the superior labrum up to the attachment of the biceps tendon without clear displacement of the anchor from the labrum. Type 1 lesions are characterized by labral degeneration and coarsening, correlating with diffusely increased SI within the labrum without acute tear. Abnormal labral signal without extension to the surface is generally considered indicative of labral degeneration rather than tear. Other potential SI patterns on conventional MRI include a hypointense labrum demonstrating blunting and fraying. Type 2 SLAP lesions consist of high SI extending to the labral surface in the presence or absence of the degenerative findings above. The tear extends through the superior labrum, involving the biceps anchor. Type 2 SLAP lesions comprise a plurality of true labral tears. Superior labrum anterior cuff and peel-back lesions are subtypes of type 2 SLAP lesions, extending predominantly in the anterior and posterior directions, respectively. A meniscoid variant labrum at its free edge may be confused in appearance for a type 2 SLAP lesion. In the former, glenoid articular cartilage extends to the area of labral attachment, whereas in a type 2 tear, displacement of the labrum from the glenoid cartilage by 3 to 4 mm is frequently seen. Fraying of the labrum and synovitis are often useful ancillary findings indicating tear. Bucket-handle type superior labral tears without and with a concurrent tear of the biceps tendon constitute type 3 and 4 lesions, respectively. Bucket-handle tears are typically well visualized in the sagittal plane where three hypointense structures are seen—the two bucket-handle components and the biceps tendon. Bucket-handle tears may extend into the anterior or anteroinferior labrum. The latter case, in which a concurrent Bankart and SLAP lesion are present, constitutes a type 5 lesion. Type 6 SLAP lesions consist of radial or flap tears with anchor involvement. SLAP lesions extending anteriorly to concurrently that tear the middle glenohumeral ligament constitute type 7 lesions, whereas tears resulting in posteriorly labral detachment are considered type 8 lesions. A type 9 lesion consists of concentric avulsion of the entire labrum around the glenoid. Coronal images best demonstrate detachment of the superior and inferior labrum, while axial images best display the remainder with the entire detached labrum often being visible on sagittal slices. Type 10 lesions concurrently involve the tendons of the rotator cuff via extension through the superior glenoid ligament. Although not a cause of anterior instability per se, glenolabral articular disruptions (GLAD) are a cause of shoulder pain, consisting of partial anterior labral tears with defects in the adjacent articular cartilage. Fluid sensitive sequences demonstrate hyperintense chondral divots or flaps adjacent to the nondisplaced labral tear. On direct MR arthrography, contrast infiltrates the labral tear and extends into the cartilaginous defect.

85 Avascular Necrosis of the Hip

Pelvic and hip MRI is typically obtained utilizing a body coil, enabling simultaneous bilateral imaging. Unilateral imaging with a dedicated surface coil, however, allows increased SNR and spatial resolution. The detection and treatment of early avascular necrosis (AVN) of the femoral head—the most common location for this condition in the body—is the primary indication for hip MRI. SI characteristics of femoral head AVN correspond well with underlying pathology: the commonly described double-line sign within the femoral head refers to the appearance of a hyperintense line immediately adjacent to linear hypointense signal on T2WI or PDWI. The former line correlates pathologically with granulation tissue and the latter with reactive sclerotic bone and fibrosis. Together the double line represents the interface between normal and necrotic marrow. The Mitchell system classifies the MRI progression of femoral head ischemia. Early, lesions (class A) demonstrate fat-like SI as shown in the left femoral head of **Figs. 85.1A,B**. Here, **(A)** T1WI demonstrates isointensity of the lesion to normal marrow superior to a hypointense line correlating with a nidus of fibrovascular proliferation and demarcating pathologic from normal bone. A full double-line sign is not seen, as is the case 20% of the time. On **(B)** FS T2WI, the linear border demonstrates high SI, although SI of the superomedial area of necrosis remains low (i.e., that of attenuated fat). The appearance of early AVN may, in fact, be indistinguishable from other causes of bone marrow edema, and contrast-enhanced T1WI may be necessary to differentiate ischemia from completely devitalized bone. In advanced osteonecrosis, contrast-enhanced examinations differentiate viable (although possibly ischemic), enhancing bone from necrotic, nonenhancing bone. Class B lesions are rarer and demonstrate SI changes compatible with late subacute hemorrhage (high SI on T1WI and T2WI), while a class C lesion consists of edema-like SI within the ischemic femoral head. A class D lesion is illustrated in the right femoral head of **Figs. 85.1A,B**. Superomedial to the line demarcating necrotic and normal bone, hypointensity is seen on both **(A)** T1WI and **(B)** FS T2WI, correlating with chronic fibrosis. Important ancillary findings in this patient

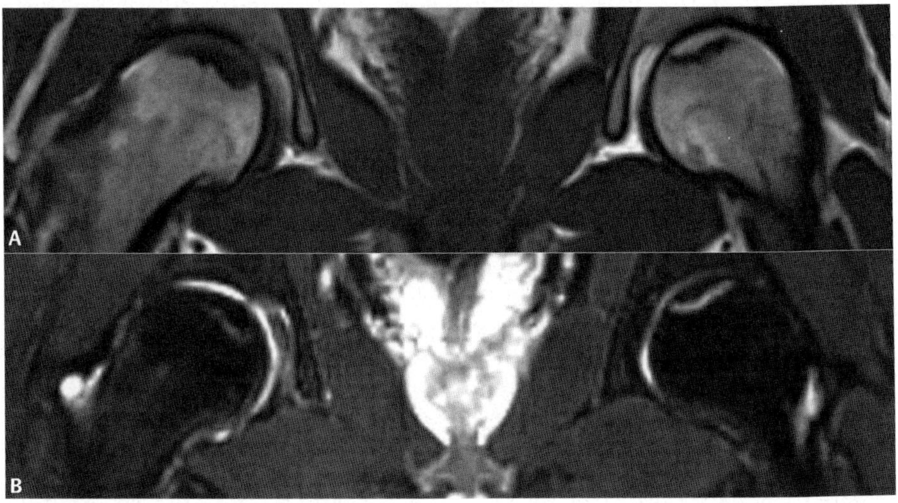

Fig. 85.1 (A,B)

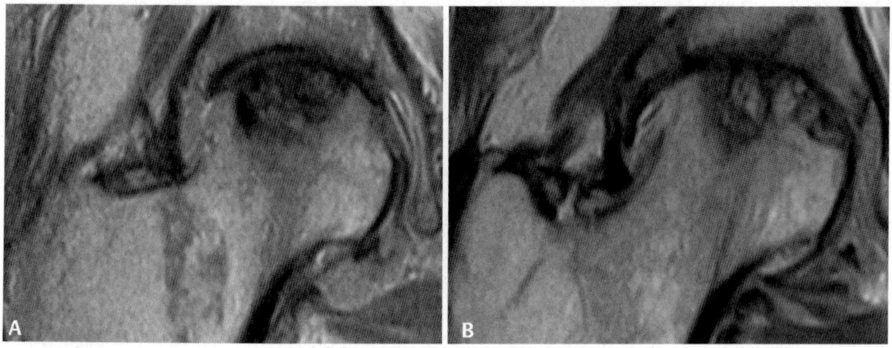

Fig. 85.2 (A,B)

include the presence of small bilateral effusions within the hip joints (right greater than left) demonstrating typical edema-like SI. As illustrated here, AVN occurs bilaterally in the majority of cases. PDWI of **Figs. 85.2A,B** demonstrate two additional cases of AVN. In both, hypointensity within the superior aspect of the femoral head denotes either a class C or D lesion. In the **(B)** second image, marrow intensity is similar, but partial femoral head collapse is noted—a condition predisposing to chondral fracture, chondromalacia, and chronic osteoarthritis. Bone remodeling and collapse are better assessed and classified on CT. Transient osteoporosis of the hip may mimic early femoral head AVN, but is distinguishable clinically by its rapid onset and a lack of AVN risk factors and on MRI by the presence of diffuse edema throughout the femoral head without a clearly differentiable area of subchondral osteonecrosis. Some believe that transient osteoporosis (transient marrow edema syndrome) may represent salvaged AVN.

In the pediatric patient (typically between 4 and 9 years old), MRI is utilized for evaluation of idiopathic AVN of the femoral head epiphysis, known as Legg-Calves-Perthes disease. The earliest MRI finding of this condition may simply consist of a joint effusion—the presence of which in an appropriately aged child with high clinical risk for the condition warrants MRI follow-up. T1WI typically reveals diminished SI of the epiphysis, whereas SI on T2WI is variable. Nonenhancing regions of the femoral head correlate with necrotic, nonviable tissue. Group 1 lesions involve only the anterior epiphysis, while later, progressive changes include physeal bridging or compression with subchondral fissure formation (group 2), diffuse metaphyseal involvement (group 3), and eventually epiphyseal collapse (group 4). Obese children are predisposed to a Salter Harris type 1 fracture of the femoral head known as a slipped femoral capital epiphysis and demonstrated on the coronal PDWI of **Fig. 85.3**. Here, as is typical, physeal widening with inferomedial epiphyseal displacement is present. Hyperintense signal compatible with edema was seen within the proximal metaphysis on STIR images (not shown). Sequelae of slipped capital femoral epiphysis include femoral head AVN, premature physeal fusion, and osteoarthritis.

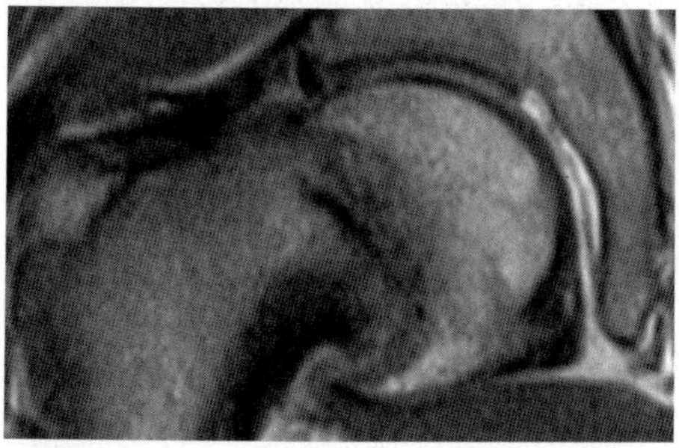

Fig. 85.3

86 Insufficiency Fractures, Acetabular Labrum

Fractures characteristically demonstrate hyperintensity on STIR and FS T2WI as well as linear hypointensity on T1WI perpendicular to the direction of force. A left pubic insufficiency fracture is illustrated on the T1WI and FS T2WI of **Figs. 86.1A,B**, respectively. The left parasymphysial area of the pubis exhibits low SI on **(A)** T1WI with a more lateral linear band of hypointensity, perpendicular to the direction of weight-bearing. **(B)** FS T2WI demonstrates hyperintensity within this region, further suggesting an insufficiency fracture. Bone contusion may appear similar, but differs in clinical history and also in the lack of linear-appearing hypointensity. **Figure 86.2A,B** illustrates a sacral insufficiency fracture on the coronal T1WI and axial FS T2WI, respectively. Vertically oriented linear hypointensity is present within the right sacrum on the former, consistent with an insufficiency fracture. Sacral fractures are often present on lumbar spine MRI, although they may be missed due to location at the periphery of the region of interest. Careful examination of sagittal images for such findings is therefore warranted.

Degenerative hip disease is predisposed by femoroacetabular impingement. In cam impingement normal femoral head-neck concavity is lost, as opposed to pincer impingement in which acetabular overcoverage (of which there are several varieties) is responsible. Sensitivity to labral tears is greatly improved by direct arthrography, although the invasiveness of this technique is a disadvantage, as is the potential for artifacts from extraarticular contrast leakage and air bubbles—the low SI of which may mimic free fragments of osseous cortex. The normal fibrocartilaginous labrum appears as a hypointense triangular band on coronal images. At the margin with the lateral acetabular rim, the labrum covers hyaline cartilage. On MR arthrography Czerny stage 1, 2, and 3 lesions consist, respectively, of abnormal labral high SI not extending to its surface, intraarticular contrast extending into the labrum, and labral detachment. The A and B substages are based on the preservation or obliteration of the perilabral sulcus, respectively. **Figures 86.3A and 86.3B** are FS T1WI obtained after intraarticular gadolinium chelate injection. The superior labrum is infiltrated with contrast (**Fig. 86.3A**, *white arrow*), although the perilabral space (*small black arrow*) is preserved—a stage 2A lesion. Inferior labral detachment is also present, stage 3A (**Fig. 86.3A**, *black arrow*). A posterior tear (stage 2B) is seen in the oblique axial plane (i.e., parallel slices to the femoral neck) (**Fig. 86.3 B**, *white arrow*). Examination in all imaging planes is important as evaluation of the anterosuperior labrum (the most common location of tear) is limited in the coronal plane due to a change in labral orientation in this region. Normal attachments to the acetabulum may mimic a tear on conventional MRI due to nearby intermediate SI of articular cartilage. On

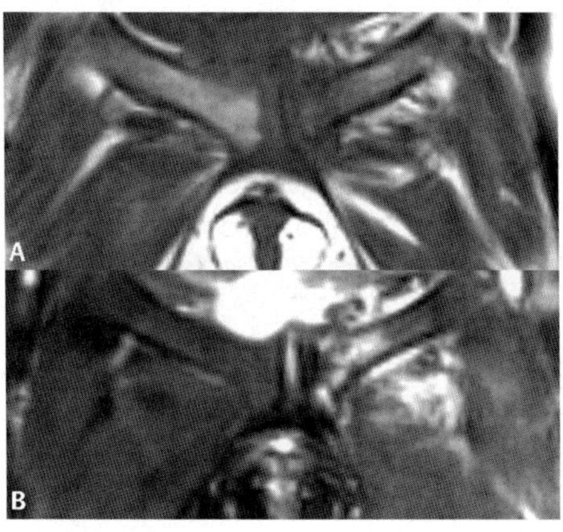

Fig. 86.1 (A,B)

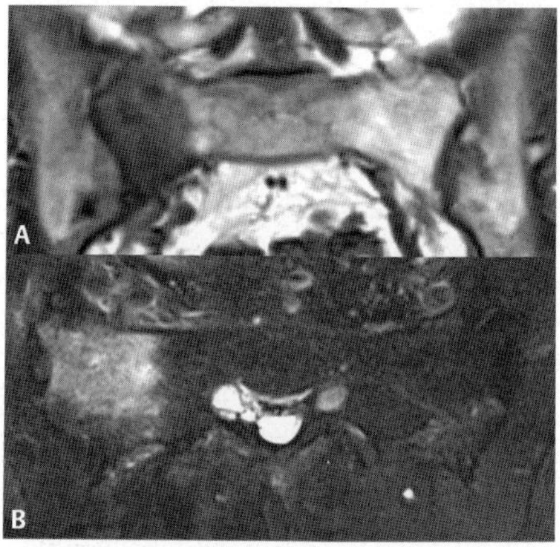

Fig. 86.2 (A,B)

arthrography no contrast should infiltrate this area, in distinction to **Fig. 86.3C,** where the anterior labrum is detached from the acetabulum. Labral thickening has also obliterated the perilabral sulcus in this stage 3B lesion. A full-thickness defect of the normally intermediate SI articular cartilage is illustrated in **Fig. 86.3D** (*white arrow*), contiguous with abnormal SI in the superolateral labrum. Adjacent supraacetabular cysts are present. Such paralabral cysts result from the dissection of synovial fluid through a labral or acetabular tear and are best visualized as hyperintensity on STIR or FS T2WI. Cyst enhancement on direct arthrography occurs only if connection to the joint space persists.

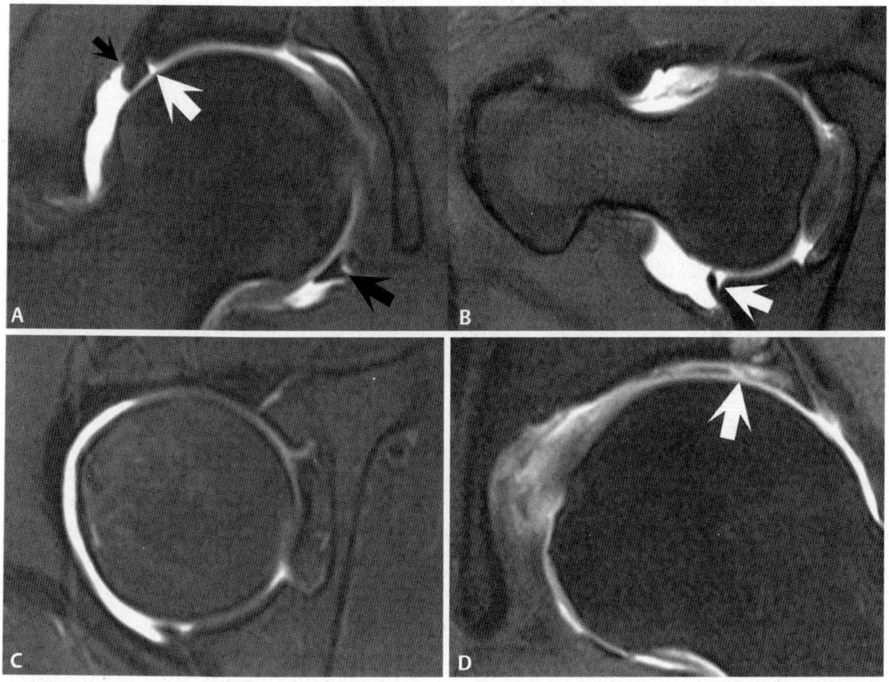

Fig. 86.3 (A–D)

87 Carpal Tunnel Disease and Wrist Fractures

The small structures involved in wrist MRI necessitate maximization of spatial resolution and SNR with dedicated surface coils and imaging at 3 T. The effect of such measures is illustrated by the ability to detect injuries to small structures like the median nerve, which is affected in carpal tunnel syndrome, illustrated in **Fig. 87.1**. Here **(A)** axial T1WI and **(B)** FS T2WI demonstrate enlargement of the nerve as it courses between flexor tendons deep to the flexor retinaculum at the level of the hamate. Calculating ratios of ipsilateral nerve diameters at the pisiform or hamate versus at the distal radius may prove more useful in documenting enlargement than contralateral size comparisons, as carpal tunnel syndrome is bilateral in more than half of cases. **Figure 87.1B** demonstrates high SI within the nerve correlating with edema and inflammation. Median nerve inflammation proximal to the actual carpal tunnel is termed pseudoneuroma. After surgical retinaculum release, nerve hyperintensity may persist; chronic fibrosis is marked by hypointensity. Additional findings at the level of the hamate in carpal tunnel include nerve flattening and palmar bowing of the low SI flexor retinaculum. Secondary causes of carpal tunnel syndrome—scar tissue, tendon sheath fibrosis, and tumors—are easily detected with MRI, as are long-term sequelae of denervation such as thenar atrophy—initially manifesting as intramuscular hyperintensity on FS PD and T2WI prior to fatty replacement leading to hyperintensity on T1WI. The ulnar nerve may demonstrate similar SI characteristics when compressed within the Guyon tunnel, formed by the hamate and pisiform. Etiologies of such compression vary based on location: ganglion cysts and hook of the hamate fractures may affect the deep (motor) or superficial (sensory) nerve; ulnar artery aneurysms tend to affect the superficial portion only.

Radiographically occult fractures of the forearm and wrist are also well evaluated on MRI. The distal radial fracture illustrated in **Fig. 87.1** on **(C)** T1 and **(D)** FS T2WI was radiographically occult. The low SI fracture line is flanked by edema-like SI on both images. In contrast to conventional radiography, imaging of a casted arm—as performed in this case—affects image quality relatively little in MRI. Angulation is better demonstrated in sagittal planes, and coronal images may help detect concurrent carpal or carpal ligament injury. Carpal instability related to ligamentous disruption is termed dissociative, in contrast to less common nondissociative instability. Scapholunate ligamentous tears constitute stage 1 perilunate instability. Progression of this spectrum consists of progressive failure of the radioscaphocapitate (stage 2) and lunotriquetral ligaments (stage 3), followed eventually by complete dislocation of the lunate from the radiolunate fossa (stage 4). The scapholunate ligament ordinarily demonstrates low SI on T1, T2, and PDWI due to its low water content, consisting of membranous, dorsal, and volar portions. These components are best distinguished with axial imaging utilizing slice thicknesses under 3 mm. Membranous perforations are clinically insignificant: the dorsal ligament is essential for stability. Complete ligamentous tears may be visible as ligamentous dissociation (well evaluated on STIR or GRE T2WI) or alternatively as areas of linear high SI within the ligament. The latter appearance is also typical for partial tears. MR arthrography may aid in detection by demonstrating contrast penetration into an injured ligament in a partial tear or in a complete tear by showing contiguity of contrast between the midcarpal and radiocarpal joints. To appreciate widening of the scapholunate gap (>3 mm) tears of both the volar and dorsal aspects of the scapholunate as well as radioscaphoid injury are

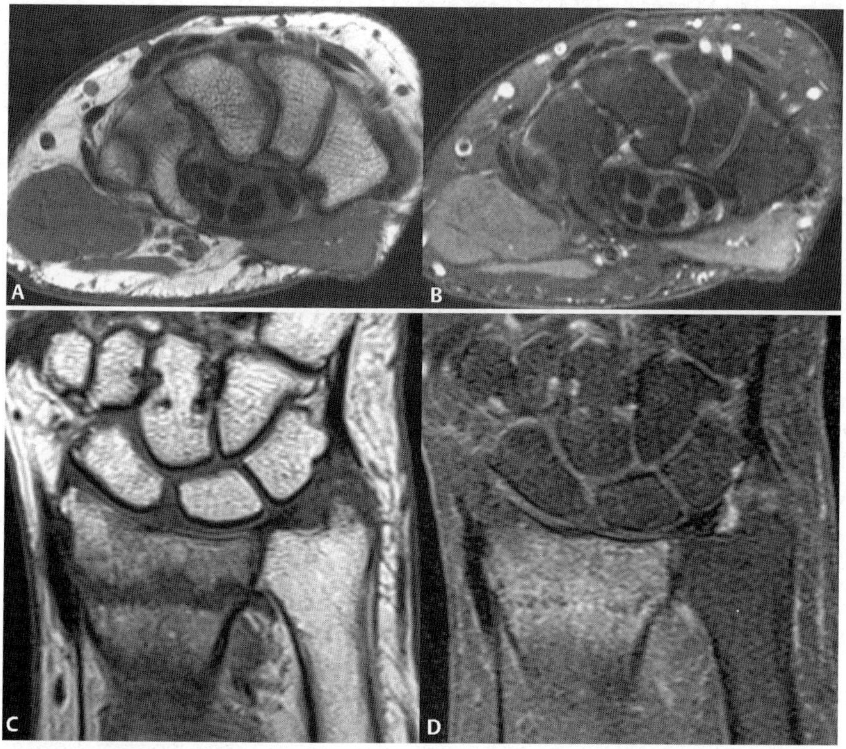

Fig. 87.1 (A–D)

necessary. Dorsal intercalated segment instability (DISI) may occur with scapholunate tears, occasionally as the presenting finding. In this lesion, the lunate is tilted dorsally leading to capitolunate and scapholunate angles over 30 and 70 degrees, respectively (as measured in sagittal planes), along with proximal capitate migration. Scapholunate advanced collapse (SLAC) may ultimately result from degenerative disease related to scapholunate instability. Tears of the ordinarily linear or delta-shaped lunotriquetral ligament are less common and poorly visualized on MRI due to the ligament's small size. Coronal imaging, especially utilizing high-resolution 3D techniques, is useful: axial images help distinguish the ligament's three components. Unlike the scapholunate, tears of the lunotriquetrum rarely lead to visible osseous separation but are most commonly visualized as a fluid-filled gap within the ligament. Normal ligamentous discontinuity without alteration of SI may be seen at the insertion of the triangular fibroosseous cartilage complex. Disruption of the proximal line of Gilula may be seen, as may contrast extension from the radiocarpal to midcarpal joint on arthrography. Volar intercalated segment instability (VISI) may occur with these tears, manifesting as distal carpal row migration proximally as well as scapholunate and capitolunate angles greater than and up to 30 degrees, respectively.

88 Triangular Fibrocartilage Complex Tears

The high-resolution thin-section imaging afforded by high-field MRI allows for accurate assessment the triangular fibrocartilage (TFC) complex of the wrist—a key stabilizer of the radiocarpal and radioulnar joints. This complex consists of the triangular fibrocartilage, the extensor carpi ulnaris tendon sheath, and the meniscal homologue (fibrous tissue between the ulnar styloid and triquetrum), as well as the dorsal and volar radioulnar and ulnocarpal ligaments. The proximal portion of the TFC complex arises from the lunate fossa of the radius and inserts at the ulnar styloid tip and fovea. Distal insertions include the triquetrum, hamate, and fifth metacarpal base. The complex inserts volarly on the triquetrum and lunate, and dorsally upon the extensor carpi ulnaris tendon sheath. The TFC proper (also known as the articular disk) cushions the radiocarpal and radioulnar joints and is the most commonly injured portion of the complex. It is best visualized as a hypointense (due to its fibrocartilaginous composition) biconcave structure on coronal images. On axial scans, the TFC appears triangular, its apex at the ulnar styloid. Its anterior and posterior boundaries are the radioulnar ligaments (dorsal and volar, respectively).

TFC defects are characterized as traumatic or degenerative under the Palmer classification. The former, often caused by a direct blow, are more likely to occur at the TFC's thicker radial attachment. Due to normal poor vascularity of this area such tears are unlikely to heal, and the injured TFC is often resected. Such defects constitute Palmer class 1 lesions, one type of which (class 1A) is illustrated on the MR arthrogram in **Fig. 88.1**. On this FS T1WI, the hypointense TFC demonstrates a 1-mm region of complete discontinuity (*black arrow*) that is filled with enhancing gadolinium chelate. This central, full-thickness disruption is present several millimeters medial to the TFC's radial insertion, as is typical. MR arthrography for suspected TFC injury is most commonly performed with a single radiocarpal joint injection followed by triplanar image acquisition with GRE to facilitate thin-slice imaging. This type of injection allows, as seen in **Fig. 88.1**, demonstration of contrast leakage from the distal radiocarpal space across the disrupted TFC into the proximal radioulnar space. Partial tears bordering the radiocarpal space exhibit intravasation of contrast. As this technique does not

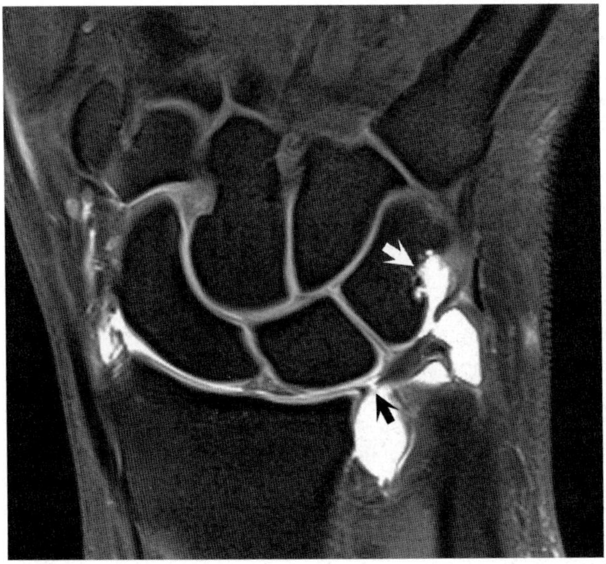

Fig. 88.1

afford evaluation of partial undersurface (proximal) TFC tears, FS T2WI are also frequently obtained. The abnormally intravasated triquetral contrast in **Fig. 88.1** is consistent with the patient's history of a remote fracture of that structure (*white arrow*). Class 1B Palmer lesions are marked by ulnar TFC avulsion with or without styloid fractures. A TFC tear at the insertion of the ulnolunate or ulnotriquetral ligament constitutes a class 1C lesion; a lesion tearing the TFC from its radial attachment (with or without osseous avulsion) is classified as class 1D.

Degenerative tears of the TFC are much more common, but may be only distinguishable by clinical history (i.e., no trauma), a predilection for the elderly, and associated findings. Of the latter, an ulna positive configuration is most common. This is demonstrated in **Figs. 88.2A,B**. The presence of joint effusion, in distinction, suggests a more acute process. Fluid due to an effusion may be distinguished from that of a normal joint by its propensity to enhance on contrast-enhanced MRI. Degenerative TFC defects affect the thinner, more central or ulnar portions of the TFC. The ulnar aspects of the TFC are vascularized, and surgical repair of such lesions is commonly attempted. High SI within the ulnar aspect of the TFC may be nonspecific due to the striations in this area or the presence of the nearby, moderate SI meniscal analogue. Arthrography may be useful in further delineating such lesions. Class 2A and 2B degenerative lesions consist of degenerative changes of the TFC without tear. Class 2B lesions include concurrent lunate or ulnar chondromalacia. Degenerative changes within the TFC may appear as hyperintensity on T1 and PDWI, correlating with myxoid or mucinous infiltration, and commonly involve the proximal TFC surface centrally. Intrasubstance TFC tears may occasionally occur and are best detected on GRE T2WI. High SI of the nearby radial articular cartilage on this sequence may, however, confuse the diagnosis. A class 2C lesion is illustrated in **Figs. 88.2A,B**. Here, the TFC is clearly torn as demonstrated by the high SI at its distal surface on (**A**, *arrow*) FS T2WI. As only one surface is involved, the tear is partial. Within the proximal lunate on the T1WI of **Fig. 88.2B**, low SI is prominent against normal hyperintense fatty marrow. The **(A)** FS T2WI more clearly depicts subchondral cysts surrounded by high SI edema, consistent with ulnocarpal abutment. Associated lunotriquetral perforation would constitute a class 2D lesion; class 2E lesions demonstrate such perforations and severe ulnocarpal arthritis. Ulnocarpal impaction differs from ulnar impingement, in which the distal portion of a shortened ulna articulates with the radius, and ulnar styloid impaction where an elongated styloid process extends and contacts the carpal bones, usually the triquetrum. Further considerations for ulnar wrist pain include avascular necrosis of the lunate, hamate fracture, triquetropisiform arthritis, and tendonitis of the extensor carpi ulnaris—the latter may also be associated with TFC injury.

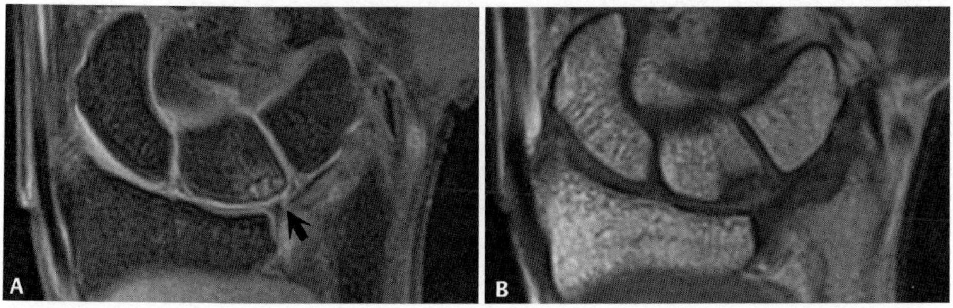

Fig. 88.2 (A,B)

89 Carpal Fractures and Other Causes of Wrist Pain

MRI is the most sensitive modality for the detection of carpal fractures. Findings are typical of nondisplaced fractures elsewhere in the musculoskeletal system, consisting of a fracture line flanked by edema-like SI. **Figure 89.1** demonstrates a transverse, nondisplaced fracture through the waist of the scaphoid. The fracture line appears as low SI on both **(A)** PDWI and **(B)** STIR T2WI, surrounded by marrow edema appearing as low and high SI on those respective sequences. Such edema may also be well demonstrated on FS PDWI. Due to the distal origin of the proximal scaphoid's blood supply, fractures of the proximal scaphoid or the waist are susceptible to AVN. Images obtained 2 weeks later again demonstrate edema-like SI on **(C)** T1WI localized primarily to the proximal pole. On **(D)** postcontrast FS T1WI, however, the proximal pole, in distinction to the distal pole, does not enhance, signifying a lack of viable tissue therein. Over time, SI of the necrotic scaphoid will decrease on T2WI, indicating fibrosis. The same factors that predispose to AVN of the scaphoid—poor vascular supply, inadequate immobilization, or displacement—also predispose to fracture nonunion, particularly of proximal scaphoid fractures and vertically oriented fractures of its middle third. The presence of fluid or fibrous-like (i.e., low SI on all pulse sequences) SI between displaced fragments on MRI signifies impending nonunion, and the lack

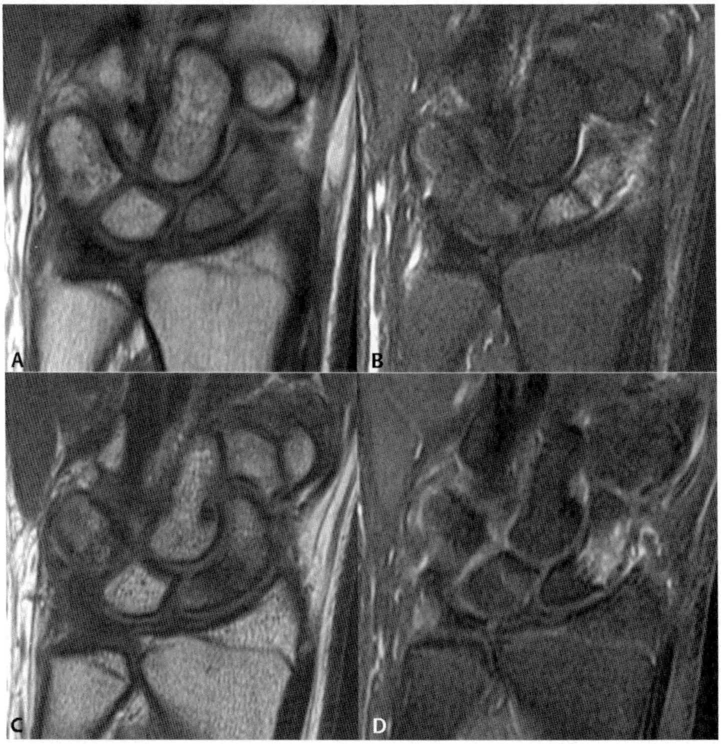

Fig. 89.1 (A–D)

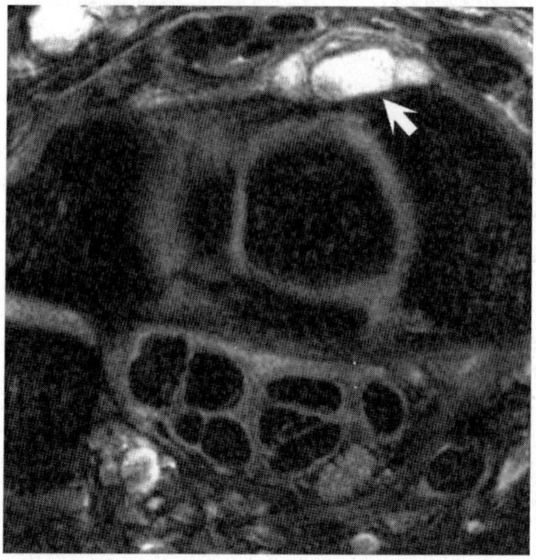

Fig. 89.2

of a bone bridge within 6 months by definition constitutes nonunion. Type 1 nonunion is characterized by nonunion of nondisplaced fragments. Type 2 nonunion involves fragment instability, displacement greater than 1 mm, or dorsal intercalated segment instability (DISI)—distal lunate tilting yielding a scapholunate angle greater than 70 degrees. The scaphocapitate angle may be increased as well. If radioscaphoid arthritis is present, lesions are classified as type 3, whereas scapholunate collapse in the setting of AVN is termed a scaphoid nonunion advanced collapse (SNAC, type 4). With time, resulting arthritis may diffusely involve the wrist (type 5). AVN of the lunate is called Kienböck malacia (or lunatomalacia). The Lichtman classification divides lunate osteonecrosis into lesions that appear radiographically occult (stage 1), demonstrate sclerosis on conventional radiographs (stage 2), and demonstrate collapse without (stage 3A) or with (stage 3B) scapholunate dissociation. Lunate elongation on sagittal MRI is frequently seen in stage 3 lesions. Diffuse osteoarthritis of the wrist constitutes a stage 4 lesion. A fracture line is less uniformly seen with lunate fractures, which are associated with ulnar negative variance. Viable tissue demonstrates typical edema-like SI. Nonviable bone—the presence of which reflects a poorer prognosis—often appears hypointense on both T1 and T2WI. Inflammatory arthritis and ganglion cysts are other possible etiologies of wrist pain. In rheumatoid arthritis, MRI reveals pannus formation around the carpal and metacarpophalangeal joints. This pannus tends to brightly enhance and, when acute, demonstrates decreased SI on T1WI and increased SI on T2WI. Chronic pannus demonstrates low SI on both T1WI and T2WI. Ganglion cysts are the most common tumors of the hand, often arising in close proximity to a major vessel. MRI is useful both in identifying these lesions and in delineating their relationship to nerves, tendons, and vascular structures; such cysts may also be intracapsular. As seen in the axial T2WI of **Fig. 89.2**, the typical appearance is one of well-demarcated, homogeneous, fluid-like SI (*white arrow*). The presence of a cystic soft tissue mass on MRI warrants contrast administration to rule out a sarcoma which will enhance, unlike benign cystic masses. Giant cell tumor of the tendon sheath may also enhance and typically exhibits low SI on T2WI (in part related to hemosiderin deposition).

90 Temporomandibular Joint Disease

The temporomandibular joint (TMJ) is a synovial joint between the mandibular condyle, glenoid fossa, and articular eminence of the temporal bone. MRI reliably evaluates joint pathology and meniscal position in most patients, with the exception of those where metallic dental hardware limits image quality secondary to susceptibility artifact. Bilateral TMJ coils are typically utilized—an important consideration given that over half of patients have bilateral dysfunction. SE T1WI are typically obtained in sagittal-oblique planes through the TMJ with both open- and closed-mouth views. FSE T2WI may be added if inflammatory disease, joint effusion, or meniscal degeneration is suspected. Coronal T1WI may be obtained to help identify meniscal displacement medially or laterally. Cine GRE images may be performed in incremental stages of mouth opening to allow for "dynamic" evaluation of joint motion. The normal appearance of the TMJ is demonstrated in the **(A)** closed- and **(B)** open-mouth FSE T1WI of **Fig. 90.1**. The mandibular condyle is located anterior to the external auditory meatus with its head articulating with the glenoid fossa and articular eminence of the temporal bone. The normal, biconcave meniscus is hypointense on both T1WI and T2WI. When **(A)** the mouth is closed, the mandibular condyle lies centered in the glenoid fossa with the meniscus (*black arrow*) lying along its anterosuperior aspect. With **(B)** mouth opening, the condyle translocates anteriorly with the meniscus moving into the 1- or 2-o'clock position. The posterior portion of the meniscus is attached to the retrodiscal bilaminar zone, which contains elastic tissue and fat and thus appears hyperintense to the meniscus. This hyperintensity is often lost in the presence of pathology. The bilaminar zone connects the meniscus to the temporal bone behind the condyle. The lateral pterygoid is located anterior to the meniscus and divides into superior and inferior heads. The former inserts onto the anteromedial aspect of the meniscus, applying traction to the structure to allow the anterior translocation of the condyle by the inferior belly of the lateral pterygoid.

The most common cause of TMJ dysfunction is an anterior reducible dislocation of the meniscus, seen in the closed-mouth FSE T1WI of **Fig. 90.1C**. Here the low SI meniscus is located anterior to the mandibular condyle with the condyle resting on the retrodiskal tissue. **Figure 90.1D** demonstrates the reducibility of this dislocation: the condyle has translocated anteriorly under the posterior band of the meniscus, allowing it to assume a normal position in open-mouth views. Without such reduction, the anterior defect is termed fixed or nonreducible. **Figures 90.1E and 90.1F** demonstrate a fixed-type of dislocation with the meniscus again seen anterior to the mandibular condyle in **(E)** closed-mouth views. In **(F)** open-mouth views, the low SI disk remains dislocated anteriorly to the condyle. Often a fixed, chronically dislocated meniscus will appear deformed or compressed due to repetitive trauma during opening and closing of the mouth. A so-called locked condyle occurs when mechanical obstruction prevents the anterior translocation of the condyle. As noted previously, medial or lateral displacement of the meniscus is often best-detected on coronal images. Chronically, disk perforations may occur, although this is better evaluated on arthrography than on MRI. Myxomatous degeneration of the meniscal cartilage may also be seen, resulting in increased SI on T2WI. Ancillary findings such as degenerative changes within the superior body of the lateral pterygoid, particularly fibrosis, atrophy, and contracture, may occur. Resultant fatty replacement within the muscle leads to an increased SI on T1WI. Thickening of the fascia within the inferior belly of the lateral pterygoid may also occur as a result of a chronic anterior disk displacement.

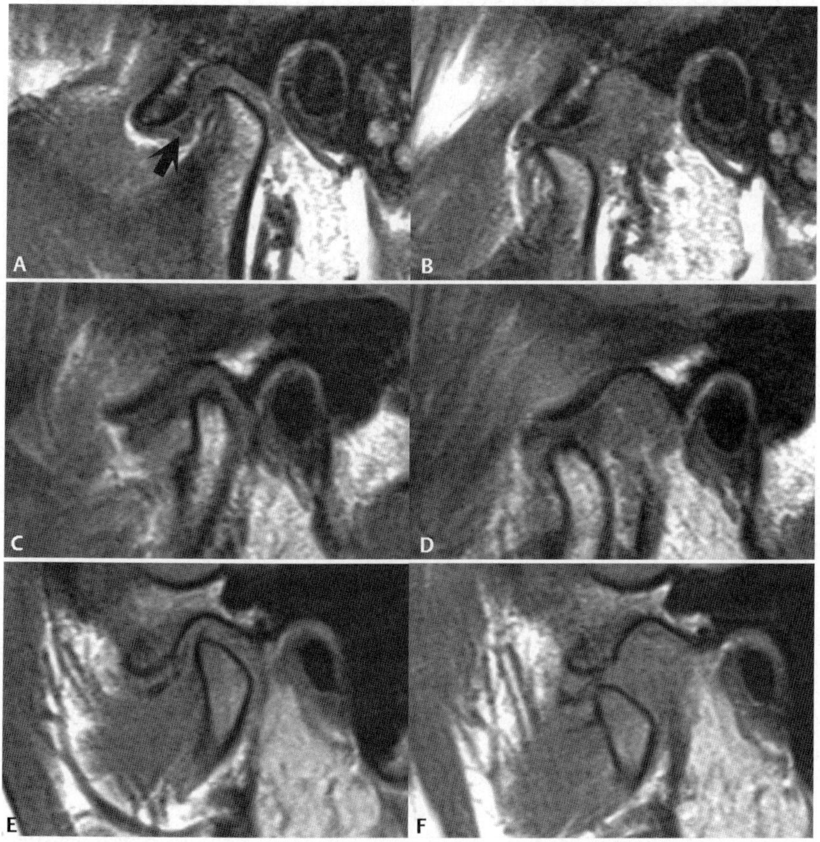

Fig. 90.1 (A–F)

A chronically dislocated disk results in the condyle articulating with the posterior attachment of the disk rather than with the disk itself, leading to inflammation and perforation of the posterior meniscal attachment. Eventually, temporal bone erosion may occur due to the direct contact between the osseous structures. Resulting osteoarthritis occurs with osteophytes and osseous deformities along the glenoid fossa and mandibular condyle. TMJ derangement may eventually lead to osteochondritis or even AVN of the mandibular condyle. Progression of MRI SI in condylar AVN is similar to that previously described in the hip (see Chapter 85). Osteochondritis appears as a focal subarticular bone defect, often with central hypointensity surrounded by hyperintensity on both T1WI and T2WI. Osteoarthritic changes within the TMJ are similar to those in other joints, and include condylar flattening along with articular fossa deformity. Accompanying subchondral sclerosis may be identified as low SI on T1 and T2WI; edema-like SI indicates inflammatory changes within the joint. Other arthritides less commonly involve the TMJ. Detection of those of inflammatory etiology, in particular, is aided by the acquisition of contrast-enhanced T1WI in which inflamed synovium will enhance against a background of low SI joint fluid.

91 Elbow Injuries

The annular, lateral ulnar collateral and the radial collateral ligaments comprise the lateral ligamentous structures of the elbow. The normal appearance of the latter is demonstrated on the coronal oblique T1WI of **Fig. 91.1A**, images acquired in a plane bisecting the epicondyles thus allowing optimal visualization of the elbow's ligaments and tendons. As illustrated, the radial collateral ligament (*black arrow*) originates from the lateral humeral epicondyle and joins with the annular ligament surrounding the radius. The common extensor tendon (*white arrow*), which gives rise to the muscles of hand and wrist extension, also originates from the lateral epicondyle and, as shown in **Fig. 91.1A**, runs superficial to the radial collateral ligament. In the FS T2WI of **Fig. 91.1B**, this tendon demonstrates abnormal fluid-like hyperintensity with discontinuity representing a tear of the common extensor tendon origin. Tendinosis with or without a partial tear also demonstrates increased tendinous SI, but does not show a full thickness defect; thickening and thinning of the tendon are most suggestive of tendinosis while focal intratendinous fluid-like signal supports the diagnosis of a partial tear. Full tendinous disruption with intervening hyperintensity on FS T2 or PDWI indicates a complete tear. The radial collateral ligament also demonstrates fluid-like hyperintensity and discontinuity in **Fig. 91.1B**, consistent with a full-thickness tear. Along with the more posteriorly located lateral ulnar collateral—which transverses the radiocapitellar joint superficial to the annular ligament—the radial collateral ligament prevents posterolateral rotatory elbow instability—a condition leading to perching of the trochlea upon the coronoid, a predisposition to further injury.

A normal medial (ulnar) collateral ligament is illustrated in the coronal T1WI of **Fig. 91.2A** (*white arrow*). This ligament typically connects the inferior medial epicondyle of the humerus to the sublime tubercle of the medial coronoid process of the ulna, running deep to the flexor tendons. Medial epicondylitis is less common than lateral. Changes in regional osseous SI warrant careful evaluation of nearby ligaments and tendons. For example, the coronal FS T2WI of **Fig. 91.2B** demonstrate bone marrow edema-like signal with minimal hyperintensity of the medial epicondyle and marked hyperintensity of the sublime tubercle of the ulna—findings suggestive of bone contusion. However, the visualized portions of (from lateral to medial) the flexor tendon origin, and the anterior and posterior medial (*white arrow*) collateral ligaments demonstrate uniform hypointensity and are apparently intact, although these structures are best evaluated with MR arthrography. Tears of the anterior bundle of the

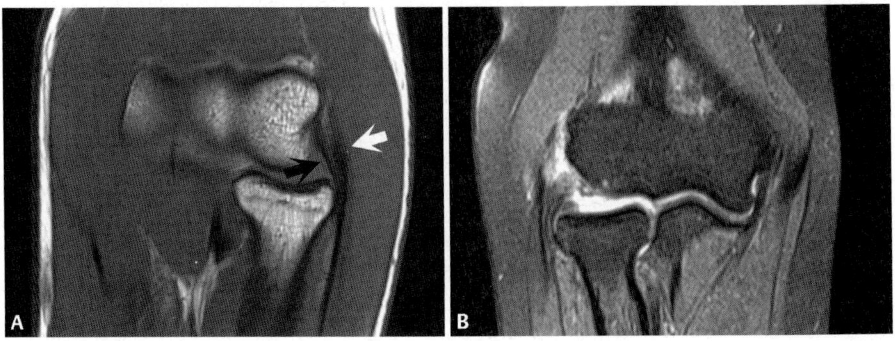

Fig. 91.1 (A,B)

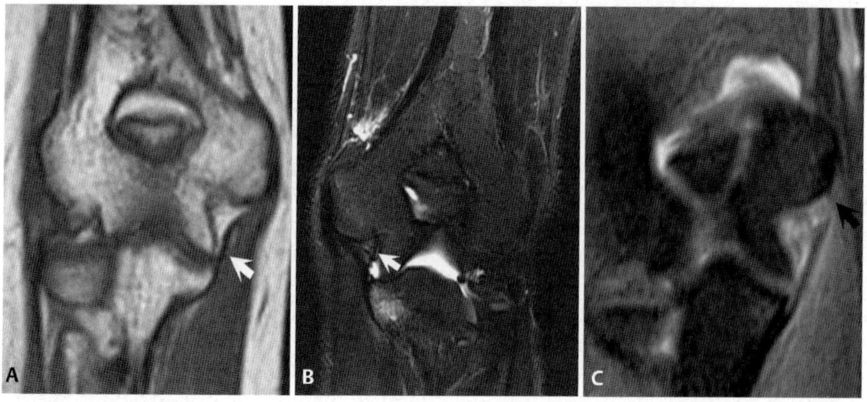

Fig. 91.2 (A–C)

medial collateral ligament are most common, classically occurring in baseball pitchers, presenting with a T-sign reflecting partial detachment from the sublime tubercle. Medial epicondylitis is typified by edema within and thickening of the flexor and pronator tendons arising at the medial humeral condyle, with adjacent bone marrow edema also common. Findings of associated ulnar neuritis such as neuronal hyperintensity and thickening are well visualized on axial images. A full-thickness ulnar collateral ligament tear is illustrated in the FS T2WI of **Fig. 91.2C**. Here, continuity of the low SI ligament is interrupted at its proximal origin by a hyperintense gap (*black arrow*). Chronic tears are associated with calcification (marked ligamentous hypointensity on all pulse sequences) or fatty ligamentous infiltration (hyperintensity on T1 and PDWI). Extravasation of contrast may be seen with MR arthrography in full-thickness tears; partial undersurface tears may be identified by the so-called T-sign. This appearance refers to contrast extending between sublime tubercle and distal attachment of the anterior band of the superficial ligament perpendicular to the contrast normally seen within the ulnohumeral joint. Medial collateral ligament tears may also avulse a portion of the medial epicondyle—a finding identifiable on the radiograph of the patient in **Fig. 91.2C,** but not on MRI. A similar condition may occur in children—known as little leaguer's elbow—consisting of stress fractures through the medial epicondylar epiphysis or medial epicondylar apophysitis. Chronically, the valgus stress causing medial epicondylitis may lead in lateral impaction and resulting radiocapitellar osteochondritis dissecans. As in other joints, fluid on T2WI or contrast with MR arthrography encircling an osteochondral fragment denotes instability. GRE T2WI may aid in identification of free joint fragments. Osteochondritis dissecans involves the epicondylar epiphysis in children between 5 to 10 years old, but does not necessarily result in osseous fragmentation. Finally, tears of the biceps tendon may be visualized on elbow MRI—best seen on images obtained in elbow flexion and abducted shoulder with supinated forearm (FABS position)—as edema-like SI often surrounding a retracted tendon. Axial MRI must thus include the radial tuberosity—the tendon's insertion—and coronal and sagittal fields of view must include sufficient portions of the superior arm so as to identify a significantly retracted tendon.

92 Tendinous Injuries of the Ankle and Foot

MRI accurately depicts the anatomy of the ankle, allowing evaluation of soft tissue masses, and cartilaginous, ligamentous, tendinous, and osseous abnormalities. Utilization of an extremity coil (or in its absence, a knee or head coil, the latter allowing for simultaneous bilateral imaging) maximizes SNR and spatial resolution, with a slice thickness of 3 mm or less desirable. T1WI and T2WI (with or without FS) are obtained, with ligaments and articular cartilage better visualized on GRE T2WI. GRE sequences may, however, suffer from bone-related susceptibility artifact (leading to intraosseous SI loss). The magic angle phenomenon is seen on T2WI, whether FSE or GRE in type, when TE is reasonably short (<60 millisecondsec). In this instance, ligaments or tendons oriented 55 degrees to the main magnetic field (z axis) may manifest an artifactual increase in signal intensity. As in other joints, tendons, ligaments, and cortical bone demonstrate hypointensity due to a lack of mobile protons, whereas hyaline cartilage SI is intermediate. Coronal images accurately depict collateral ligaments and the tibia–fibula–talar relationship; anterior and medially lying tendons are best evaluated on sagittal images.

The Achilles tendon normally demonstrates low SI on all pulse sequences—with some degree of heterogeneity possible normally on T1WI and PDWI—and is best visualized on sagittal and axial images. In axial planes, the Achilles tendon is flat with anterior concavity, posterior convexity, and rounding of its lateral and medial portions. Achilles injuries most commonly occur proximal (2–3 cm) to its calcaneal insertion—a region of sparse vascularity—as in the complete tear illustrated in **Fig. 92.1A**. Here, FS T2WI demonstrates clear, complete disruption in tendinous contour with a ~2 cm fluid-filled (high SI) gap between its proximal and distal portions. Hemorrhagic components may also fill this gap with SI characteristics varying with blood product ages. Imaging of such tears in plantar flexion allows approximation of tendon ends. A vertically oriented, interstitial, partial thickness tear of the Achilles tendon is seen in the FS T2WI of **Fig. 92.1B**. In this case, the low SI tendon is clearly thickened with hyperintense fluid seen within its posterior aspect, but not extending to the surface. Anterior and posterior to the interstitial hyperintensity, the tendon clearly remains intact. A partially torn tendon will demonstrate low to intermediate SI on T1WI. Early Achilles tendonitis, which predisposes to the above entities, may initially appear as increased SI within the anterior fat pad on FS T2WI. With time, tendinous thickening and eventually increases in intratendinous SI are seen on both T1WI and T2WI. This correlates with mucoid degeneration and predisposes to further injury. The Achilles tendon illustrated in **Fig. 92.1C** is thinned compared with that of **Fig. 92.1B**. More moderate hyperintensity present is also consistent with tendinosis. In addition, this case also illustrates replacement of the normal posterior fatty marrow of the calcaneus (suppressed on FS T2WI) with edema. This was felt to represent a stress reaction at the Achilles insertion and is, along with fluid in the retrocalcaneal bursa, typical in appearance for Haglund syndrome.

Other tendons of the foot and ankle are well evaluated with MRI. Tears of the laterally located peroneal tendons are classified as degenerative, partial, or complete, and most are partial and longitudinally oriented. Of the medial tendon group—consisting of the tibialis posterior, flexor hallucis longus, and flexor digitorum longus—the posterior tibial tendon is most frequently injured. Type 1 tears are interstitial, manifesting with thickening and scattered areas of vertically oriented hyperintensity. Type 2 tears

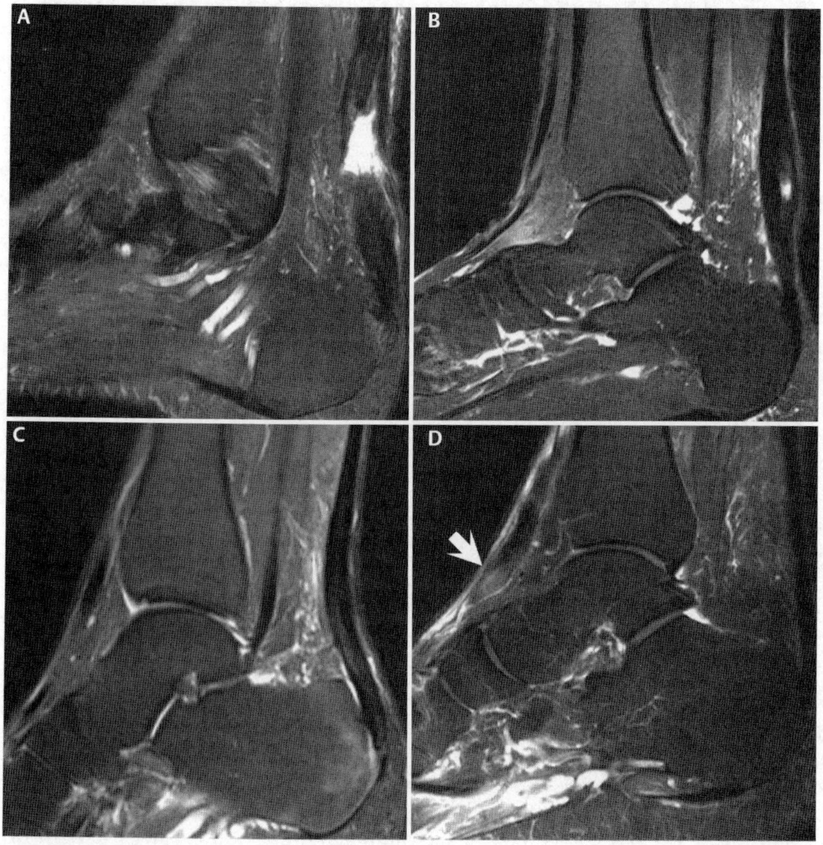

Fig. 92.1 (A–D)

are partial (i.e., extend to only one tendinous surface) and exhibit areas of tendinous attenuation (thinning); type 3 lesions consist of a complete tear. The latter tend to occur in women and young athletes. Tears of the flexor hallucis longus also occur in athletes, but may also result from tendinous compression due to posterior ankle impingement or a prominent os trigonum posteriorly (an accessory retro-talar bone) or from repetitive injury at the first metatarsal (turf toe). Injuries to tendons of the anterior tendon group—the tibialis anterior, peroneus tertius, extensor hallucis longus, and extensor digitorum longus—occur rarely often as a result of direct injury. Peroneal tendon injuries may also arise secondary to calcaneal fractures or in the presence of an os peroneum (an accessory ossicle within the distal peroneus longus near the cuboid). **Figure 92.1D** illustrates a case of complete, retracted tibialis anterior tear (*white arrow*) in a patient with chronic tendinosis. The latter findings are exhibited by the intermediate SI seen within the tendon as it courses adjacent to the distal anterior portion of the talus. Near the talonavicular joint the tendon tapers, and distal to this demonstrates high SI fluid and only a few low SI fibers. Any injured tendon may eventually become entrapped by surrounding callus and scar tissue. Tendinous dislocations and subluxations are also readily visible on MRI.

93 Ligamentous Injuries of the Ankle

Ligamentous injuries of the ankle are quite common and well visualized on MRI. Ligamentous structures appear as uniform low SI on all conventional pulse sequences, although magic angle effects can produce a focus of high SI on short TE sequences (T2WI). Familiarity with the normal ligamentous anatomy of the ankle is crucial. The ankle can be divided into medial and lateral ligamentous compartments. The lateral collateral ligamentous complex is most commonly injured and consists of the anterior talofibular, posterior talofibular, and calcaneofibular ligaments. The normal appearance of the anterior talofibular ligament is illustrated in **Fig. 93.1A**, an axial FS T2WI illustrating this low SI ligament spanning from the anterior portion of the fibular lateral malleolus to the talar neck. The posterior talofibular ligament is also best visualized on axial or coronal images and spans from the fibular malleolar fossa to the posterior talar tubercle. The anterior talofibular ligament, due to its relative lack of strength compared with other lateral compartment ligaments, is the first and often only ligament torn in inversion injuries of the plantar-flexed foot. Ligamentous stretching constitutes a grade 1 lateral ankle sprain; a partial tear represents a grade 2 lesion. Grade 3 lateral ankle sprains consist of complete tearing of anterior talofibular and calcaneofibular ligaments. The axial FS T2WI of **Fig. 93.1B** demonstrate thickening, intermediate SI, and discontinuity of the fibers of the anterior talofibular ligament, findings consistent with a partial tear (*white arrow*). A complete tear of the anterior talofibular ligament is seen in **Fig. 93.1C** in which the ligament is simply absent. Other appearances of complete tears include a fluid-filled gap or focal ligamentous discontinuity with fraying of its ends. Soft tissue edema and joint effusions are reliable findings that indicate lesion acuity, resolving in the setting of chronic tears. A thick, irregular ligament also signifies chronicity. MR arthrography may be used to assess lateral ankle injuries. In complete anterior talofibular tears, contrast will extend to surround the talar neck. If a calcaneofibular tear is present, contrast will enter the peroneal tendon sheath.

The deltoid or the medial collateral ligament is commonly sprained but infrequently torn. This ligament consists of four superficial and two deep components. The superficial components all originate at the medial malleolus, extending to the navicular (tibionavicular), sustentaculum tali (tibiocalcaneal), medial talar tubercle (superficial tibiotalar), and spring ligament (tibiospring). The spring or plantar calcaneonavicular ligament is a deep ligament stabilizing the arch and spanning from the

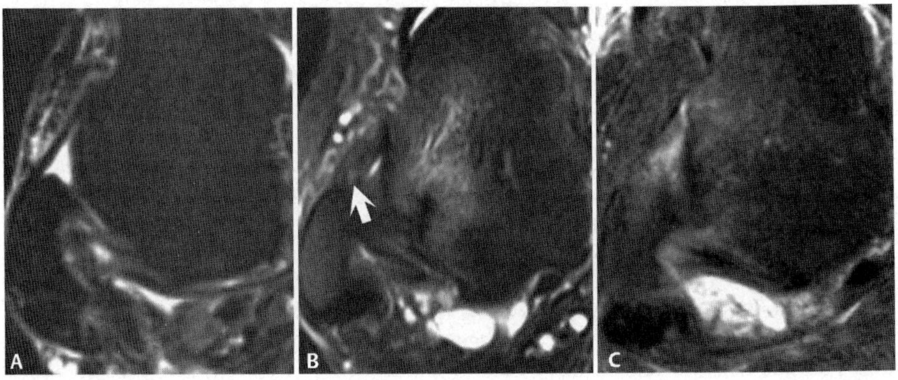

Fig. 93.1 (A–C)

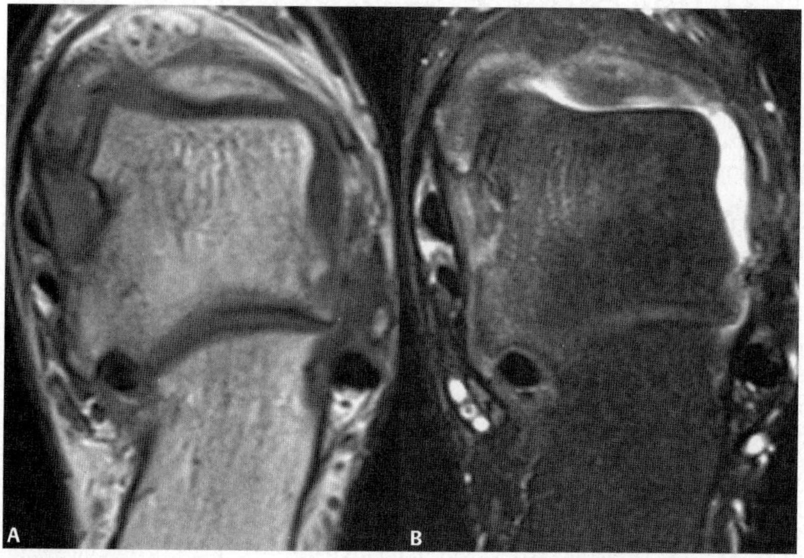

Fig. 93.2 (A,B)

sustentaculum tali to the medial navicular. The deep ligaments arise at the anterior colliculus of the medial malleolus and attach to the anterior and posterior portions of the talus (anterior and posterior deep tibiotalar ligaments). **Figures 93.2A and 93.2B** demonstrate a tear of the deltoid ligament, specifically of its posterior tibiotalar component. On **(A)** paraxial T1WI, the ligament is thickened, has lost its striated appearance, and demonstrates moderate SI. There is also the suggestion of scattered hypointensity within the medial talus and medial malleolus, consistent with bone contusion. Avulsion fracture of the latter may occur with some deltoid tears. **(B)** A paraxial FS T2WI demonstrates interstitial hyperintensity within the ligament and also hyperintensity within the talus and medial malleolus, again correlating with marrow edema. At the insertion of the ligament at the medial talus, there is curvilinear hyperintensity suggestive of a nondisplaced avulsion fracture. Coronal imaging identified tears of both superficial and deep talotibial components—the latter are typically more resistant to injury. Concomitant syndesmotic injury is common with medial ligamentous complex injuries. The tibiofibular syndesmosis consists of the anteroinferior and posteroinferior tibiofibular ligaments as well as the interosseous tibiofibular ligament. Syndesmotic injuries constitute the so-called high ankle sprain, resulting from external rotation of the dorsiflexed foot. The anteroinferior tibiofibular ligament often exhibits a fluid-filled gap or discontinuity suggesting a complete tear, whereas the stronger posteroinferior tibiofibular ligament is rarely completely torn. Widening of the syndesmosis may be seen as a result of injury.

In the foot, the Lisfranc ligament connects the base of the medial cuneiform to the medial base of the second metatarsal, substituting for the absent intermetatarsal ligament between the first and second metatarsal. Sprains of the Lisfranc ligament, the so-called midfoot sprain, constitute the second most common foot injury in athletes (after metatarsophalangeal injuries). Signs of Lisfranc sprains on MRI include fluid SI surrounding or extending within the ligament or first metatarsal, as well as a visibly enlarged, irregular ligament.

94 Other Ankle and Foot Disorders

Osteochondral lesions of the talus may arise as a result of direct injury or repetitive microtrauma. **Figure 94.1A** is an example of such a lesion with a displaced fragment clearly seen within the posterosuperior aspect of the posterior subtalar facet on sagittal FS T2WI. Homogeneous hyperintensity within the calcaneus and talus correlates with associated bone contusion (better appreciated as hypointensity on T1WI). Talar osteochondral lesions are divided into five categories by the MRI criteria devised by Hepple. Stage 1 lesions are radiographically occult, consisting of damage to only the articular cartilage. Concomitant cartilaginous and osseous fractures with and without edema comprise stage 2A and 2B lesions, respectively. A detached but nondisplaced fragment is seen in stage 3. Fragment displacement constitutes a stage 4 lesion. Stage 5 lesions are marked by subchondral cyst formation. **Figures 94.1B and 94.1C** demonstrate an osteochondral lesion within the posteromedial talus. Inferior and superior portions of the medial cortical surface are disrupted on both coronal **(B)** T1WI and **(C)** FS T2WI. Superiorly, formation of a subchondral cyst is best appreciated on **(C)** FS T2WI, consistent with a grade 5 lesion. Edema—hypo- and hyperintense on the T1WI and FS T2WI, respectively—is seen throughout the talus. In the midst of this edema on the **(C)** FS T2WI there is a smaller focus of hypointensity. Although such areas often represent reactive sclerosis, here the hypointensity correlated with an area of necrotic bone associated with AVN. AVN most frequently involves the talar dome, the typical appearance consisting of a low SI ischemic foci surrounded by hyperintense (on FS images) marrow edema. Chronically, the surrounding edema resolves with the osteonecrotic focus persisting. More diffusely infarcted bone often exhibits serpiginous hypointensity on T1WI. Edema in AVN is more prominent compared with that typically seen in osteochondral lesions. The latter lesions tend to exhibit edema emanating to a more localized area around the lesion. The typical pattern of an osteochondral lesion is exhibited in the sagittal T1WI and FS T2WI of **Figs. 94.1D,E**: patchy hyperintensity on **(E)** FS T2WI extends peripherally from an osteochondral defect seen along the lateral surface of the talar dome. Cortical disruption is again seen along the articular surface with accompanying subchondral cyst formation—demonstrating high SI on **(E)** FS T2WI and low SI on **(D)** T1WI—denoting a stage 5 lesion. Contrast-enhanced MRI aids in detecting viable (enhancing) bone fragments, hypertrophic synovium, and subchondral edema. MR arthrography directly identifies detached fragments: contrast (or synovial fluid in nonenhanced MRI) extending completely beneath an osteochondral fragment, for example, indicates the presence of a detached stage 3 lesion; irregular, incomplete hyperintensity suggests a stage 2 lesion. Unfortunately, nearby hyperintense or enhancing granulation tissue (indicative of healing) may mimic the appearance of underlying joint fluid or contrast, respectively. Underlying hypointensity is more specific for healing. In this figure, the articular cartilage of the talus, typically of moderate SI on T1 and T2WI although best identified as hyperintensity on GRE T2WI, also demonstrates irregularity and hyperintensity on **(E)** FS T2WI. Other cartilaginous abnormalities include structural deformity, bowing, or joint fluid infiltrating within or beneath.

An assortment of other abnormalities may affect the foot and ankle. Freiberg infraction—osteonecrosis of the 2nd metatarsal head—is best visualized on sagittal MRI, demonstrating subchondral marrow edema on FS T2WI and flattening of the anterosuperior aspect of the metatarsal head. Osteochondrosis of the navicular is termed Köhler disease. Stress fractures are detected earlier on MRI than on conventional

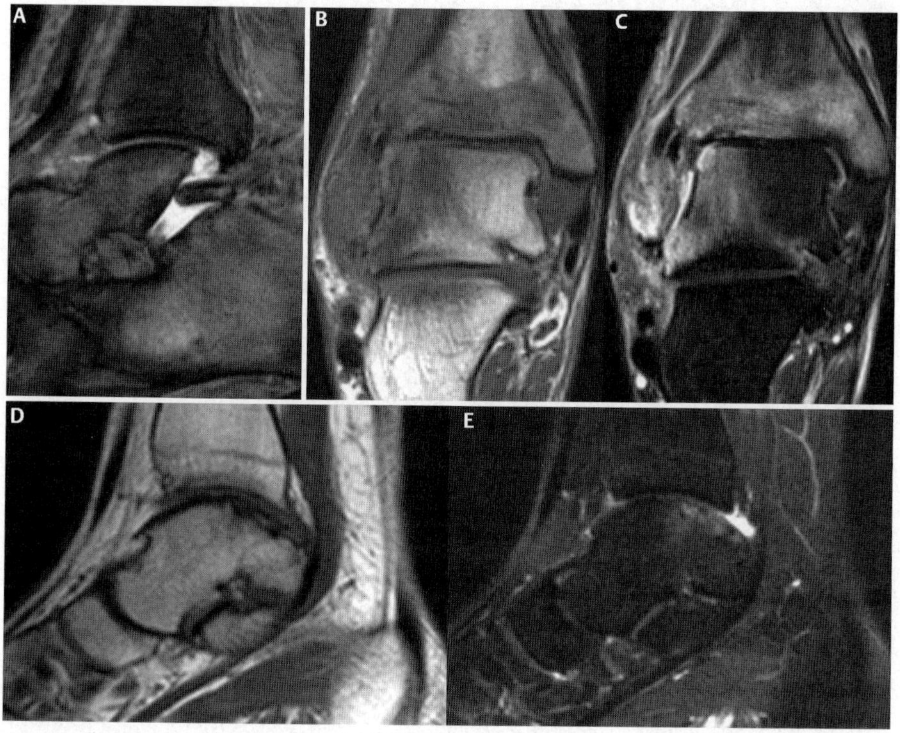

Fig. 94.1 (A–E)

radiography with SI changes that are similar to that of bone contusions (described above), consisting of edema-like SI surrounding an irregular hypointense fracture line, although the latter is not uniformly identified. Various named fractures of the distal tibia and fibula appear similar. Also on the differential for diffuse marrow edema is migratory osteoporosis, distinguishable only by its transience. Diabetic arthropathy and osteomyelitis appear similar. Surrounding cellulitis, sinus tracts, and abscesses typify the latter, whereas the former tends to fragment bone and lack overlying ulcers. Both are accompanied by marrow enhancement and joint effusions. Neuropathic joints, in distinction, affect multiple joints and are typified by a lack of pure edema SI, often demonstrating low SI on both T1WI and T2WI. Morton neuroma presents as a dumbbell-shaped mass between any of the metatarsal heads but most commonly the 3rd and 4th. This lesion exhibits moderate SI on conventional MRI and variable enhancement. In distinction, true neuromas are typically hyperintense on T2WI. Plantar fascitis (predisposed by a plantar enthesophyte) is visualized as edema-like SI within the plantar aponeurosis, which contrasts well against SI of more superficial fat. Pigmented villonodular synovitis is best identified by hypointense (owing to paramagnetic hemosiderin) joint deposits on conventional MRI. Inflammatory arthritis exhibits a characteristic enhancing pannus.

95 Musculoskeletal Neoplasms

The distinction between benign and malignant bone tumors is frequently not possible on MRI, although benign lesions generally possess well-defined peripheral margins and lack adjacent soft tissue masses and spare cortical bone. The high SI of cartilage on T2WI aids in the identification of chondroid lesions. Osteochondromas are the most common benign osseous tumor, the cortex of these lesions being continuous with the parent bone. A hyperintense (on T2WI) cartilaginous cap greater than 1.5 cm in thickness in the presence of a closed physis suggests chondrosarcomatous degeneration as do low SI foci—correlating with calcification—therein. A surrounding dark rim of perichondrium may be visualized on T2WI. Enchondromas may also degenerate into chondrosarcomas—indicated by adjacent soft tissue, epiphyseal, or cortical invasion—although those outside the appendicular long bones and axial skeleton tend to be benign. Lobules of chondroid matrix distinguish such lesions from a bone infarction. The classic fluid-fluid level of an aneurysmal bone cyst involving the talus is illustrated on FS T2WI (**A**) and T1WI (**B**) of **Fig. 95.1**. The fluid-fluid level is a result of differences in densities and MRI SI appearances of cystic fluid contents, relating to the stage of blood products within. This finding is also associated with telangiectatic osteosarcoma, but can be seen in other entities as well, including giant cell tumors. A fluid-fluid level is present on the sagittal T2WI of the lumbar spine in **Fig. 95.1C**. Here, it is associated with an expansile, enhancing osteoblastoma arising from the right vertebral pedicle on the contrast-enhanced T1WI of **Fig. 95.1D**. Osteoid osteomas appear similar, only smaller and classically containing a well-defined nidus with high and low SI on T2WI and T1WI, respectively, and copious amounts of surrounding marrow edema. Giant cell tumors and chondroblastomas are best characterized by their location within epiphyseal equivalents, the latter also exhibiting prominent marrow edema. The MRI appearance of benign soft tissue tumors may be more specific for certain lesions: hemangiomas, lipomas, and subacute hematomas demonstrate hyperintensity on T1WI, reflecting fat in the former two and methemoglobin in the latter. Hemangiomas also rapidly enhance due to their high vascularity. Hemosiderin in pigmented villonodular synovitis leads to low SI within the synovium on all pulse sequences. Amyloid depositions are also hypointense, but not as well seen on GRE T2WI due to amyloid's lack of paramagnetism. Periarticularly, synovial sarcoma is an additional consideration and may be confused for a ganglion cyst without contrast administration, the former brightly enhancing. Scar tissue and various fibromatoses appear hypointense on conventional sequences, with only the latter enhancing.

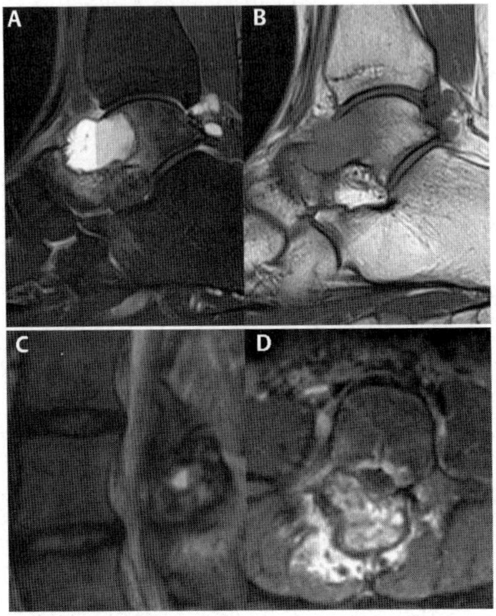

Fig. 95.1 (A–D)

Osteosarcoma is the second most common primary tumor of bone after multiple myeloma. The FS T1WI of

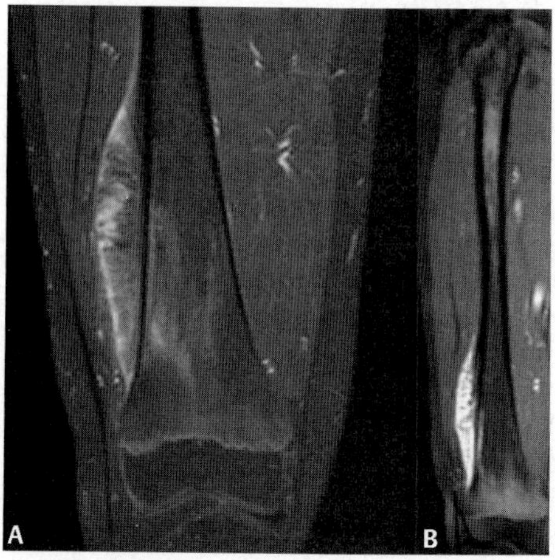

Fig. 95.2 (A,B)

Fig. 95.2A demonstrate hypointense linear bone oriented perpendicular to the low SI osseous cortex, well visualized against the background of enhancing abnormal soft tissue. As seen here, MRI is useful at demonstrating extension of osseous neoplastic lesions into nearby tissues and delineating intramedullary extension—indicated by disruption or hyperintensity within the normally low SI bone cortex on T2WI or contrast-enhanced T1WI. The presence of skip lesions may be documented on MRI and as such the entirety of the involved bone should be imaged. The contrast-enhanced T1WI of **Fig. 95.2B** was obtained one year after (and with a larger FOV than) that in **Fig. 95.2A**, and demonstrates a skip lesion within the proximal femur. Ewing sarcoma may originate from bone or soft tissue. A particularly aggressive, heterogeneously enhancing lesion is illustrated in the contrast-enhanced T1WI of **Fig. 95.3**. Multiple enhancing lesions are seen throughout the visualized pelvis and proximal femurs, consistent with widespread metastatic disease. The origin of the lesion in **Fig. 95.3** could not be definitively localized and thus, in this child, the primary differential consideration was metastatic rhabdomyosarcoma (the most common malignant soft tissue tumor in children), which demonstrates similar nonspecific SI characteristics. In an adult similar-appearing soft tissue masses include malignant fibrous histiocytomas—an infiltrative-appearing tumor that is relatively hypointense on T2WI (as are its benign analogue and fibrosarcomas) due to the presence of copious fibrous tissue. Other soft tissue malignancies with unique MRI appearances include well-differentiated liposarcoma and melanoma, which are both hyperintense on T1WI owing to the presence of fat and free radicals within melanin, respectively.

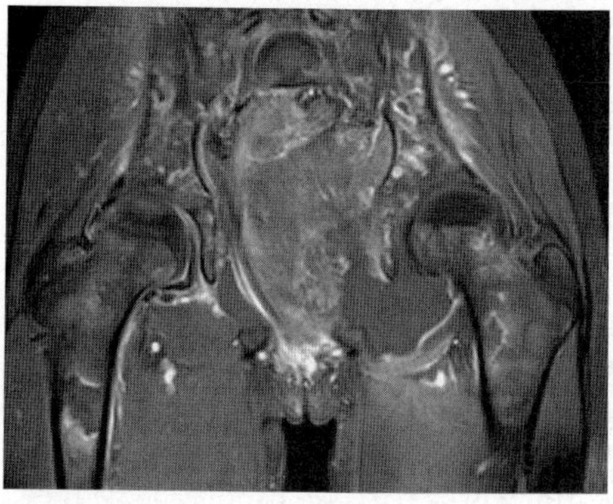

Fig. 95.3

96 Diseases of Marrow

The rationale for the SI characteristics of normal adult bone marrow on SE and FSE T1 and T2WI has been described in previous chapters. Marrow SI on MRI must be interpreted in the context of a patient's age. At birth, hematologically active red marrow is widespread, its higher water content yielding a lower SI appearance than fatty marrow on T1WI. In the infantile stage of marrow development, fatty replacement begins at the phalanges, apophyses, and epiphyses. From that point on, fatty replacement progresses proximally, ending in complete replacement within the appendicular skeleton and a predominance of yellow over red marrow in the axial skeleton. Diffuse reconversion of yellow to red marrow may occur in pathologic conditions and normally in some individuals. The latter is erythropoietin-mediated and often present in endurance athletes and obese smokers, with a female predilection overall. Reconversion typically proceeds from the axial skeleton, where some residual hematopoietic marrow normally remains, to the appendicular system. Pathologic conditions leading to marrow hypointensity on T1WI include disorders leading to proliferation of cell line precursors such as leukemia, multiple myeloma, or polycythemia vera. The latter may progress to myelofibrosis, which appears as hypointensity on both T1WI and T2WI. Use of erythro- and granulocyte-stimulating chemotherapeutic agents may result in a similar appearance. The most common cause of hematogenous marrow reconversion is chronic anemia such as thalassemia or sickle cell. A case of the latter is illustrated in **Fig. 96.1A**. The normal high SI marrow of the femur and tibia demonstrate diffuse hypointensity on T1WI, correlating with proliferation of hematopoietic marrow in response to the associated anemia. In the setting of multiple blood transfusions (i.e., hemosiderosis), susceptibility effects from deposited iron lead to markedly low SI on FSE and GRE T2WI. Bone infarction is a possible sequela of sickle cell disease, presenting with focal hypointensity. Other factors may lead to bone infarction, synonymous with AVN discussed in previous chapters, including corticosteroid use, alcoholism, and collagen vascular disease. The patient in **Fig. 96.1B** was on long-term steroid therapy for asthma: T1WI demonstrate focal areas of linear hypointensity outlining more moderate SI regions within the distal femur and proximal tibia. The hypointense outline correlates with sclerosis and is characteristic for a bone infarct as is the double-line sign on T2WI, whereby a hyperintense line is seen just within the hypointense sclerotic outline, correlating with granulation tissue. The area circumscribed by sclerosis in bone infarctions may demonstrate variable SI consistent with that of fatty marrow, hemorrhage, edema, or collagenous infiltration.

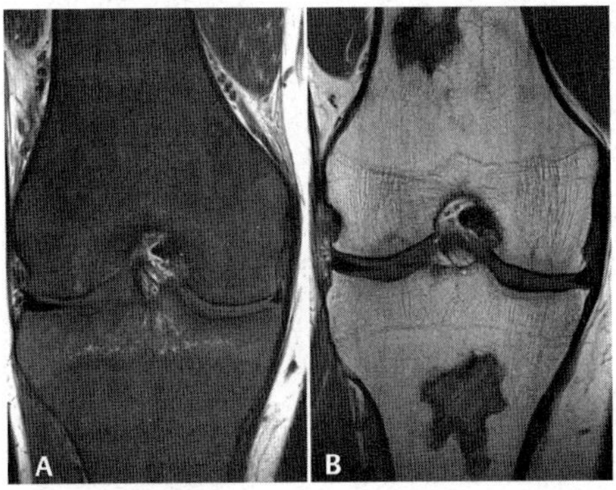

Fig. 96.1 (A,B)

The spectrum of MRI appearances for multiple myeloma—the most common primary bone neoplasia—has been described in previous chapters. Of note, multifocal hypointensity on T1WI may be seen in monoclonal gammopathy of undetermined significance; however, diffuse marrow replacement is more typical of myeloma. If unapparent on MRI, myeloma is associated with a more delayed progression. A solitary plasmacytoma within a vertebral body can have

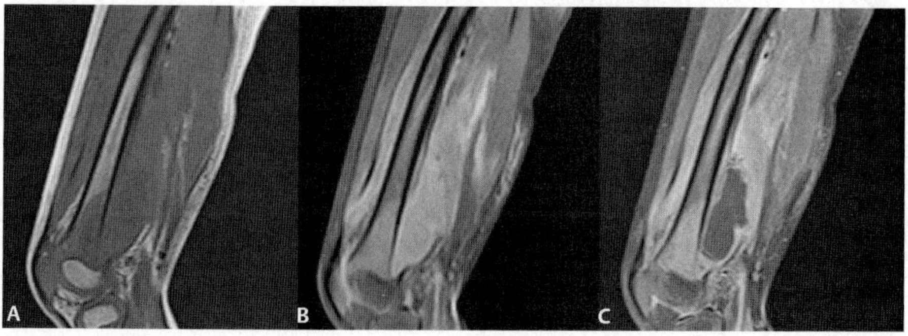

Fig. 96.2 (A–C)

an appearance visually similar to the human brain. Following chemotherapy for myeloma, resolution of lesion enhancement or confinement of enhancement to a peripheral distribution is a marker of therapeutic response, as is the transformation of a diffuse pattern of involvement into a focal or variegated pattern. Focal areas of T1 hypointensity may also represent metastatic disease. The halo sign—in which a ring of hyperintensity on T2WI surrounds the lesion—is indicative of a metastatic process, although a focus of high SI in the center of an osseous lesion is a marker of benignity. Metastatic lesions often enhance, although this may be confused with enhancement of vestiges of hematopoietic marrow normally present in the axial skeleton. The former tend to enhance much more briskly, and demonstrate low ADC values if DWI is performed. Osteomyelitis is an additional cause of marrow edema. Although radionucleotide bone scans are often performed to evaluate osteomyelitic foci, MRI offers superior sensitivity, better sinus tract delineation, and improved detection of associated abscesses while allowing for operative planning. Typical SI characteristics are illustrated in **Figs. 96.2A,B,C**. Here, extensive, confluent low and high SI on **(A)** T1WI and **(B)** FS T2WI, respectively, involves the distal femur. Surrounding myositis and fascitis are also present. Marrow SI changes in reactive marrow edema secondary to overlying soft tissue infections are generally less confluent than the changes seen here. **(C)** Contrast-enhanced FS T1WI conclusively demonstrates the presence of a posterior subperiosteal abscess with an enhancing rim surrounding a low SI fluid collection. The distal femur enhances as well. Bone neoplasia, both primary and metastatic, are differential considerations for this appearance, but tend not to have a subperiosteal collection in the absence of treatment history. An osteoid osteoma may evoke extensive edema that obscures detection of its hypointense central nidus on FS T2WI. The distinction between osteomyelitis, diabetic arthropathy, and neuropathic joints is particularly difficult within the lower extremity as further discussed in Chapter 94.

97 Overview of MR Contrast Agents

Extracellular gadolinium chelates are the most common contrast agents utilized in clinical MRI. Gadolinium is a heavy metal, extremely toxic in its elemental form. The safety basis of gadolinium-based contrast agents thus lies in the ability of a chelate to tightly bind the gadolinium ion, ensuring rapid, near complete excretion (see Chapter 98). The paramagnetic effect of the gadolinium ion reduces T1 and T2 of nearby mobile protons, changes manifest as increased and decreased SI on T1WI and T2WI, respectively. The latter effect—attributable to susceptibility or T2* effects—is used in first-pass perfusion imaging, but effects on tissue T1 are more commonly exploited clinically. In the CNS, BBB disruption allows passage of the extracellular chelate into pathologic tissue, resulting in lesion enhancement on T1WI, improving detection and lesion characterization. Illustrated in **Fig. 97.1** is a lung cancer metastasis to the brain on **(A)** pre- and **(B)** postcontrast T1WI, with enhancement improving both conspicuity and definition of the lesion margin in this instance. On postcontrast images, vascular structures such as the choroid plexus and nasal turbinates normally enhance, allowing identification of contrast-enhanced scans. Similar principles allow depiction of vascular anatomy with contrast-enhanced MRA as in Chapters 99 through 101. Contrast-enhanced lesion detection in other regions of the body is reliant on metal chelate passage through leaky capillaries of granulation tissue or neoplastic lesions. The latter mechanism is demonstrated in **Fig. 97.2**, where the conspicuity of a squamous cell carcinoma metastasis is markedly improved from that on **(A)** precontrast T1WI with (B) contrast-enhanced FS T1WI. Talar and calcaneal enhancement in **Fig. 97.2B** illustrates the importance of utilizing fat suppression to aid in visualization of enhancing osseous pathology, a point further emphasized in **Fig. 97.3**. Here, **(A)** sagittal T1WI demonstrates replacement of the normal high SI fatty marrow of T12 and L1 with metastatic tumor. Because subtle enhancing lesions are difficult to detect against high SI marrow on contrast-enhanced T1WI, spectral fat suppression is used to null the normal hyperintense signal of fatty bone marrow. This is illustrated in the **(B)** contrast-enhanced FS T1WI of **Fig. 97.3** in which the T12 and L1 vertebral bodies brightly enhance compared with the suppressed SI of the other visualized vertebrae. STIR fat suppression nulls SI from all protons with short T1, and as such may suppress tissues with T1 reduced by the presence of gadolinium chelates. The approved nonprotein binding gadolinium chelates in the United States (**see Fig. 98.1**) have similar efficacy—as measured by T1 relaxivity—all less than that of the single approved agent with transient protein-binding, MultiHance (Bracco Diagnostics, Inc., Princeton, NJ). Large proteins like albumin tumble or spin at a slower rate than gadolinium chelate molecules. The benzyloxymethyl group (**see Fig. 98.1**) of MultiHance, however, allows transient interactions with albumin and other proteins, reducing the chelate's tumbling. This reduced rate allows more efficient interactions with bulk water, improving relaxivity. The standard dose of all agents in the U.S. for nonangiographic applications is 0.1 mmol/kg.

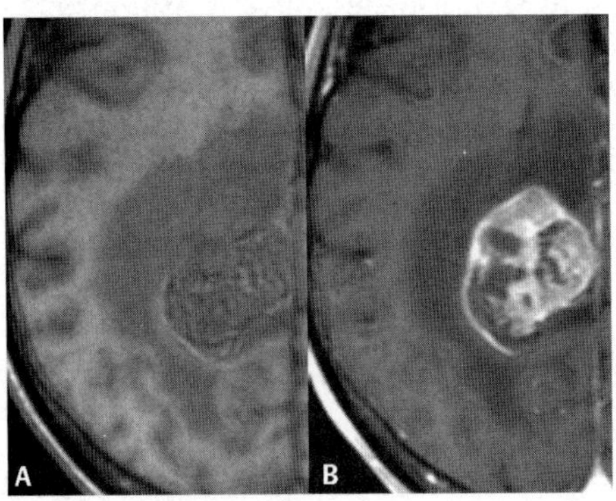

Fig. 97.1 (A,B)

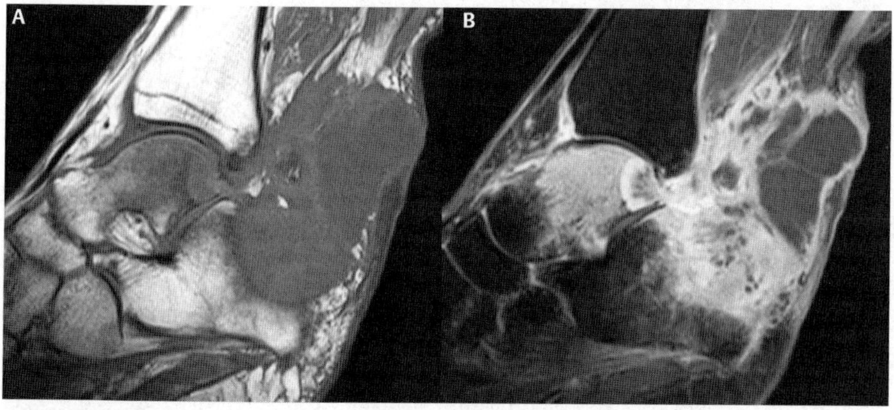

Fig. 97.2 (A,B)

Although agent relaxivity decreases at 3 versus 1.5 T, improved lesion enhancement is seen at 3 T. This is due, in part, to the theoretical doubling in SNR seen at 3 versus 1.5 T and to the prolongation in T1 of surrounding tissues (i.e., normal brain parenchyma in contrast-enhanced neuroimaging or background tissue in contrast-enhanced MRA) at 3 T, leading to, on contrast-enhanced T1WI, less background SI.

With the exception of MultiHance and an additional agent used strictly for liver imaging, Eovist (Primovist; Bayer Healthcare, LLC, Shawnee Mission, KS), all gadolinium chelates are excreted 100% renally. The partial hepatobiliary excretion of the two above agents allows acquisition of images with hepatic enhancement due to hepatocellular uptake. Detection of metastases and intrinsic pathologies associated with poorly functioning hepatocytes is facilitated by the hypointensity of these entities against the enhancing background (see Chapter 66). Lesion detection with large, superparamagnetic (nongadolinium) iron oxide-based particles, like Feridex (AMAG Pharmaceuticals, Lexington, MA), is based on similar principles. Uptake within hepatic Kupffer cells results in normal hepatic tissue exhibiting a low SI on T2WI due to susceptibility (T2*) effects. The safety profile of the approved iron-based agents is in general worse than that of the gadolinium chelates, with a higher percentage of minor adverse events. Blood pool agents like gadofosveset have only been recently approved, and may prove useful in angiographic applications. Such agents bind strongly to albumin improving relaxivity and containing the compound within the intravascular space. Such agents also exhibit a prolonged steady-state phase, allowing time to perform high-resolution peripheral or coronary MRA. Oral contrast agents are rarely used in MRI. Substances high in fat or manganese (i.e., milk and blueberry juice) provide high SI contrast on T1WI, whereas iron-containing preparations can be used to provide low luminal SI on T1WI and T2WI. Barium may also be used, but is a poor agent for MRI, leading to low and high luminal SI on T1WI and T2WI, respectively.

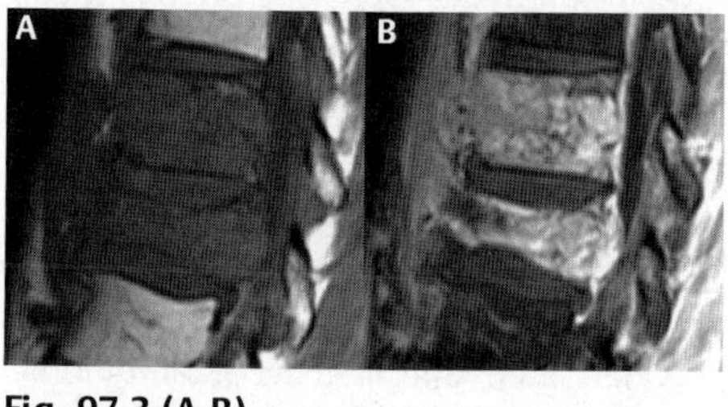

Fig. 97.3 (A,B)

98 Adverse Reactions

Despite marketing strategies implying the contrary, no rigorous study has ever demonstrated a difference in the frequency of mild adverse reactions—which include nausea (1.5%) and urticaria (0.5%)—among the various gadolinium chelate contrast agents. Severe anaphylactoid reactions with such agents are rare and even more rarely result in death. Treatment is similar to that for reactions induced by iodinated contrast media, initially consisting of cessation of agent injection and inhaled oxygen. Urticaria alone may only require use of diphenhydramine for treatment, whereas laryngeal edema and/or bronchospasm require administration of intramuscular epinephrine (1:1,000), supplemented for bronchospasm by an inhaled bronchodilator. The treatment of hypotension (alone or with tachycardia) is fluid resuscitation. Hypotension with bradycardia (vagal reaction) may require IV atropine as well. Gadolinium chelates do cross the placenta and persist in amniotic fluid. The effects of this are unknown, although no teratogenic consequences have been observed to date in humans. Gadolinium chelates should only be administered in pregnancy if the desired information can be obtained by no other means and if such information is crucial to the fetus or patient imminently during pregnancy. In this case, macrocyclic agents should be administered at the smallest dose possible. Breast feeding should be avoided within 24 hours of gadolinium chelate administration.

Gadolinium chelates are not nephrotoxic. However, in patients with renal failure (glomerular filtration rate [GFR] $<$30 mL/min per 1.73 m^2) such agents have been associated with nephrogenic systemic fibrosis (NSF), a potentially fatal disease first reported in 1997. NSF often manifests first in the legs with pain and swelling, progressing to skin thickening and eventual contracture. Internal organ fibrosis may be seen later in the disease. The proposed pathophysiology of NSF relates to in vivo dechelation with subsequent deposition of gadolinium ions in tissue inducing fibroblast proliferation. Most cases have occurred in renal failure patients who have received multiple, often high doses (such as those used in contrast-enhanced MRA) of gadolinium chelates over time (with administration specifically of the less stable chelates)—the latter observation suggesting a cumulative dose dependence. Prompt repeated dialysis may lower the risk of NSF. Unlike rates of minor contrast reactions, the gadolinium chelates agents do differ in their association with NSF. The incidence of NSF depends on chelate stability and relates to the fundamental safety basis of the gadolinium chelates—that the gadolinium ion (a toxic transitional metal) must be tightly bound to the chelate providing for near complete renal clearance. The strength of this binding is related to chelate molecular structure. Specifically, macrocyclic agents are more stable than their linear counterparts, and among the latter, those bearing an ionic charge are more stable than those without. This correlates well with experience regarding the five major U.S. Food & Drug Administration (FDA-) approved gadolinium chelates, whose chemical structures are shown in **Fig. 98.1**. Omniscan (GE Healthcare, Waukesha, WI)—a nonionic, linear agent—has been implicated in the majority of unconfounded (i.e., cases where only one agent has been administered) worldwide NSF cases. The rate of NSF with Omniscan in patients with stage 5 kidney disease (GFR $<$15 mL/min per 1.73 m^2) has been estimated at 18%. Optimark, another nonionic, linear agent, is responsible for a smaller number of cases than Omniscan and Magnevist (Bayer Schering Pharma, Berlin, Germany) the latter a more widely used, intermediate-stability ionic, linear chelate. When accounting for the less-frequent utilization of Optimark (Mallinckrodt, Inc., St. Louis, MO), however, the overall rate of NSF is higher versus

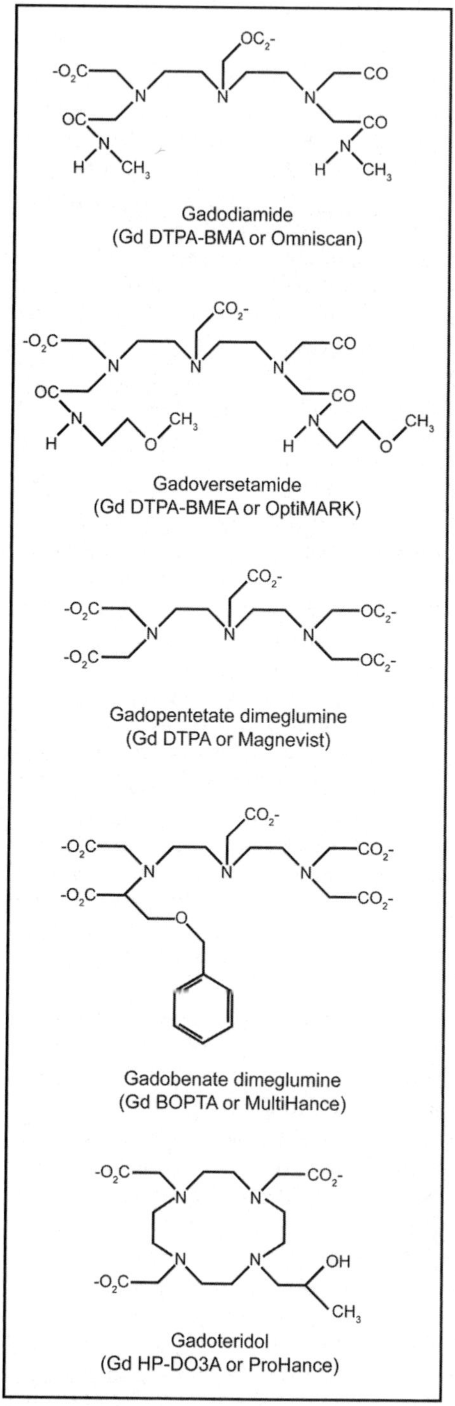

Fig. 98.1

Magnevist. In **Fig. 98.1**, the agents are presented in order by incidence of NSF, with the highest first, and the final two agents without known unconfounded cases. Soon after the association between NSF and gadolinium chelate administration became known, the European Union banned the use of Omniscan and Magnevist in patients with a GFR below 30 mL/min per 173 m^2. The manufacturer of Optimark (which was not available at that time in Europe) subsequently voluntarily added a contraindication in patients at risk for NSF. In September 2010, the FDA issued new warnings with Magnevist, Omniscan, and Optimark described as "inappropriate for use among patients with acute kidney injury or chronic severe kidney disease." Given such safety concerns, neither linear nonionic chelate is likely to remain on the market long term. In distinction to these agents, ProHance (Bracco Diagnostics)—a nonionic, macrocyclic compound—has never been associated with a biopsy proven case of NSF. Gadovist (gadobutrol; Bayer Schering Pharma), another nonionic macrocyclic agent, has been approved for many years in Europe and has recently completed clinical trials in the United States. This agent exhibits greater T1 relaxivity than all other nonprotein-binding extracellular agents and is available in a higher concentration formulation (1 Molar). Dotarem (Guerbet, Villepinte, France), an ionic macrocyclic agent, is likewise undergoing clinical trials in the United States. In distinction to the linear agents, the difference between ionic and nonionic does not appear to be important for stability of the macrocyclic agents.

99 MRA Principles and Carotid MRA

As described in Chapter 12, TOF MRA is commonly utilized in the evaluation of the circle of Willis. TOF MRA allows depiction of vasculature without the utilization of gadolinium-chelate contrast agents, relying instead on flow-related enhancement. The appearance of flowing blood in TOF MRA is dependent upon the technique employed. SE and FSE sequences consist of slice selective 90- and 180-degree RF pulses, requiring a given proton to be subjected to both pulses to produce signal. As such, protons flowing into a given slice with sufficient speed to experience only one pulse are manifest as a flow void on FSE images. Such imaging is thus termed a “black blood” technique. Slowly flowing blood, on the other hand, may experience both RF pulses, thus appearing of higher SI. In distinction, in GRE imaging excitation by only one slice-selective RF pulse is required because the echo is refocused using the gradients. GRE may thus be utilized for “bright blood” TOF imaging. Laminar flow dynamics, wherein the velocity of flowing fluid within a vessel diminishes by the square of the distance from the center, are disrupted in areas of tortuosity, stenosis, or vessel bifurcation. Reductions in SI thus may occur in such areas in bright blood TOF MRA. In bright blood TOF MRA, background tissue is suppressed using slice-selective RF pulses in short succession, at much shorter intervals than the T1 of typical stationary tissue. When subjected to such pulses, stationary protons within a slice have inadequate time to recover longitudinal magnetization, resulting in a low background SI. In distinction, protons from blood flowing into a slice between slice-selective pulses possess a full complement of longitudinal magnetization, thus appearing of high SI on GRE T1WI. In 2D TOF techniques, slices are acquired sequentially one-by-one perpendicular to the direction of flow. When suppression of antiparallel flow from venous structures is necessary, additional saturation pulses may be applied adjacent to the slice of interest so as to suppress signal from inflowing venous blood. 2D TOF techniques suffer misregistration artifacts if patient motion occurs between slice acquisitions. Elimination of such artifacts is possible with 3D TOF where an entire imaging slab is excited without interslice gaps. Such techniques also allow for improved spatial resolution. In 3D TOF, however, blood travels a larger distance within the imaging volume, resulting in loss of SI from saturation effects, effects more pronounced with slower-flowing structures. Thus, 2D TOF is primarily utilized for imaging of slower-flowing venous structures; 3D TOF is the preferred technique for evaluating intracranial arterial structures. Achieving a balance between saturation effects and background tissue suppression necessitates careful selection of RF pulse repetition time (TR) and flip angles in 3D TOF MRA. With larger flip angles, longitudinal recovery of background tissue protons takes more time, improving background suppression and thus image contrast. However, the rate at which signal from flowing blood reaches steady-state suppression is also greater, decreasing depth of penetration (specifically visualization of vessels) within a slab. Lower flip angles allow better penetration, but at the expense of background suppression. Flip angles may actually be varied across the imaging slab, with lower flip angles being used proximally and larger flip angles distally in an attempt to lessen saturation effects. Considerations with TR are similar—a long TR resulting in less penetration. Magnetization transfer, whereby the commonly low SI (due to very short T2) protons bound to macromolecules are excited and transfer their magnetization to their unbound counterparts, reducing their SI, may alternatively be used to decrease background SI. This technique reduces the SI from fat (i.e., periorbital fat) to a lesser degree, however. TE selection is also an important consideration. On MRA, turbulence results in phase dispersion, and is manifest as a loss of SI. Effects of such phase dispersions are more pronounced on scans obtained with longer TEs, exaggerating vessel stenoses. The minimum TE that can be achieved with 3D TOF MRA is substantially less than with 2D, leading to less artifactual exaggeration of vessel stenoses. Reduced voxel sizes also lessen variation in phase within such voxels, further diminishing the effects of turbulent flow on 3D TOF. TOF MRA images may be stacked with postprocessing to produce MIP images, which appear similar to images obtainable by conventional angiography. Such may lead to prominent misregistration artifacts caused by patient motion between sequential slice acquisitions. Even with 3D TOF such artifacts may be seen at slab interfaces (typically three such slabs are acquired for a circle of Willis MRA). Because TOF MRA is obtained using GRE T1WI, entities with short T1—such as methemoglobin-containing clot—also appear as high SI on such images. Review of source images improves identification of such clot and of artifacts from motion and metallic susceptibility. Isometric voxel acquisition allows further flexibility due to the ability to reconstruct projections in any desired plane. Examples are given in Chapter 12.

Due to decreased acquisition times, contrast-enhanced MRA has replaced TOF MRA for most clinical applications, the main exceptions being circle of Willis (3D) and intracranial venous thrombosis (2D) evaluations. Contrast-enhanced MRA allows direct visualization of blood via utilization of extracellular gadolinium chelate contrast agents. Most such agents exit the intravascular space within minutes, thus necessitating rapid image acquisition. Images are acquired utilizing fast 3D spoiled GRE T1WI with short TR and TE, both aiding in saturation of background tissue SI. A decrease in blood T1 from the contained gadolinium chelates leads to an increased SI of vascular structures on such scans. To aid in distinction from background tissue, the T1 of arterial blood must be reduced to below that of fat, with the degree of T1 relaxation related to contrast agent relaxivity and infusion rate. Digitally subtracted images, whereby postcontrast images are subtracted from precontrast data further aid in suppression of background SI. Image acquisition is typically timed so as to fill the center of k-space (which encodes data related to image contrast) during the time at which arterial contrast is at a peak. Centric ordering (i.e., center filled first then the periphery) is commonly employed in contrast-enhanced MRA. The choice of k-space, however, must be matched with the timing and length of the bolus. Accurate determination of circulation time from the site of injection to the area of imaging interest is essential for bolus timing. For example, if the central portion of k-space is acquired too early before maximum arterial SI, ringing artifacts may be generated, whereas artifactual venous enhancement and suboptimal arterial SI may be present if images are acquired with too much of a delay. As discussed in subsequent chapters, timing of image acquisition may be achieved by a variety of techniques, including administration of a test bolus, real-time MR fluoroscopy, and acquisition of dynamic scans. Breath holding is generally necessary for carotid (to achieve good visualization of the vessel origins from the aortic arch), thoracic, and abdominal contrast-enhanced MRA.

Contrast-enhanced MRA of the neck is typically performed during a 20-second breath-hold with image acquisition occurring 8 to 10 seconds following bolus injection (at 2 mL/s) of IV gadolinium chelate. Imaging must be performed rapidly given the fast transit of the contrast agent from the carotid arteries to the jugular veins. MIP projections of contrast-enhanced MRA images of the neck are displayed in **Figs. 99.1A,B,C.** On the **(A)** right side, there is high-grade, near complete stenosis of the right internal carotid artery at the bulb. **(B)** Coronal MIP images illustrate two stenoses in total (*white arrows*) with an additional high-grade stenosis seen in the internal carotid

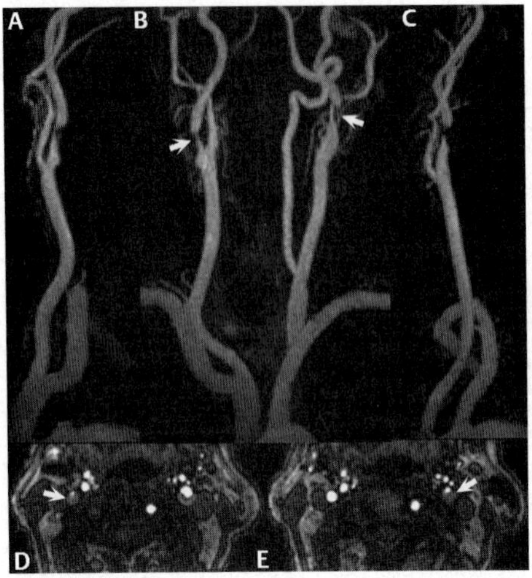

Fig. 99.1 (A–E)

artery on the left, better visualized on (**C**) additional MIP images. The left vertebral artery is dominant. Axial source images in **Figs. 99.1 D,E** allow direct visualization of the occlusive atherosclerotic disease present in both the (**D**, *white arrow*) right and (**E**, *white arrow*) left sides. Source images, as evident here, provide improved delineation of surrounding soft tissue structures. Per the NASCET (North American Symptomatic Carotid Endarterectomy Trial) criteria, percentages of stenosis are computed by dividing the luminal diameter at the area of stenosis by the diameter of a normal, more distal portion of the evaluated artery. Proximal estimates of normal vessel caliber are less accurate given compensatory dilatation often present in such regions. Hemodynamically significant stenoses (>50%) are graded as moderate (50 to 70%) or severe (70 to 99%). Stenoses greater than 95% may result in complete SI loss even on contrast-enhanced MRA. Slow flow distal to such stenoses must be assessed, as should collateral flow within the circle of Willis in addition to the patency of the ophthalmic artery either on neck contrast-enhanced MRA or often concurrently performed 3D TOF MRA of the head. Vascular paragangliomas may often be visualized as enhancing carotid space masses on contrast-enhanced MRA.

In the past few years, it has been possible to acquire contrast-enhanced MRA images with high temporal (and to a lesser degree, spatial) resolution utilizing dynamic techniques. The most common approaches to this include TWIST (time-resolved angiography with interleaved stochastic trajectories) and TREAT (time-resolved echo-shared angiographic technique). Such techniques are based on the fact that contrast information in MRI is primarily derived at the center of k-space. Such techniques rapidly sample the center of k-space multiple times allowing for acquisition of dynamic contrast information, the periphery being sampled less frequently. Because multiple images are acquired at different temporal intervals, test boluses are not needed to time image acquisition. Furthermore, gadolinium chelate dosage may also be diminished by a factor of 2 to 4 with such techniques. The direction of flow may be determined by such imaging as may separation of arterial and venous components of flow. Such sequential images obtained with TWIST technique are displayed in **Figs. 99.2A–F**. The contrast bolus progressively fills the brachiocephalic artery in **Figs. 99.2A,B,C** with progressive filling of the remainder of the great vessels in **(D,E)** later images. The **(F)** final image demonstrates complete opacification of the circle of Willis and right internal jugular vein. Delayed filling of the right internal carotid artery, demonstrates the hemodynamic significance of the high-grade right internal carotid artery stenosis. Dynamic contrast-enhanced MRA is also useful in the evaluation of subclavian steal, the technique readily identifying reversal of vertebral artery flow to supply the subclavian artery distal to an area of stenosis or occlusion.

Contrast-enhanced MRA may aid in delineation of other less common pathologies of the great vessels including traumatic carotid or vertebral artery dissections. In such

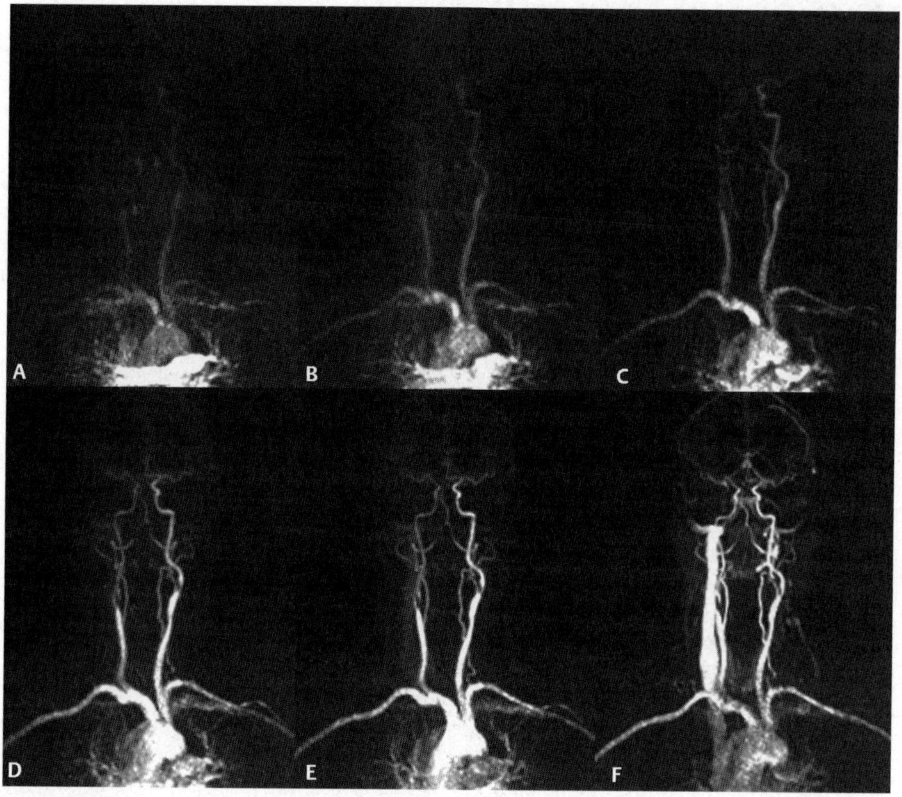

Fig. 99.2 (A–F)

cases, the false lumen fails to fill with contrast on contrast-enhanced MRA. On dynamic imaging, high SI from methemoglobin-containing luminal clot persists prior to and following passage of the contrast bolus. Clot containing blood products of other stages appears of low SI against the enhancing patent vessel lumen. In comparison to atherosclerotic narrowing, narrowing of the vessel due to a dissection typically involves a longer segment, and spares the carotid bulb. Ulcerated plaque is identifiable on contrast-enhanced MRA by the presence of focal outpouching among mural thrombus and plaque, whereas fibromuscular dysplasia exhibits a characteristic "string of beads" appearance on contrast-enhanced MRA. Normal carotid arteries on TOF MRA may occasionally mimic this appearance due to misregistration artifacts. Vasculitis is manifest on contrast-enhanced MRA as alternating stenoses and dilatations in the involved arteries.

100 Peripheral MRA

MRA, specifically contrast-enhanced MRA—the dominant clinical technique—offers a rapid, noninvasive evaluation of the peripheral vasculature with sensitivity and specificity for the detection and grading of stenoses near that of catheter angiography. The other major noninvasive technique, CT angiography, is limited in this application due to the lack of dynamic flow information obtainable and by its reduced accuracy in the presence of calcified plaque. Contrast-enhanced MRA sequences are typically obtained utilizing a heavily T1W 3D spoiled GRE sequence. Contrast-enhanced MRA images are also acquired with a short TE so as to reduce flow-related signal loss and susceptibility artifacts. Before the actual contrast injection the same sequence later used for the contrast-enhanced scan is acquired as a mask for subsequent subtractions.

Coordination of the arrival of the contrast bolus with image acquisition (i.e., bolus timing) is a critical consideration in contrast-enhanced MRA. Inadequate timing resulting in delays acquiring the center of k-space leading to venous contamination or scans acquired too early to achieve maximal obtainable intraarterial SI. Specifically, the center of k-space—the portion encoding data important for image contrast—should be filled when arterial enhancement is at its peak. Several methods are employed for coordinating central k-space acquisition and bolus arrival. Bolus timing consists of acquiring a series of axial T1WI at the level of interest while a small test bolus (1–2 mL) is injected at the same rate as the actual bolus. This is used to calculate a circulation time so as to estimate the timing of bolus arrival during the actual examination. In certain applications, such as whole-body MRA, more than one test bolus is needed. In distinction, with MR fluoroscopy, the full contrast dose is given, and serial coronal 2D images obtained until the bolus has arrived within the desired region, as determined through region of interest analysis by the system or manually by the technologist. Upon arrival, the full scan is then acquired. Using rapid, time-resolved MRA techniques such as TRICKS (time-resolved imaging of contrast kinetics), TWIST (time-resolved angiography with interleaved stochastic trajectories), and TREAT (time-resolved echo-shared angiographic technique), the need for bolus timing is eliminated. These techniques undersample the periphery of k-space, while repeatedly sampling the center of k-space, allowing acquisition of image-contrast information at a high rate. Due to the subsequent data acquisition at a high frame rate both arterial and venous phase images are acquired. This is especially useful in eliminating problems stemming from venous overlay in patients with altered hemodynamics due to inflammation and collateral flow.

To optimize bolus timing and thus image contrast with respect to the total area of anatomic coverage, several different techniques can be used. For peripheral MRA with the step-by-step approach, coronal images are typically obtained at three to four different stations (meaning the technologist must plan three to four different FOVs) so as to fully visualize all vessel stations from the diaphragm to the distal calves. Automated table positioning is then used to track the bolus and image the region of interest. For the purposes of avoiding venous contamination in the calves, this region is typically scanned first utilizing a centric k-space acquisition strategy with the other evaluated FOVs (pelvis and thigh) evaluated subsequently. The advent of dedicated multielement coil systems as well as SNR gains achievable at 3 T has enabled the implementation of continuous table movement (CTM) MRA. Using CTM-MRA, only one large FOV, encompassing the vasculature from the diaphragm to the calves, need be planned.

Effective contrast-enhanced MRA techniques require both adequate temporal and spatial resolution, the latter due to the small caliber vessels that must be visualized in the calf. The increased SNR afforded by imaging at 3 T as well as the prolonged T1-relaxivity of the background tissue at that field strength (reducing background SI on T1WI), increases vessel conspicuity to the point where images may be obtained utilizing parallel imaging factors of 3 without significant SNR detriment. Reductions in acquisition times obtainable through parallel imaging can alternatively be used to provide further increases in spatial resolution.

Although contrast-enhanced MRA can be performed with any gadolinium chelate, agent efficacy and safety, especially with regard to NSF, must be considered. Macrocyclic agents reduce the potential risk of NSF due to their chemical structure, which more tightly binds the toxic Gd^{3+} ion. Combined with the SNR gains at 3 T, high relaxivity agents like gadobutrol have been further shown to produce adequate image quality even when a lower agent dose is utilized, the latter offering a further reduction in the theoretical risk of NSF. Gadobenate dimeglumine, an agent with transient protein-binding (and thus improved T1 relaxivity), is an additional option for decreasing imaging dose, particularly at 3 T.

Contrast-enhanced MRA images are commonly presented for interpretation as MIP images, which due to acquisition of scans with an isotropic voxel size (i.e., size equal in three dimensions), can be rotated into any desired plane, thus increasing diagnostic accuracy of stenosis grading. Volume-rendered images are less diagnostically useful. Source images should always be viewed alongside the MIP images, with examination of unsubtracted source images potentially improving vessel wall evaluation. A coronal MIP image from a contrast-enhanced MRA patient exam is illustrated in **Fig. 100.1**. Severe peripheral arterial occlusive disease of the runoff vasculature is present, with high-grade stenoses (*arrows*) of the left femoral and posterior tibial arteries. **Figures 100.2** and **Fig. 100.3A** (*white arrow*) are coronal contrast-enhanced MRA MIP images illustrating complete occlusion of the right common iliac artery and high-grade left iliac artery stenosis (findings associated with Leriche syndrome). The length of stenoses is important to ascertain, as is the degree. With respect to the latter, assessment of the left external iliac artery is aided by visualization in multiple planes and obliquities, including (**Fig. 100.3B**) sagittal and **(C)** axial images. The identification of collaterals—present extensively from the inferior mesenteric and epigastric arteries in this case (**Fig. 100.2 and Fig. 100.3A**)—vessel reconstitution, and patency of the distal vasculature are important findings to describe in evaluation of any vascular process. The length of a stenosis may further determine whether endovascular (if short segment) or open surgical repair is

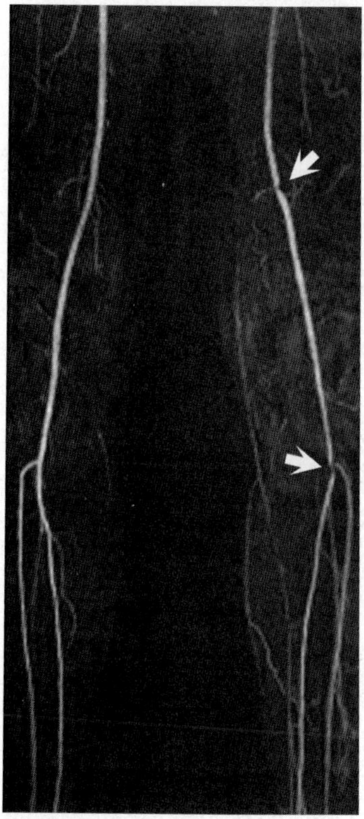

Fig. 100.1

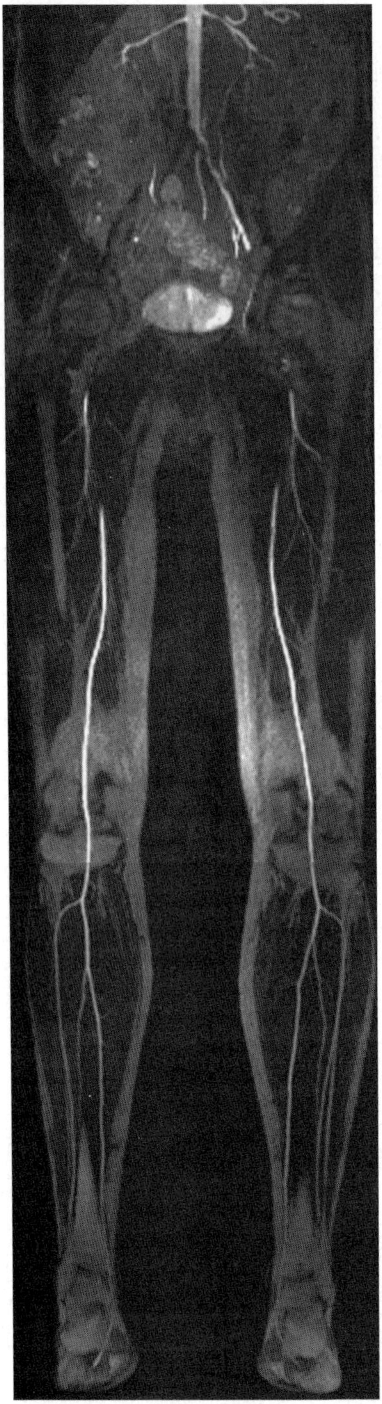

Fig. 100.2

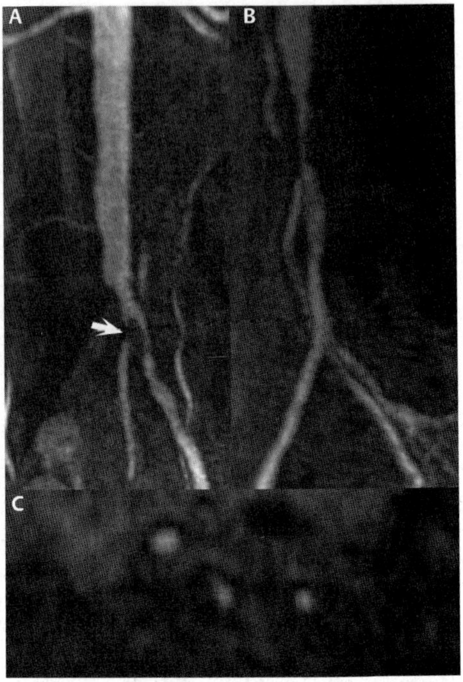

Fig. 100.3 (A–C)

indicated. In superficial femoral artery disease, it is further crucial to localize vessel reconstitution to above—where synthetic graft material may be used—or below the knee—where native veins are more suitable.

Dynamic time-resolved MRA images in **Fig. 100.4** illustrate **(A,B,C)** early preferential filling of the left lower arterial system with poor and no flow demonstrated through the right fibular and left posterior tibial arteries, respectively. Delayed images **(D,E,F)** exhibit venous filling—a finding often more prominent in the presence of a concomitant soft tissue infection. The mechanism for improved left-sided flow is an aortofemoropopliteal bypass (**A**, *white arrows*) to the left popliteal artery. Synthetic grafts themselves do not typically cause susceptibility artifact on MRA, although clips at anastomotic sites may. Artifact from stainless steel may be severe and mimic a short segment occlusion. History and prior studies can aid in detecting such a false stenosis, a

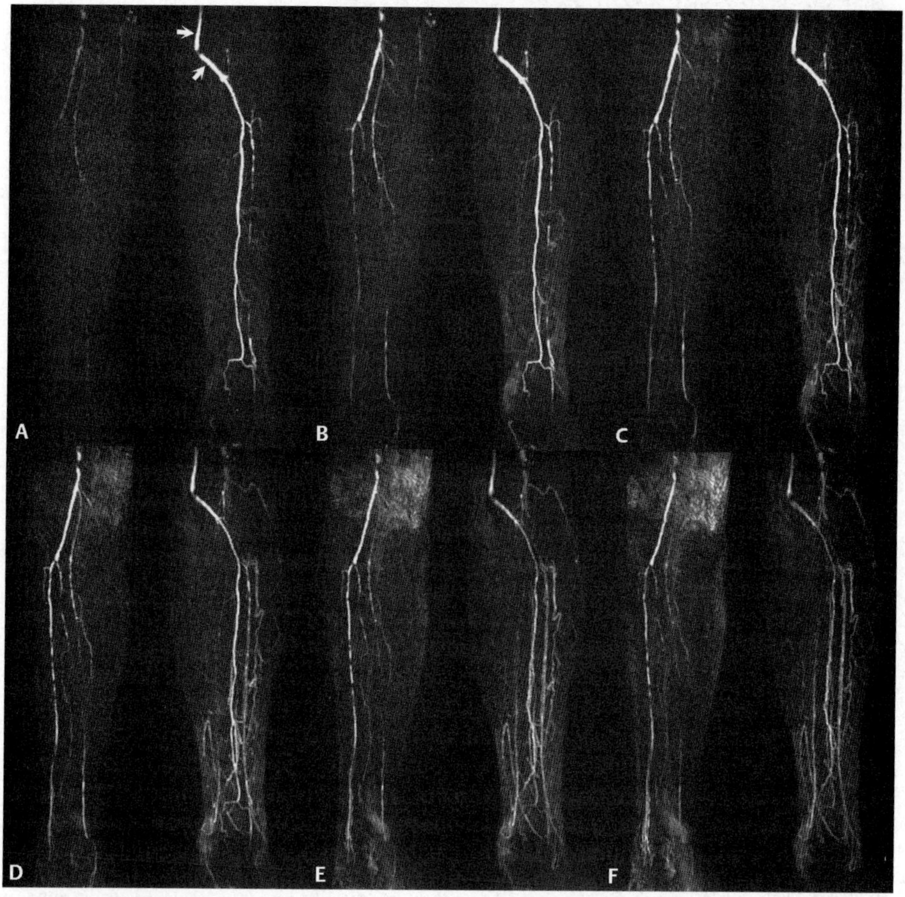

Fig. 100.4 (A–F)

finding also identifiable by the sharp transition from the normal to stenotic vessel and lack of collateral blood flow. Nitinol stents typically do not produce severe artifacts. In less commonly performed MRA evaluations for acute embolic disease, the aorta and proximal vessels should be evaluated as potential sites of embolus. If extensive distal occlusive stenosis of small- and medium-sized vessels is present concurrently with corkscrew-like collateral vasculature, Buerger disease (i.e., thromboangiitis obliterans) is a consideration.

101 Renal Artery MRA

Contrast-enhanced MRA is also commonly utilized for the noninvasive evaluation of renal artery stenosis—the most common cause of secondary hypertension. **Figure 101.1** demonstrates focal high-grade stenosis of the right renal artery on **(A)** coronal contrast-enhanced MIP MRA images. Focal, less-severe narrowing at the left renal artery origin is also present. Typically, only renal artery stenoses greater than 50% respond to surgical therapy; however, significant drops in arterial blood flow may not occur until stenoses exceed 75% in degree. Some stenoses occur without associated parenchymal dysfunction as evidenced by the fact that not every patient with moderate- or high-grade stenosis responds to surgical treatment. Atherosclerotic causes of renal artery stenosis predominate, preferentially involving the proximal third of the renal artery and the ostium. Measurements of renal artery stenoses are conveniently performed on coronal source images but suffer intraobserver variability and assess the stenosis in only one dimension. Image acquisition with isometric voxels allows reconstruction in any desired plane, as illustrated by the **(B)** sagittal, showing the origins of the superior mesenteric and celiac arteries, and **(C)** axial MIP reconstructions, both obtained from the same coronal source image dataset as was the coronal MIP in **Fig. 101.1A**. A more reproducible approach to stenosis measurement thus involves initial identification of potential stenoses on coronal MIP images with subsequent measurements performed on reconstructions perpendicular to the region of suspected stenosis and also in the sagittal plane.

Fibromuscular dysplasia (FMD) is the second most frequent cause of renal artery stenosis, responsible for ~30% of cases. Contrast-enhanced MRA reliably (93–97% sensitivity) detects the characteristic findings of FMD including multiple aneurysms resulting in the pathognomonic string-of-beads sign (**Figs. 101.2A,B**, *white arrow*), but identifies disease with subtle morphologic changes less sensitively than catheter angiography due to motion artifacts including random diaphragmatic motion as well as poor spatial resolution near the smaller, distal two-thirds of the vessel in which such lesions tend to occur. In addition, utilization of lower spatial resolution (>1 mm^3) or lower field strengths (i.e., 1 or 1.5 T) may further diminish sensitivity of contrast-enhanced MRA for the diagnosis of the above pathologies.

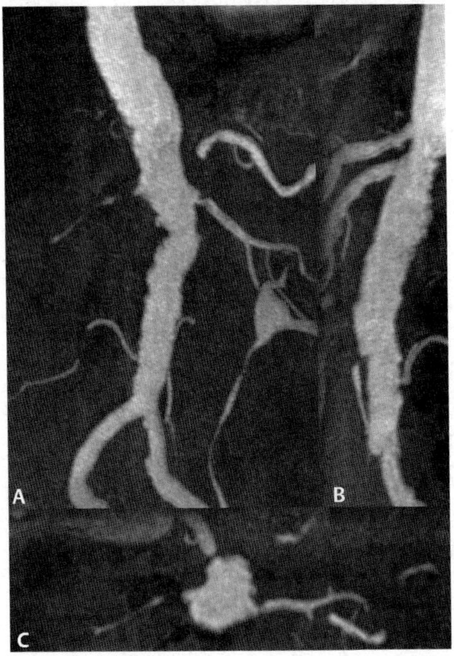

Fig. 101.1 (A–C)

Contrast-enhanced MRA is also utilized, along with MRI to evaluate the suitability of living kidney donors. The first assessment must be whether an accessory renal artery is present. Detection of renal arteries and of the origins of the small accessory arteries supplying the uretero-pelvic junction requires acquisitions with large FOVs as such arteries may arise from any portion of the aorta or iliac vessels. Imaging with

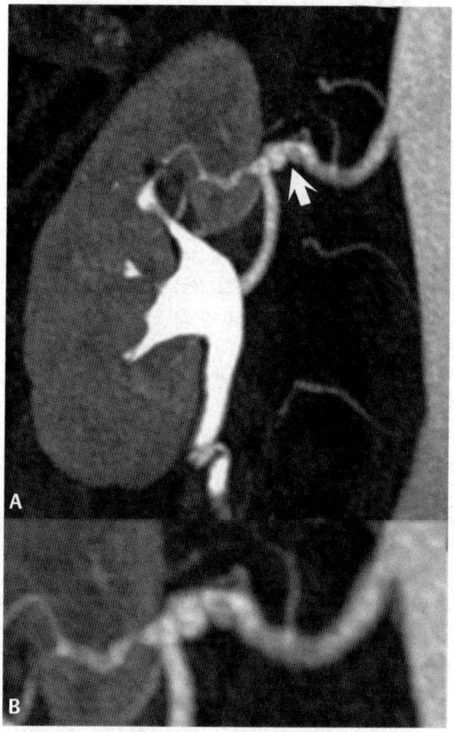

Fig. 101.2 (A,B)

high resolution is also important, as arteries supplying these junctions must be adequately evaluated.

In posttransplant patients, contrast-enhanced MRA may be used to detect vascular abnormalities such as renal artery kinking or stenosis. Susceptibility artifacts from surgical clips in the renal fossa are often present, degrading scans of all types. Renal MR perfusion studies may be utilized for functional assessment, including measurements of renal plasma flow. Renal MRV is utilized to assess not only the renal veins in perioperative transplant patients, but also to evaluate subtle venous invasion by renal carcinoma.

As alluded to above, the versatility of MRI can be harnessed to evaluate a stenosis for hemodynamic significance and to detect nonvascular parenchymal disease through use of techniques assessing parenchymal perfusion, the latter also proving useful in the evaluation of transplanted kidneys. Although techniques not based on gadolinium chelate administration such as blood-oxygen-level-dependent MRI (BOLD) and acquisition of diffusion parameters may eventually be utilized to clinically assess parenchymal function, dynamic contrast-enhanced MRI, utilizing quantitative renal perfusion parameters such as renal blood flow, glomerular filtration rate, and cortical and medullary blood volume, is currently the most frequently utilized approach. Although postprocessing techniques are not yet firmly standardized, calculation of such parameters is typically based on temporal evolution in renal enhancement in relation to the arterial input function. Integration of perfusion assessments with traditional MRA offer potential for a comprehensive evaluation of renal disease, which has shown early promise in identifying hemodynamically significant stenoses and localizing the source of parenchymal renal dysfunction to either a renovascular or nonrenovascular source.

A discussion of renal contrast-enhanced MRA would be remiss without mention of the association of NSF with gadolinium chelate contrast administration in patients with GFR's less than 30 mL/min per 1.73m^2. This topic was further addressed in Chapters 97 and 98. TOF MRA is not commonly utilized for renal MRA due to poor sensitivity to small stenoses. Breath-hold or navigator gated 3D steady-state free precession (SSFP)—a "bright blood" technique used in cardiac imaging with T2W/T1W—sequences with fat suppression, although not yet widely studied, present a potential alternative to contrast-enhanced MRA in renal failure patients in which NSF risk would otherwise prevent administration of gadolinium chelates. Such sequences are relatively resistant to differences in flow dynamics and exhibit sensitivity for renal artery stenosis only slightly less than that obtainable with contrast-enhanced MRA.

102 Other MRA Applications

Beyond its most established uses, contrast-enhanced MRA can aid in the assessment and evaluation of other vascular diseases, especially aneurysms. Abdominal aortic aneurysms are defined as dilatations greater than 3 cm, and can be classified with respect to their location relative to the renal arteries. Suprarenal aneurysms lie above the origin of the renal arteries, juxtarenal aneurysms within 1 cm of the renal arteries, and infrarenal arteries below the renal arteries. Aneurysms greater than 5 cm are typically repaired either by surgery or stenting. In such cases, the distance between the aneurysm neck and the more distal renal artery should be reported, along with the aneurysm length (on coronal images), the distance from the aneurysm to the common iliac arteries, and the diameter of the external iliac arteries. In the case of intraaneurysmal thrombosis, the diameter of the thrombosis and the patent lumen itself should be measured. An aneurysm of the ascending thoracic aorta is defined as being 4 cm or greater in diameter, a common iliac artery aneurysm as greater than 1.5 cm, and a popliteal aneurysm as greater than 0.7 cm. Multiple lesions are not uncommon with abdominal aneurysms increasing the probability of concomitant femoral or popliteal aneurysms, the latter of which commonly thrombose.

Dissections consist of separation of the arterial media from the adventitia, often originating in the thoracic aorta and propagated distally. Stanford type A lesions are those involving the ascending aorta and type B lesions are those without ascending aortic involvement. **Figure 102.1** illustrates a volume-rendered image of an aortic dissection extending into the right common iliac artery. Such images often help elucidate whether a given vascular structure is fed from the true or false vessel lumen—an important finding particularly with respect to the renal arteries. In **Fig. 102.1**, the false and true dissection lumens feed the right and left renal arteries, respectively. A coronal MIP image in **Fig. 102.2A** provides similar information, while an axial MIP image (**Fig. 102.2B**) confirms extension of the dissection into the left renal artery—a more subtle finding not well visualized on volume-rendered imaging and illustrating the importance of viewing structures in multiple planes. Time-resolved studies can further help to distinguish the true and false lumen in the presence of dissection and to identify the origin of the renal vasculature, in addition to allowing visualization of renal perfusion and excluding renal infarctions. Findings associated with inflammatory arteritis may also be visualized on MRA. Takayasu arteritis preferentially involves medium and large arterial structures. Takayasu arteritis is associated with concentric

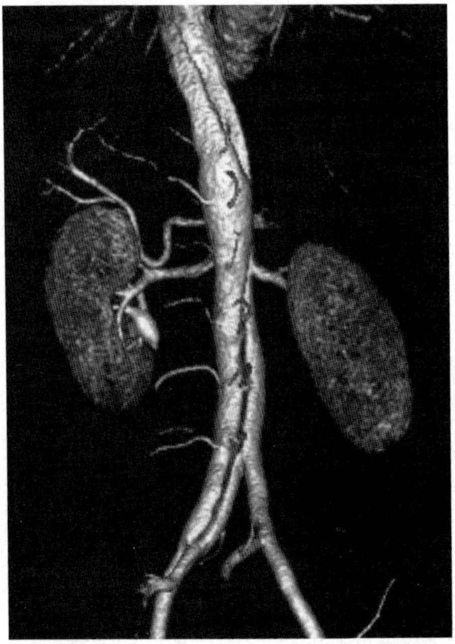

Fig. 102.1

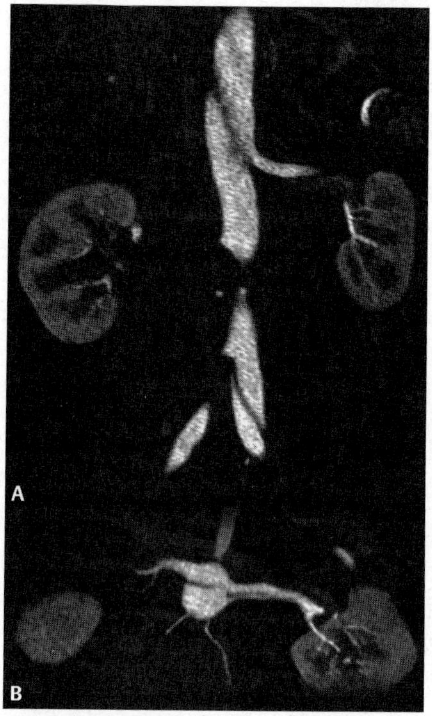

Fig. 102.2 (A,B)

vessel wall thickening with wall enhancement indicating active disease. Contrast-enhanced MRA in this case may help identify associated stenoses, occlusions, or aneurysms. Polyarteritis nodosa affects small- and medium-sized vessels in a similar manner with DSA remaining the gold standard for diagnosis due to the frequent small size of associated findings.

Magnetic resonance venography (MRV) is commonly utilized to evaluate extent of tumor thrombus into venous structures, particularly in the setting of renal vein invasion in renal cell carcinoma. Transient protein-binding "blood-pool" agents such as gadofosveset trisodium extend the window of time available for MRV, making peripheral MRV evaluations more feasible. The development of peripheral MRV for the assessment of deep venous thrombosis offers the possibility of a combined thoracic MRA and peripheral MRV protocol, allowing comprehensive evaluation for venous thrombosis and pulmonary embolism in a single examination. **Figures 102.3A and 102.3B** provide a depiction of bilateral pulmonary emboli (*white arrows*) on coronal and axial contrast-enhanced MRA. Detection of venous and arterial thrombi might also be improved by use of thrombin-binding contrast media, with one such agent, EP-2104R, evaluated in limited clinical trials.

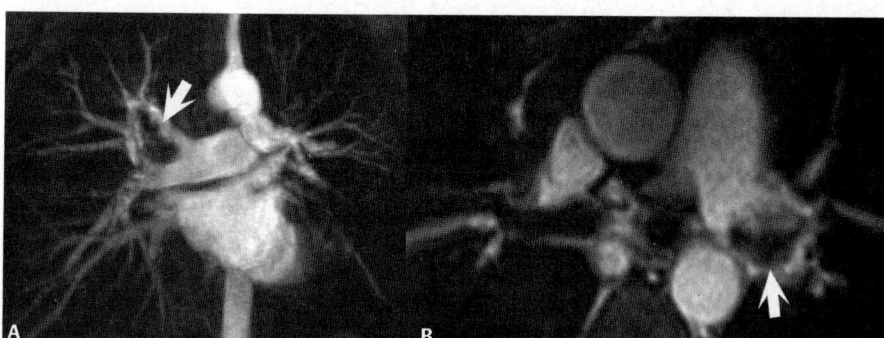

Fig. 102.3 (A,B)

Index

Note: Page numbers followed by *f* indicate figures.

A

Abdominal aortic aneurysm(s), 218
Abscess
  in brain, 31, 36, 38, 39*f*, 40, 41*f*, 44–45
  epidural, lumbar spine, 101, 101*f*
  hepatic
    amebic, 141
    pyogenic, 141
  peritonsillar, 120*f*, 121
  salivary gland, 121
AC. *See* Acromioclavicular
ACA. *See* Anterior cerebral artery
Achilles tendon
  injury, 194, 195*f*
  tendonitis, 194, 195*f*
ACL. *See* Anterior cruciate ligament
Acquired immunodeficiency syndrome. *See* HIV-infected (AIDS) patients
Acromioclavicular joint, 174–175, 175*f*
Acute disseminated encephalomyelitis, 37
Acute lymphocytic leukemia, lumbar spine in, 104, 104*f*
Adamantinoma(s), 13, 13*f*
ADEM. *See* Acute disseminated encephalomyelitis
Adenocarcinoma
  hemorrhagic, of head and neck, 119
  mucinous, of head and neck, 119, 119*f*
  pancreatic. *See* Pancreatic adenocarcinoma
Adenoid cystic carcinoma, of head and neck, 117, 118
Adenomyoma, uterine, 159, 159*f*
Adenomyosis, uterine, 159, 159*f*
Adenosine, 124
Adrenal gland(s)
  adenoma, 146, 146*f*
  carcinoma, 146–147, 147*f*
  cysts, 147, 147*f*
  disease, 146–147, 146*f*, 147*f*
  hemorrhage, 147
    in child, 153, 153*f*
  masses, 146, 147, 147*f*
  metastatic disease, 147, 147*f*
  myelolipoma, 146, 147*f*
Adrenocortical carcinoma, 146–147, 147*f*
Adrenoleukodystrophy, 52, 53, 53*f*
Agyria, 50, 51*f*
AICA. *See* Anterior inferior cerebellar artery
AIDS. *See* HIV-infected (AIDS) patients
Alcoholism, cerebellar atrophy caused by, 34
Alexander disease, 53
Allergic fungal sinusitis, 116
ALPSA. *See* Anterior labral ligamentous periosteal sleeve avulsion injury
Alzheimer disease, 34, 34*f*
AMBRI, 176
Amyloid deposits, 200
Amyloidosis, myocardium in, 122
Anaphylactoid reactions, contrast agent–induced, 206
Anemia, bone marrow in, 105, 202

Aneurysm(s)
abdominal aortic, 218
berry, 24, 48
common iliac artery, 218
coronary, 125
fusiform, 24
giant, 24–25, 25*f*
arteries involved in, 24
intracranial, 24–25, 25*f*
clot in, 25
rupture, 25
intraventricular, 125, 125*f*
popliteal, 218
saccular (spherical), 24, 25*f*
thoracic aorta, 218
vein of Galen, 21
Aneurysmal bone cyst, 200, 200*f*
Angiomyolipoma, renal, 149, 149*f*
Ankle
abnormalities, 198–199
bone contusion, 197, 197*f*, 198–199
fractures, 197, 197*f*
inflammatory arthritis, 199
lateral ligamentous complex, 196, 196*f*
ligamentous anatomy, 196, 196*f*
ligamentous injuries, 196–197, 196*f*, 197*f*
medial ligamentous complex, 196–197
osteochondral lesions, 198
syndesmotic injury, 197
tendinous injuries, 194–195, 195*f*
Ankle sprain(s), 196–197
grading, 196
high, 197
Annular ligament (elbow), 192, 192*f*
Anterior cerebral artery, 31
infarction, 27–28, 29
Anterior choroidal artery, 29
Anterior communicating artery, aneurysm, 24, 25*f*
Anterior cruciate ligament
surgical reconstruction, 168–169
tears, 168–169, 169*f*
Anterior inferior cerebellar artery, 29–30
Anterior labral ligamentous periosteal sleeve avulsion injury, 178
Anterior longitudinal ligament
injury, 61
MRI appearance, 61
Anterior spinal artery, 85
Anterior talofibular ligament, 196, 196*f*
tears, 196, 196*f*
Antrochoanal polyps, 116
Aorta, thoracic
aneurysms, 130, 218
fusiform, 130
saccular, 130
dissection, 130–131, 131*f*, 218, 218*f*, 219*f*
DeBakey type 3, 131
DeBakey type 1 and 2, 131
type A, 131, 218
type B, 131, 218
false aneurysms, 130
thrombus, 130–131, 131*f*
Aortic valve
insufficiency, 126–127
stenosis, 126, 127*f*
Arachnoid cyst(s), 11, 18, 48–49, 49*f*
differential diagnosis, 48
distribution in brain, 48
infratentorial, 48
intraspinal, 58
with mass effect, 48
retrocerebellar, 48, 49*f*
in thoracic spine, 80*f*, 81
Arachnoid granulation(s), 14
Arachnoiditis, lumbar spine, 101
Arcuate ligament (knee), 171
Arcuate sign, 169
Arrhythmogenic right ventricular dysplasia, 123, 123*f*
Arterial switch, 128–129
Arteriovenous fistula, spinal, 84–85, 84*f*
cord, 84–85
dural, 84–85, 84*f*
Arteriovenous malformation(s)
cerebrovascular, 20–21, 21*f*
congenital, 20, 21*f*
dural-based, 21
feeding arteries, 20, 21*f*
aneurysms, 24
nidus size, 20, 21*f*
pulmonary, 130, 131*f*
spinal, 84
intramedullary, 84
juvenile, 84
Arteritis, inflammatory, 218–219
Artery of Adamkiewicz, 85
ASA. *See* Anterior spinal artery
ASD. *See* Atrial septal defect
Astrocytoma(s). *See also* Glioblastoma multiforme
anaplastic (grade 3), 2, 3
in brain, 2, 3*f*
mass effect, 2, 3*f*
cerebellar, 4–5, 5*f*
in cervical spine, 74
in children, 2
circumscribed (grade 1), 2

diffusely infiltrating, 5
fibrillary, 4–5
giant cell, subependymal, 56–57, 56*f*
low-grade (grade 2), 2, 3*f*
in thoracic spine, 74
WHO classification, 2
Atherosclerosis
in carotid arteries, 209–210, 210*f*
ulcerated plaque in, 211
Atlantoaxial subluxation, in rheumatoid arthritis, 67
Atlanto-occipital dislocation, 60
Atrial septal defect, 128, 129*f*
Atrial switch, 128–129
Avascular necrosis, talar, 198, 199*f*
AVF. *See* Arteriovenous fistula
AVM. *See* Arteriovenous malformation(s)

B

Bankart fracture, 176, 177*f*
Bankart lesion, 176–177, 177*f*, 178
"medialized," 178
reverse, 177, 177*f*
Bartholin gland cysts, 157, 157*f*
Basilar artery
infarction, 29
tip, and giant aneurysm, 24
Basilar invagination, 58, 67
Beckwith-Wiedemann disease, 153
Benign prostatic hypertrophy, 155, 155*f*
Bennett lesion, 177
Bernoulli equation, 126
Bile, 144
Biliary disease, 144–145, 144*f*, 145*f*
Binswanger disease, 29, 35
Black blood sequences, 122, 208
Bladder cancer, 154, 154*f*
metastases, 154
staging, 154
Blood-oxygen-level dependent MRI, 217
Blood product degradation, 16–17. *See also* Deoxyhemoglobin; Hemosiderin; Methemoglobin
BOLD. *See* Blood-oxygen-level dependent MRI
Bone infarction, 105, 202, 202*f*
Bone marrow
age-related changes in, 105, 202
chemotherapy and, 104–105, 202
chronic anemia and, 105, 202
diseases, 202–203
edema, 203, 203*f*
imaging characteristics, 202
infarct, 105, 202, 202*f*
in lumbar spine
disorders, 104–105, 104*f*
MRI appearance
in metastatic disease, 102, 102*f*
normal, 102, 102*f*
neoplastic replacement, 104, 104*f*, 105
physiologic reconversion, 105, 202
radiation therapy and, 80, 80*f*
Bradycardia, contrast agent–induced, 206
Brain
abscess, 31, 36, 38, 39*f*, 40, 41*f*, 44–45
age-related changes in, 34
aneurysms in, 24–25, 25*f*. *See also* Aneurysm(s); *specific vessel*
arteriovenous malformations, 20–21, 21*f*
atrophy, widened subarachnoid space secondary to, 48
callosal lesions, 36, 37*f*
cystic lesions, differential diagnosis, 48
diffuse axonal injury, 33, 33*f*
dilated perivascular spaces, 29
ex vacuo dilatation in, 32, 32*f*
gray matter
cobblestoning, 50, 51*f*
heterotopic, 50, 51*f*, 56
lesions, 34–35
MRI appearance in neonates, 52
hemorrhage, 31
extraaxial, 18, 18*f*, 19*f*
intraparenchymal, 16–17, 17*f*
aneurysmal, 24–25
with dural AVMs, 21
intraventricular, 19
subarachnoid, 18–19, 19*f*, 24, 42
with dural AVMs, 21
in HIV-infected (AIDS) patients, 44–45, 45*f*
in immunocompromised patient, 44–45, 45*f*
infarction, 26–28, 29–31, 30*f*
arterial thrombotic, 30*f*, 31
embolic, 31
hemodynamic, 31
hemorrhagic, 31, 41
lacunar, 29–31, 30*f*
in meningitis, 43
venous, 41
ischemia, 26–28, 29–31, 30*f*, 57
lymphoma, 3
meningiomas, 8–9, 8*f*
meningitis, 42–43, 43*f*
metastases to, 3, 6–7, 6*f*, 44–45
cystic appearance, 6*f*, 7
hemorrhagic, 6*f*, 7
as ring-enhancing lesions, 6*f*, 7, 38

Brain (*Continued*)
MS plaques in, 34–35, 36–37, 37*f*
neoplasms, 31, 38. *See also specific neoplasm*
hemorrhagic, 17, 17*f*
infratentorial, 4–5, 5*f*
as ring-enhancing lesions, 6*f*, 7, 38
supratentorial, 2–3, 3*f*
neurodegenerative disorders in, 34–35, 34*f*, 35*f*
parenchymal infections, 38–39, 39*f*
periventricular lesions, 36
periventricular leukomalacia, 32, 32*f*
postsurgical changes, 42
posttraumatic changes, 42
sinus disease, 40–41, 41*f*
small vessel ischemia, 34, 35*f*, 36
sulcal island, 57
sulcal widening, 34, 35*f*, 36, 37*f*
vascular malformations, 22–23, 22*f*, 23*f*, 57
venous thrombosis, 40–41, 41*f*
watershed areas, 31
white matter
inherited diseases, 52–53, 53*f*
MRI appearance in neonates, 52
white matter lesions, 34–35, 35*f*
Brainstem, neoplasms, 4–5
Branchial cleft cysts, 117
Breast(s)
biopsy, MRI-guided, 135
cancer, 134–135, 134*f*, 135*f*
cerebral metastases, 6
cervical spinal metastases, 110, 110*f*
lumbar spinal metastases, 110, 110*f*
ductal carcinoma in situ (DCIS), 135
implants, 136–137, 136*f*, 137*f*
neoplasia, 134–135, 134*f*, 135*f*
in patient with implants, 137
silicone granuloma, 137
Bright blood sequence, 122, 208, 217
Bronchogenic carcinoma, 132, 133*f*
Bronchospasm, contrast agent–induced, 206
Buford complex, 178
Buphthalmos, in neurofibromatosis, 55
Butterfly glioma, 2

C

Canavan disease, 53
Capillary telangiectasia(s), in brain, 23, 23*f*
Capitolunate angle, 185
Caput medusae, 23
Carcinoid, 150
Cardiac imaging, 122, 123*f*
Cardiac output, calculation, 126
Cardiomyopathy, 122–123, 123*f*
congenital, 123
Carotid artery(ies). *See also* Internal carotid artery
atherosclerosis, 209–210, 210*f*
displacement, by tumor, 9
dissection, 210–211
normal, 211
Carpal instability
dissociative, 184
nondissociative, 184
Carpal tunnel syndrome, 184, 185*f*
Cartilage
articular, 172
imaging technique for, 172
postoperative evaluation, 172
trilaminar appearance, 172
truncation artifact and, 172
microvascular repair, 173
osteoblastic differentiation, 173
Caudal regression, 86, 86*f*
Caudate, vascular supply to, 29
Caudate nuclei, atrophy, 34, 35*f*
Cavernous angioma(s)
in brain, 22, 22*f*
hemorrhagic, 22–23
in cervical spine, 74, 75*f*
Cavernous hemangioma, infantile, in liver, 153
Cerebellar herniation, 58, 58*f*
Cerebellar peg, 46, 47*f*, 58, 58*f*
Cerebellar tonsil(s), 58, 58*f*
Cerebellar vermis, absence, with Dandy-Walker malformation, 47
Cerebellomedullary cistern, prominent, 48
Cerebellopontine angle
masses, in neurofibromatosis, 55, 55*f*
schwannoma, 10–11, 11*f*
Cerebellum
abnormalities, with Chiari malformation, 47, 47*f*
atrophy, 34
infarctions, 31
vascular supply to, 30
Cerebral edema
with abscess, 38, 39*f*
cytotoxic, 26
with juvenile pilocytic astrocytoma, 4, 5*f*
with meningioma, 8, 8*f*
vasogenic
with astrocytomas, 2
in brain ischemia, 26
with metastases, 7

Cerebral gyri, abnormalities, with Chiari malformation, 47, 47*f*
Cerebral infarction, 26–28, 29–31, 30*f*, 41
Cerebral ischemia, 26–28, 29–31, 30*f*
Cerebritis, 40, 41*f*
Cerebrospinal fluid
  pulsation artifacts, 84, 85, 96
    and thoracic spinal imaging, 79, 79*f*
  transependymal resorption, 4, 5*f*
Cervical cancer, 161, 161*f*
  staging, 161, 161*f*
Cervical nerve(s), impingement, disk herniation and, 62–63, 62*f*
Cervical spine
  age-related changes in, 68
  astrocytomas, 74
  cavernous angioma, 74, 75*f*
  compression (burst) fractures, 61, 61*f*
  congenital abnormalities, 58–59, 58*f*, 59*f*
    osseous, 58
  degenerative disease, 64–66, 64*f*–66*f*, 68
    with disk herniation, 65, 65*f*
  disk herniation, 62–63, 62*f*, 63*f*
    in degenerative disease, 65, 65*f*
    traumatic, 60, 61*f*
  diskitis, 68
  ependymoma, 74, 75*f*
  epidural hematoma, 60, 60*f*
  fusion surgery, postoperative changes, 67–68, 68*f*
  hemangioblastoma, 74
  imaging
    artifacts, 62
    technique for, 62, 96
  laminectomy, postoperative changes, 67–68, 68*f*
  ligamentous injury, 61, 61*f*
  lymphoma metastatic to, 110–111, 111*f*
  meningioma, 74–76, 76*f*
  metastatic disease in, 72–73, 72*f*, 73*f*, 110, 110*f*
  in multiple sclerosis, 69–70, 69*f*, 70*f*
  neoplasms, 74–76, 75*f*, 76*f*
  nerve sheath tumors, 74, 76
  neural foraminal narrowing, 64–65, 65*f*
  orthopedic hardware in, 67, 68*f*
  osseous injuries, 60–61, 61*f*
  osteophytes, 63, 63*f*, 64, 64*f*, 65, 65*f*, 68, 68*f*
  perched facet in, 60, 61*f*
  postoperative changes, 67–68, 68*f*
  rheumatoid arthritis in, 67, 67*f*
  scar in, 68
  spondylotic disease, 65–66, 66*f*
  subacute combined degeneration, 71, 71*f*
  transverse ligament laxity, 67
  transverse myelitis, 71
  trauma, 60–61, 60*f*–61*f*
  vertebral fusion in, 59, 59*f*
Chamberlain's line, 58, 67
Charcot-Marie-Tooth disease, 112
Chemotherapy, and bone marrow, 104–105, 202
Cherubism, 14
Chiari malformations
  type 1, 46, 46*f*, 58, 58*f*, 77, 77*f*
  type 2, 46–47, 47*f*, 50, 58, 58*f*, 86, 86*f*
    and tethered cord, 86–87
  type 3, 47
Child(ren). *See also* Pediatric
  adrenal hemorrhage in, 153, 153*f*
  avascular necrosis of femoral head in, 181
  ganglioneuroblastoma in, 152, 153*f*
  ganglioneuroma in, 152
  Legg-Calve-Perthes disease in, 181
  liver masses in, 153, 153*f*
  malignant soft tissue tumors in, 201
  mesoblastic nephroma in, 152–153, 153*f*
  nephroblastoma in, 152–153, 152*f*
  nephroblastomatosis in, 153
  neuroblastoma in, 152, 152*f*
  osteochondritis dissecans in, 172–173
  renal imaging in, 152–153, 153*f*
  renal metastatic disease in, 153
  retroperitoneal mass in, 152, 152*f*
  slipped capital femoral epiphysis in, 181, 181*f*
Child abuse, subdural hematomas in, 18, 19*f*
Cholangiocarcinoma, 144–145, 145*f*
  extrahepatic, 145, 145*f*
  hepatic, 140
  intrahepatic (peripheral), 144–145
Cholangitis
  infectious, 145
  primary sclerosing, 145, 145*f*
Cholecystitis
  acute, 144
  chronic, 144
Cholelithiasis, 144, 144*f*
Cholesteatoma(s), 121
Cholesterol granuloma, 121
Chondrosarcoma, 200
  of skull base, 117
Chordoma, of skull base, 117
Choriocarcinoma, metastases, to brain, 7
Choroidal fissure, cyst, 48–49
Choroid plexus
  enlargement, 57
  papilloma, 5

Chronic inflammatory demyelinating polyneuropathy, 111–112, 112*f*
Chylothorax, 132–133
Cingulate gyri, radial, 50, 51*f*
Cirrhosis
  hepatic, 143, 143*f*, 145
  primary biliary, 145
Cisterna magna, prominent, 48
Clay shoveler's fracture, 60
Cleft sign, with meningioma, 8*f*, 9
Colloid cyst(s), in brain, 49
Colon cancer, hepatic metastases, 141, 141*f*
Common iliac artery, aneurysm, 218
Congenital heart disease, 128–129, 129*f*
Congestive heart failure, 143
Conjoint tendon (knee), 171, 171*f*
Constrictive pericarditis, 122
Contrast agents, 204–205. *See also* Gadolinium chelates; *specific agent*
  adverse effects, 206–207
  blood pool agents, 205, 219
  iron-based, 205
  oral, 205
  thrombin-binding, 219
Contrast-enhanced imaging
  of aortic dissection, 131, 131*f*
  of breast neoplasia, 134–135, 134*f*, 135*f*
  of cerebral AVMs, 20, 21*f*
  of cerebral ischemia/infarction, 28
  of cervical cancer, 161, 161*f*
  of cervical disk herniation, 62*f*, 63, 63*f*
  of cervical spine neoplasia, 74
  of craniopharyngiomas, 13, 13*f*
  of female pelvis, 157–159, 157*f*–159*f*
  of heart, 122
  of intracranial aneurysms, 24–25, 25*f*
  in ischemic heart disease, 124–125, 125*f*
  of liver, 138, 205
  in magnetic resonance cholangiopancreatography, 144
  of melanoma, 118
  in meningitis, 42, 43*f*
  of metastatic disease
    in brain, 7, 204, 204*f*
    in diploic space, 14, 15*f*
    in lumbar spine, 102–103, 103*f*
  of MS plaques in brain, 36, 37*f*
  of multiple myeloma with vertebral involvement, 102–103, 103*f*
  in multiple sclerosis, 70, 71*f*
  of osseous pathology, 204, 205*f*
  of ovarian pathology, 162–163, 163*f*
  pancreatic, 151, 151*f*
  of paranasal sinusitis, 120, 120*f*
  of pericardium, 122
  of pituitary microadenomas, 12, 12*f*
  of postoperative lumbar spine, 94–95, 94*f*, 95*f*
  principles, 204
  of pulmonary embolism, 130, 131*f*
  of retinoblastoma, 119, 119*f*
  of schwannomas, 10, 11*f*
  of sinus disease in brain, 40, 41*f*
  of squamous cell carcinoma metastases, 204, 205*f*
  of thoracic neoplasia, 82, 83*f*
  of uterine cancer, 160, 160*f*
  of venous angiomas, 23, 23*f*
  of vertebrae, 204, 205*f*
  of vertebral body hemangioma, 88, 88*f*
  of vertebral metastases, 72–73, 73*f*
Coronary artery(ies), ectasia, 125
Cor pulmonale, 130, 131*f*
Corpus callosum
  agenesis, 47, 47*f*, 50, 51*f*, 86, 86*f*
    with Dandy-Walker malformation, 47
  malformations, 50, 51*f*
Corpus luteum cyst(s), 162, 163*f*
Cortical heterotopias, with Dandy-Walker malformation, 47
CPA. *See* Cerebellopontine angle
Craniocervical junction, malformations, 58
Craniopharyngioma(s), 13
Cyst(s). *See also* Aneurysmal bone cyst
  adrenal, 147, 147*f*
  Bartholin gland, 157, 157*f*
  in brain. *See also* Arachnoid cyst(s)
    differential diagnosis, 48–49
  cerebellar, 4, 5*f*
  corpus luteum, 162, 163*f*
  esophageal, 133
  ganglion, 200
    in wrist, 189, 189*f*
  hepatic, 138, 138*f*
    echinococcal, 138
    hemorrhagic, 138
    mucinous, of foregut origin, 138
  meniscal, 167, 167*f*
  ovarian, 162, 162*f*
    hemorrhagic, 162
  paralabral, in hip, 183, 183*f*
  renal, 148, 148*f*
    Bosniak types, 148, 149*f*
  seminal vesicle, 154
  subarachnoid, arachnoiditis and, 101
  testicular, 156
  tracheobronchial, 133

Cystadenocarcinoma, pancreatic, 150
Cystadenoma
  ovarian
    mucinous, 162
    serous, 162, 163*f*
  pancreatic
    mucinous, 150
    serous, 150
Cystic hygroma, 117
Cystitis, 154
Cytotoxic edema, 26

D

DAI. *See* Diffuse axonal injury
Dandy-Walker malformation, 47, 50
  differential diagnosis, 48
  extracranial abnormalities associated with, 47
  intracranial abnormalities associated with, 47
Deep venous thrombosis, 219
Degenerative disk disease, in lumbar spine, 96–99, 96*f*–99*f*
Deltoid ligament (ankle), 196–197, 197*f*
Demyelination. *See also* Multiple sclerosis
  in acute disseminated encephalomyelitis, 37
  in progressive multifocal leukoencephalopathy, 44, 45*f*
Dens, erosions, 67, 67*f*
Deoxyhemoglobin, 16, 17, 17*f*, 33
Dermal sinus, dorsal, 87
Dermoid
  cerebellopontine angle, 11
  in internal auditory canal, 11
  lumbosacral, 109, 109*f*
  ovarian, 162, 163*f*
Dermoid plug, 162, 163*f*
Diabetes insipidus, 15
Diabetic arthropathy, 203
  of ankle/foot, 199
Diastematomyelia, 59, 59*f*
Diffuse axonal injury, 33, 33*f*
Dilated cardiomyopathy, 122
Dilated perivascular spaces, 29
Diploic space
  lesions, 14–15, 15*f*
  metastases to, 14, 15*f*
Dipyridamole, 124
DISI. *See* Dorsal intercalated segment instability (wrist)
Disk bulge(s), 92
  with annular tear, 96, 96*f*
Disk extrusion(s), 92
Disk fragment(s), 92, 93
Disk herniation(s)
  central, 92, 93
  cervical spine, 62–63, 62*f*, 63*f*
    in degenerative disease, 65, 65*f*
    traumatic, 60, 61*f*
  foraminal, 92, 93
  lumbar spine, 89, 92–93, 92*f*, 93*f*
  paracentral, 92–93, 92*f*
  thoracic spine, 77–79, 77*f*–79*f*
Diskitis, 68
  lumbar spine, 98–99
Disk protrusion(s), 92
Dobutamine, 124
Donut sign, 141, 141*f*
Dorsal intercalated segment instability (wrist), 184–185, 189
Dotarem, 207
Double-duct sign, 150, 150*f*
DPVSs. *See* Dilated perivascular spaces
Drop metastases, 110
Dural tail, with meningioma, 8–9, 8*f*, 11
Dysmyelination, 52

E

Echinococcal cyst(s), hepatic, 138
Echinococcosis, hepatic alveolar, 138
EG. *See* Eosinophilic granuloma
Ejection fraction, calculation, 126
Elbow
  biceps tendon tears, 193
  injuries, 192–193
  lateral epicondylitis, 192
  ligamentous structures, 192, 192*f*
  medial epicondylar apophysitis, 193
  medial epicondylitis, 192–193
  radiocapitellar osteochondritis dissecans, 193
  tendons, 192, 192*f*
Elbow flexion and abducted shoulder with supinated forearm, 193
Electrocardiographic gating, 122
  prospective, 122
  retrospective, 122
Empyema, in meningitis, 42–43, 43*f*
Encephalitis, 38–39, 39*f*
  herpes simplex virus type 1, 38–39, 39*f*
  herpes simplex virus type 2, 39
  neonatal, 39
Encephalocele, cervical-occipital, with Chiari malformation, 47
Encephalomalacia, post-stroke, 26–27, 27*f*
Enchondroma, 200
Endocarditis, 127

Endometrioma(s), 162, 163*f*
Endometriosis, 162, 163*f*
Endometrium
  carcinoma, 160
    staging, 160–161, 160*f*
  ectopic, 159
  hyperplasia, 160
  polyps, 160
Endomyocardial fibrosis, 122
Eosinophilic granuloma, 14–15
Eovist. *See* Primovist/Eovist
Ependymoma, 4
  cellular, 108
  in cervical spine, 74, 75*f*
  lumbar spine, 106–108, 108*f*
  in lumbar spine, 74
  myxomatous, 108
  myxopapillary, 108, 108*f*
Epidermoid
  in brain, differential diagnosis, 48
  cerebellopontine angle, 11
  in internal auditory canal, 11
  lumbosacral, 109, 109*f*
Epidural hematoma(s), 18, 19*f*
  in cervical spine, 60, 60*f*
EP-2104R, 219
Esophageal cyst(s), 133
Esthesioneuroblastoma, of skull base, 117
Ethmoid sinus
  mucocele, 116, 116*f*
  mucosal thickening, 113
Ewing sarcoma, 201

F

FABS position, 193
Falx cerebri, abnormalities, with Chiari malformation, 47, 47*f*
FASI. *See* Foci of abnormal signal intensity
Fatty liver, 142, 142*f*
Femoral head
  avascular necrosis, 180–181, 180*f*, 181*f*
    in child, 181
    double-line sign, 180
    Mitchell classification, 180–181, 180*f*, 181*f*
  ischemia
    double-line sign, 180
    Mitchell classification, 180–181, 180*f*, 181*f*
Femoroacetabular impingement, 182
Feridex, 205
Ferumoxides, for hepatic imaging, 140
Fetal alcohol syndrome, 153
Fibroma(s), ovarian, 162
Fibromuscular dysplasia, 211
  and renal artery stenosis, 216, 217*f*
Fibrothecoma, ovarian, 162
Fibrous dysplasia
  craniofacial, 14, 15*f*
  malignant transformation, 14
  monostotic, 14
  polyostotic, 14
Flexor hallucis longus tendon, tears, 195
FNH. *See* Focal nodular hyperplasia
Focal nodular hyperplasia, hepatic, 139, 139*f*
Foci of abnormal signal intensity, in neurofibromatosis, 54, 54*f*
Foot
  abnormalities, 198–199
  bone contusion, 198–199
  inflammatory arthritis, 199
  ligamentous injuries, 197
  osteochondral lesions, 198, 199*f*
  tendinous injuries, 194–195, 195*f*
Forearm fractures, 184, 185*f*
Fragile-X syndrome, 34
Freiberg infraction, 198
Friedreich ataxia, 34
Fused vertebrae, 59

G

Gadobenate dimeglumine, 213. *See also* MultiHance
Gadobutrol, 213
Gadofosveset, 205, 219
Gadolinium chelates
  adverse effects, 206–207
  in breast milk, 206
  excretion, 205
  extracellular, 204
  macrocyclic, 206, 213
  and nephrogenic systemic fibrosis, 206–207, 207*f*, 213, 217
  safety, 204, 206
  stability, 206
  transplacental passage, 206
  use in pregnancy, 206
Gadolinium ethoxybenzyl diethylenetriamine pentaacetic acid. *See* Primovist/Eovist
Gadovist, safety, 207
Gallbladder
  adenomyomatosis, 144
  carcinoma, 144
  normal, 144
  wall thickening, 144
Gallstone(s), 144, 144*f*
Gamna-Gandy bodies, 143

Ganglion cyst, 200
  in wrist, 189, 189*f*
Ganglioneuroblastoma, 82, 152, 153*f*
  lumbar metastases, 103, 103*f*
Ganglioneuroma, 82, 152
Gangliosidosis
  GM1, 52, 53*f*
  GM2, 52
Gardner syndrome, 153
Gartner cysts, 157
Gastrinoma, 150
Gastrointestinal cancer
  cerebral metastases, 6
  metastases, 163
Gastrointestinal stromal tumor(s), hepatic metastases, 141
GBM. *See* Glioblastoma multiforme
Gd BOPTA. *See* MultiHance
Gd EOB-DTPA. *See* Primovist/Eovist
Giant cell tumor, 200
  of tendon sheath, in wrist, 189
GLAD. *See* Glenolabral articular disruptions
Glenohumeral joint
  anterior labral ligamentous periosteal sleeve avulsion injury, 178
  Bankart fracture, 176, 177*f*
  Bankart lesion, 176–177, 177*f*, 178
    "medialized," 178
    osseous, 176, 177*f*
    repair, postoperative imaging, 177
    reverse, 177, 177*f*
  Bennett lesion, 177
  capsular structures, 176
  double lesion, 176
  Hill-Sachs lesion, 176, 177*f*
    reverse, 177
  imaging technique for, 176
  instability, 176–177, 177*f*, 178–179, 178*f*, 179*f*
    AMBRI (atraumatic, multidirectional, bilateral), 176
    anterior, 176
    causes, 176
    posterior, 177, 177*f*
    posttraumatic, 176
  Perthes lesion, 178, 178*f*
  posterior labral ligamentous periosteal sleeve avulsion injury, 178
  triple lesion, 176
Glenohumeral ligament
  failure, 176
  humeral avulsion (HAGL), 176, 178
    bone involvement in (BHAGL), 178
    posterior (PHAGL), 178
  tears, 176
Glenoid labrum, 176
  Buford complex, 178
  degeneration, 179
  meniscoid variant, 179
  SLAP lesions, 178–179, 179*f*
  sublabral foramen, 178
  tears, 178–179, 178*f*, 179*f*
    bucket-handle, 179
    posterior, 177
    superior, 178
Glenolabral articular disruptions, 179
Glioblastoma multiforme, 2–3, 3*f*
Glioma(s)
  brainstem, 5
  hypothalamic, in neurofibromatosis, 54, 55*f*
  optic, in neurofibromatosis type 1, 54
  pontine, 5
Gliosis, 57
  in multiple sclerosis, 36–37, 37*f*
  post-stroke, 26–27, 27*f*
Glomus jugulare, 118, 118*f*
Glomus tympanicum, 10, 11*f*
Glomus vagale, 118
Graves disease, 121
Guillain-Barré syndrome, 111, 112*f*

H

Haglund syndrome, 194
Halo sign, 203
Hamartoma(s), biliary, 138
Hand-Schüller-Christian disease, 15
Hangman's fracture, 60
Hashimoto thyroiditis, 121
HCC. *See* Hepatocellular carcinoma
Head and neck
  incidental findings in, 113–115, 113*f*–115*f*
  infections, 120–121, 120*f*
  neoplasia, 116–121, 116*f*–120*f*
Heart
  malignant tumors, 132
  metastases to, 132
Heart disease
  congenital, 128–129, 129*f*
  ischemic, 124–125, 125*f*
  rheumatic, 126, 127
  valvular, 126–127, 127*f*
Heart valve(s)
  congenital defects, 127
  pressure gradients, measurement, 126
  regurgitant flow, measurement, 126
  stenosis, grading, 126

Hemangioblastoma(s), 5
  in cervical spine, 74
  lumbar spine, 108–109, 108*f*
  in thoracic spine, 74
  in von Hippel-Lindau disease, 55
Hemangioendothelioma
  in child, 153
  hepatic, 141
Hemangioma, 200
  hepatic, 138, 138*f*, 141
    in child, 153
  of skull, 15
  vertebral body, 88, 88*f*
Hemangiosarcoma, hepatic, 141
Hematoma(s)
  adrenal, 147
  epidural, 18, 19*f*
    in cervical spine, 60, 60*f*
  subacute, 200
  subdural, 18, 18*f*
    in child abuse, 18, 19*f*
Hematopoiesis, extramedullary, 105
Hemisphere(s), cerebellar, abnormalities, with Chiari malformation, 47, 47*f*
Hemivertebrae, cervical, 59, 59*f*
Hemochromatosis
  dilated cardiomyopathy in, 122
  primary, iron deposition in, 143
  secondary, hepatic findings in, 142–143, 143*f*
Hemoglobin, degradation products, 16–17
Hemorrhage
  acute, 16–17
  adrenal gland, 147
    in child, 153, 153*f*
  in brain, 31
  in cervical spine, 60
  chronic stage, 16–17, 17*f*
  extraaxial, 18–19, 18*f*, 19*f*
  hyperacute, 16, 17*f*
  intraparenchymal, 16–17, 17*f*, 24
    aneurysmal, 24–25
    associated with neoplasm, 17, 17*f*
    with dural AVMs, 21
  intraventricular, 19
  in paranasal sinuses, 120
  subacute, 16–17, 17*f*
  subarachnoid, 18–19, 19*f*, 24, 42
    with dural AVMs, 21
Hemosiderin, 16, 20, 22, 22*f*, 33, 74, 200
Hemosiderin cleft, 16, 17*f*
Hemosiderosis
  hepatic findings in, 143
  superficial, in brain, 19
Hepatic mass(es)
  benign, 138–139, 138*f*, 139*f*
  malignant, 140–141, 140*f*, 141*f*
Hepatitis, acute, 143
Hepatoblastoma, in child, 153, 153*f*
Hepatocellular carcinoma, 140, 140*f*, 143, 144–145
  in child, 153
  diffuse, 140, 141
  fibrolamellar, 140, 140*f*
Hereditary hemorrhagic telangiectasia. *See* Osler-Weber-Rendu syndrome
Hereditary spherocytosis, extramedullary hematopoiesis in, 105
Herpes simplex virus
  type 1, encephalitis, 38–39, 39*f*
  type 2, neonatal encephalitis, 39
Hill-Sachs lesion, 176, 177*f*
  reverse, 177
Hip
  avascular necrosis, 180–181, 180*f*, 181*f*
    double-line sign, 180
    Mitchell classification, 180–181, 180*f*, 181*f*
  bone marrow, edema, 180–181
  degenerative disease, 182
  fractures, 182, 182*f*
  labral disorders, 182–183, 183*f*
  osteoporosis, transient, 181
  paralabral cysts, 183, 183*f*
  transient marrow edema syndrome, 181
Histiocytosis, adrenal involvement, 147
Histiocytosis X. *See* Eosinophilic granuloma
HIV encephalopathy, 44, 45*f*
HIV-infected (AIDS) patients, CNS manifestations in, 44–45, 45*f*
Holoprosencephaly, 50, 51*f*
  alobar, 50
  lobar, 50
  semilobar, 50, 51*f*
Human immunodeficiency virus (HIV). *See* HIV-infected (AIDS) patients
Hunter syndrome, 52, 53*f*
Huntington chorea, 34
Hurler syndrome, 52
Hydrocele, testicular, 156, 156*f*
Hydrocephalus
  with Chiari malformation, 46, 47
  with Dandy-Walker malformation, 47
  ex vacuo, 34
  in meningitis, 43
  obstructive, tumor-related, 4, 5*f*
  with venous infarction, 41

Hydromyelia, 46, 46*f*, 58, 58*f*
Hydrosyringomyelia, with Chiari malformation, 46
Hypertensive encephalopathy, 29, 35
Hypertrophic cardiomyopathy, 122–123, 123*f*
Hypotension, contrast agent–induced, 206

I

Immunocompromise, CNS manifestations in, 44–45, 45*f*
Infection(s)
  of head and neck, 120–121, 120*f*
  of skull base, 117
Inferior glenohumeral ligament, 176
Insulinoma, 150
Internal auditory canal, neoplasms, 10–11, 11*f*
Internal carotid artery
  distal, thrombosis, 28
  and giant aneurysm, 24
Intraventricular area (cardiac), calculation, 126
Intraventricular hemorrhage, 19
Intraventricular volume (cardiac), calculation, 126
Inverted papillomas, of head and neck, 116, 116*f*
Ischemic heart disease, 124–125, 125*f*

J

Jefferson fracture, 60
JPA. *See* Juvenile pilocytic astrocytomas
Juvenile nasal angiofibromas, 116–117, 117*f*
Juvenile pilocytic astrocytomas, 4, 5*f*

K

Kidney(s). *See also* Polycystic kidney disease; Renal cell carcinoma
  cysts, Bosniak types, 148, 149*f*
  masses, 148–149, 148*f*, 149*f*
  mesoblastic nephroma, 152–153, 153*f*
  pediatric, 152–153, 153*f*
  transplantation
    donor assessment, 216–217
    posttransplant assessment, 217
Kienböck malacia, 189
Klatskin tumor(s), 145
Klippel-Feil syndrome, 59, 59*f*
Knee
  arcuate ligament complex, 171
  bony contusions, 168, 169*f*
  bursae, 170–171
  bursitis, 171
  button (stud) osteophyte, 172, 173*f*
  cartilage
    autologous chondrocyte implantation, 173
    autologous grafts, 173
    lesions, 172–173, 173*f*
  cartilaginous injury, 172–173, 173*f*
    grading, 172–173, 173*f*
  collateral ligaments, 170–171, 170*f*, 171*f*
  cruciate ligaments, 168–169, 169*f*, 171
  imaging, technique for, 164–165
  meniscal contusion, 167
  meniscal intrasubstance myxoid degeneration, 167
  meniscal pathology, 165, 165*f*
    differential diagnosis, 167
  meniscal tears, 165, 165*f*, 171
    bucket handle, 166–167, 167*f*
    complex, 166, 166*f*, 167, 167*f*
    flap, 166
    horizontally oriented (cleave), 165*f*, 166
    longitudinal, 166
    nonpure horizontal, 166, 166*f*
    postoperative, 167
    radial, 166
    and synovial cyst, 167, 167*f*
    vertical, 166, 166*f*, 167
  osteochondral lesions, 172–173, 173*f*
  pediatric, meniscal appearance, 167
  postolateral complex, 171
  postoperative, 167
  subchondral degenerative changes, 172, 173*f*
Köhler disease, 198
Krabbe disease, 53
Krukenberg tumor, 163
Kupffer cells, 140, 205

L

Lacunar infarcts, 29–31, 30*f*
Langerhans cell granulomatosis. *See* Eosinophilic granuloma
Laryngeal edema, contrast agent–induced, 206
Lateral collateral ligament (knee), 171
  tears, 171, 171*f*
Lateral ulnar collateral ligament, 192, 192*f*
LCL. *See* Lateral collateral ligament (knee)
Left atrium, dilation, 126, 127*f*
Legg-Calve-Perthes disease, 181
Leiomyoma, uterine, 158–159, 159*f*
Leiomyosarcoma, 159
  hepatic metastases, 141

Lenticulostriate artery(ies), 29
Lentiform nucleus, ischemia, 29, 30*f*
Leptomeningeal carcinomatosis, lumbar spine involvement in, 110–112, 110*f*–112*f*
Leptomeninges, metastases to, 7, 110
Leukemia
  bone marrow in, 202
  renal metastases, in child, 153
Leukodystrophy(ies), 52–53, 53*f*
Libman-Sacks endocarditis, 126
Ligament of Humphrey, 167
Ligament of Wrisberg, 167
Lipoma(s), 200
  brainstem, with Dandy-Walker malformation, 47
  cardiac, 132
  chest wall, 132
  intracranial, 49
  lumbar spine, 87, 87*f*
Lipomyelocele, 87
Lipomyelomeningocele, 87
Liposarcoma, 201
Lisfranc ligament, 197
  sprains, 197
Lissencephaly, 50, 51*f*
Little leaguer's elbow, 193
Liver. *See also* Hepatocellular carcinoma
  abscess
    amebic, 141
    pyogenic, 141
  adenomas, 139
  benign masses, 138–139, 138*f*, 139*f*
  central hyperintense scar, 139
  cirrhosis, 143, 143*f*, 145
  cysts, 138, 138*f*
  diffuse pathology, 142–143, 142*f*, 143*f*
  fatty, 142, 142*f*
  focal nodular hyperplasia, 139, 139*f*
  hemangioma, 138–139, 139*f*
  iron deposition in, 142–143, 143*f*
  malignant masses, 140–141, 140*f*, 141*f*
    in children, 153, 153*f*
  metastatic disease, 138, 140–141, 141*f*, 150
  neoplasms, 138–139, 139*f*
Lumbar spine
  annular tears, 96, 96*f*
  anterolisthesis, 97, 97*f*
  arachnoiditis, 101
  bone marrow
    disorders, 104–105, 104*f*
    MRI appearance
      in metastatic disease, 102, 102*f*
      normal, 102, 102*f*
  canal stenosis, 98, 98*f*, 99*f*, 103, 103*f*
  compression fractures, 90–91, 90*f*, 91*f*
    benign, 90*f*, 91
    malignant (pathologic), 91
    osteoporotic, 90–91, 90*f*
  congenital abnormalities, 86–87, 86*f*, 87*f*
  congenitally shortened pedicles, 98, 98*f*
  cystic lesions, 88–89, 89*f*
  degenerative disk disease, 96–99, 96*f*–99*f*
    end plate changes in, 97, 97*f*, 98, 98*f*
    and gas in disk, 97, 97*f*
    Modic type 1, 98
    Modic type 2, 98, 99*f*
  degenerative facet disease, 88–89, 99
  disk, MRI appearance
    age-related changes in, 96
    normal, 97, 97*f*
  disk bulge, 92, 98, 98*f*, 99*f*
    with annular tear, 96, 96*f*
  disk desiccation, 96, 98, 98*f*
  diskectomy, postoperative MRI appearance, 95
  disk fragments, 92, 93
  disk height
    loss, 97, 97*f*, 98, 99*f*, 103, 103*f*
    normal, 97, 97*f*
  disk herniation, 62
    central, 92, 93
    foraminal, 92, 93
    paracentral, 92–93, 92*f*
  disk herniations, 89, 92–93, 92*f*, 93*f*
    after prior surgery, 94–95, 95*f*
  diskitis, 98–99
  dysraphism, with Chiari malformation, 58
  ependymoma, 74
  epidural abscess, 101, 101*f*
  epidural lipomatosis, 98, 99*f*
  facet arthropathy, 99
  facet synovitis, 99
  with ferromagnetic hardware, 95
  imaging
    artifacts, 96
    technique for, 96
  incidental findings in, 88–89, 88*f*, 89*f*
  infections, 100–101, 100*f*, 101*f*
  laminectomy, postoperative MRI appearance, 95
  leptomeningeal carcinomatosis, 110–112, 110*f*–112*f*
  lipomas, 87, 87*f*
  lymphoma metastatic to, 110–111, 111*f*
  metastatic disease, 93, 102–103, 102*f*, 103*f*
    hemorrhagic, 102

in multiple myeloma, 102, 103*f*, 104, 104*f*
neoplasms, 106–109, 106*f*–109*f*
extradural, 106
intradural extramedullary, 106
medullary, 106
nerve root enhancement, 111–112, 112*f*
neuroforaminal stenosis, 99, 99*f*
osteoblastoma, 200, 200*f*
osteophytes, 99, 99*f*
pars defects, 97, 97*f*
perineural root sleeve cyst, 112
postoperative, 94–95, 94*f*, 95*f*
with disk herniation, 94–95, 95*f*
epidural fibrosis, 94, 94*f*
infection in, 95
scar, 94, 94*f*
pseudo bulge, 97, 97*f*
pseudomeningocele, 95
radiculitis, 95
spondylodiskitis, 100, 100*f*
contiguous spread, 101, 101*f*
synovial cysts, 88–89, 89, 93, 93*f*
vertebroplasty, complications, 90
Lumbosacral nerve root anomalies, 89, 89*f*
Lunate
avascular necrosis, 189
injury, 184–185
osteonecrosis, Lichtman classification, 189
Lunatomalacia, 189
Lung(s)
cancer, cerebral metastases, 6
malignant tumors, 132
MRI, technique for, 132
Lunotriquetral ligament, tears, 185
Lymphoma(s)
CNS, 3, 44–45
hepatic metastases, 141
mediastinal, 132, 133
renal metastases, in child, 153
of skull base, 117
spinal metastases, 110–111, 111*f*
vertebral marrow replacement in, 104, 104*f*
Lysosomal storage disorders, 52, 53*f*

M

Macroadenoma(s), pituitary, 12–13, 12*f*
Magic-angle phenomenon, 167
Magnetic resonance angiography
carotid, 209–210, 210*f*
continuous table movement (CTM) technique, 212
contrast agents for, 205, 213
contrast-enhanced, 209–210, 210*f*
of aneurysms, 218
dynamic techniques, 210
of great vessels, 210–211
of neck, 209–210, 210*f*
peripheral, 212–215, 213*f*–215*f*
principles, 204
renal, 216–217
time-resolved, 210, 212
peripheral, 214–215, 215*f*
TREAT technique, 210, 212
TRICKS technique, 212
TWIST technique, 210, 211*f*, 212
MIP images, 209–210, 210*f*, 213–214, 213*f*, 214*f*
peripheral, 212–215, 213*f*–215*f*
phase-contrast, 25
principles, 208–209
renal artery, 216–217, 216*f*, 217*f*
TOF, 20–21, 25, 25*f*, 208–209
Magnetic resonance cholangiopancreatography
of biliary disease, 144–145, 144*f*, 145*f*
of chronic pancreatitis, 151, 151*f*
of pancreatic carcinoma, 150, 150*f*
Magnetic resonance venography, applications, 219, 219*f*
Magnevist, and nephrogenic systemic fibrosis, 206–207, 207*f*
Malignant fibrous histiocytoma, 201
Mamillary body(ies), atrophy or enhancement, 34, 35*f*
Mammography, magnetic resonance
indications for, 134
protocols, 134
Mangafodipir, 140
Marfan syndrome, 127
Massa intermedia, abnormalities, with Chiari malformation, 47, 47*f*
Mastoiditis, 121
Maxillary sinus
antrochoanal polyps, 116
mucosal thickening, 113, 114*f*, 120, 120*f*
mucous retention cysts, 113, 113*f*
MCA. *See* Middle cerebral artery
McCune-Albright syndrome, 14
MCL. *See* Medial collateral ligament (knee)
Medial collateral ligament (knee)
deep, 170, 170*f*
lesions, 169, 170–171, 170*f*
normal, 170, 170*f*
superficial, 170, 170*f*
Medial talar tubercle, 196–197
Medial ulnar collateral ligament, 192, 193*f*
tears, 193, 193*f*

Median nerve, in carpal tunnel syndrome, 184, 185*f*
Mediastinum
 benign lymph nodes, 133
 infectious lymphadenopathy, 133
 inflammatory lymphadenopathy, 133, 133*f*
 malignant lymphadenopathy, 133
 primary tumors, 132–133, 133*f*
 tumor invasion, 132, 133*f*
Medulla, lateral, infarction, 29–30, 30*f*
Medulloblastoma, 4, 5*f*
Mega cisterna magna, 48, 50, 51*f*
Meigs syndrome, 162
Melanoma, 201
 amelanotic, 119
 cerebral metastases, 6, 7
 metastases, to brain, 6, 7
 ocular, 118–119
Meningeal carcinomatosis, 42
Meningioma(s)
 in brain, 8–9, 8*f*
 in cervical spine, 74–76, 76*f*
 in childhood, 9
 differential diagnosis, 10–11
 lumbar spine, 106, 107*f*
 malignant, 9
 multiple, 9
 in neurofibromatosis, 55, 55*f*
 perioptic, 54
 of skull base, 117
 spinal, 82–83, 83*f*
Meningitis, 35, 40, 41*f*, 42–43, 43*f*
 bacterial, 7
 clinical presentation, 42
 complications, 42–43, 43*f*
 etiologies, 42
 nerve root enhancement in, 101
 tuberculous, 7
 viral, 7
Meningocele, 112
Meningomyelocele, and tethered cord, 86–87, 87*f*
Meniscal tear(s). *See* Knee, meniscal tears
Meniscofemoral ligament, 167
Metachromatic leukodystrophy, 52–53
Metastatic disease
 adrenal gland, 147, 147*f*
 in brain, 3, 6–7, 6*f*, 44–45
  cystic appearance, 6*f*, 7
  hemorrhagic, 6*f*, 7
  as ring-enhancing lesions, 6*f*, 7, 38
 in diploic space, 14, 15*f*
 in heart, 132
 hepatic, 138, 140–141, 141*f*, 150
 leptomeningeal, 7, 110
 in lumbar spine, 93, 102–103, 102*f*, 103*f*
 orbital, 119
 of skull base, 117
 in thoracic spine, 80, 80*f*
 vertebral, 72–73, 72*f*, 73*f*
Methemoglobin, 16, 18, 24, 25, 40–41
Microadenoma(s), pituitary, 12, 12*f*
Midbrain
 abnormalities, with Chiari malformation, 47, 47*f*
 infarction, 29
Middle cerebral artery, 31
 aneurysm, 24, 25*f*
 and giant aneurysm, 24
 infarction, 27–28, 27*f*, 29
 segments, 28
Midfoot sprain, 197
Migraine disorders, 35
Mitochondrial leukoencephalopathy, 53
Mitral valve
 area, 126
 insufficiency, 126, 127*f*
 prolapse, 126
 regurgitation, 126
 stenosis, 126, 127*f*
Mn DPDP. *See* Mangafodipir
Moderator band, 129, 129*f*
Monoclonal gammopathy of undetermined significance, 202
Morton neuroma, 199
MRA. *See* Magnetic resonance angiography
MRCP. *See* Magnetic resonance cholangiopancreatography
MRV. *See* Magnetic resonance venography
MS. *See* Multiple sclerosis
Mucocele
 ethmoid sinus, 116, 116*f*
 of paranasal sinus, 120
Mucoepidermoid, of head and neck, 118
Mucopolysaccharidosis (MPS), 52, 53*f*
Mucopyocele, 116
Müllerian duct(s)
 fusion, 157
  congenital defects, 157, 157*f*, 158*f*
 hypoplasia/agenesis, 157
MultiHance, 204–205
 hepatic imaging, 138, 140
 in magnetic resonance cholangiopancreatography, 144
 safety, 207*f*
Multiple myeloma, 200, 202–203
 bone marrow in, 202

lumbar spine involvement in, 102, 103*f*, 104, 104*f*
metastases, 203
therapeutic response in, 203
thoracic spine involvement in, 81, 81*f*
vertebral involvement in, 81, 81*f*, 102, 103*f*, 104, 104*f*
Multiple sclerosis, 29, 34, 36–37, 37*f*
diagnosis
imaging technique for, 70, 71*f*
MRI criteria, 36, 69
optic neuritis in, 36–37
progression, 36–37, 37*f*
spinal cord involvement in, 36, 69–70, 69*f*, 70*f*
tumefactive lesions, 36, 37*f*
Musculoskeletal system. *See also specific anatomic entity*
imaging technique for, 164
neoplasms, 200–201, 200*f*, 201*f*
benign, 200
Myelination, 52
pseudo-early, 57
Myelocele, 87
Myelomalacia, cervical, 60
Myelomeningocele, 86–87, 87*f*
with Chiari malformation, 46, 58
Myelosclerosis, extramedullary hematopoiesis in, 105
Myocardial infarct/infarction, 124, 125*f*
Myocardial ischemia, 124–125, 125*f*
Myocardial noncompaction of ventricle, 123
Myocardial perfusion imaging, 122, 124
Myocardial scarring, 125, 125*f*
Myocardial viability, assessment, 122, 124, 125*f*
Myocarditis, 122, 123*f*
Myocardium
hibernating, 124
stunned, 124
Myxoma(s), left atrial, 132, 133*f*

N

Nabothian cysts, 157
Nasal cavity, antrochoanal polyps, 116
Nasal polyps, 116
Nausea, contrast agent–induced, 206
Navicular, osteochondrosis, 198
Neoplasms (primary)
adrenal, 146–147, 147*f*
of brain
infratentorial, 4–5, 5*f*
supratentorial, 2–3, 3*f*
breast, 134–135, 134*f*, 135*f*
of cervical spine, 74–76, 75*f*, 76*f*
head and neck, 116–121, 116*f*–120*f*
of internal auditory canal, 10–11, 11*f*
liver, 138–139, 139*f*
of lumbar spine, 106–109, 106*f*–109*f*
musculoskeletal, 200–201, 200*f*, 201*f*
pancreatic, 150, 150*f*
sellar/parasellar, 12–13, 12*f*, 13*f*
testicular, 156
thoracic, 132–133, 133*f*
of thoracic spine, 82–83, 83*f*
Nephroblastoma, 152–153, 152*f*
Nephroblastomatosis, 153
Nephrogenic systemic fibrosis, gadolinium chelates and, 206–207, 207*f*, 213, 217
Nerve sheath tumors, 82, 89
cervical spine, 74, 76
lumbar spine, 106, 112
Neural tumors, of head and neck, 118
Neuroblastoma, 82, 152, 152*f*
Neurocysticercosis, 38, 39*f*
Neurodegenerative disorders, 34–35, 34*f*, 35*f*
Neuroendocrine tumor(s), hepatic metastases, 141
Neurofibroma(s)
lumbar spine, 106, 107*f*
of thoracic spine, 82
Neurofibromatosis, 54–55, 54*f*, 55*f*
diagnostic criteria for, 54
foci of abnormal signal intensity in, 54, 54*f*
type 1, 4, 54, 82, 106, 112
type 2, 9, 10, 55, 55*f*, 82
Neuroma(s), plexiform, in neurofibromatosis, 54, 112
Neuropathic joint(s), 203
of ankle/foot, 199
Neurosarcoidosis, 42
NF. *See* Neurofibromatosis
No-reflow phenomenon, 124
NSF. *See* Nephrogenic systemic fibrosis

O

Occipitalization, 58
Odontoid fracture, 59, 60
Oligoastrocytoma, 2, 3*f*
Oligodendroglioma, 2, 3*f*
Omniscan, and nephrogenic systemic fibrosis, 206–207, 207*f*
Oncocytoma, renal, 149
Optic neuritis, in multiple sclerosis, 36–37
Optimark, and nephrogenic systemic fibrosis, 206–207, 207*f*

Orbit. *See also* Retinoblastoma
  melanoma, 118–119
  metastatic disease, 119
Orbital cellulitis, 121
Orbital inflammatory disease, 121
  idiopathic (pseudotumor), 121
Os acromiale, 175
Osler-Weber-Rendu syndrome, 20, 84, 130, 131*f*
Os odontoideum, 58–59
Os peroneum, 195
Osseous abnormalities, with Chiari malformation, 46, 58
Osteoblastoma, 200, 200*f*
Osteochondritis dissecans, 172–173
  radiocapitellar, 193
Osteochondroma(s), 200
Osteoid osteoma, 200, 203
Osteomyelitis, 203
  of ankle/foot, 199
  mandibular, 121
Osteophytes
  button/stud (knee), 172, 173*f*
  cervical, 63, 63*f*, 64, 64*f*, 65, 65*f*, 68, 68*f*
  knee, 172, 173*f*
  lumbar spine, 99, 99*f*
  shoulder, 175
  in thoracic spine, 77, 78*f*
Osteoporosis, migratory, of ankle/foot, 199
Osteosarcoma, 200–201, 201*f*
  telangiectatic, 200
Os trigonum, 195
Otitis externa, malignant, 121
Otitis media, 121
Ovarian cancer, 162–163, 163*f*
  hepatic metastases, 141
  metastases, 163
  staging, 163
Ovarian cyst(s), 162, 162*f*
Ovarian hyperstimulation syndrome, 162
Ovarian infarction, 162
Ovarian pathology, 162–163, 162*f*, 163*f*
Ovarian torsion, 162
Oxyhemoglobin, 16

P

Pachygyria, 50, 51*f*
Pancoast tumor, 132
Pancreas
  disease, 150–151, 150*f*, 151*f*
  imaging technique for, 150
  inflammatory disease, 151
  neoplasms, 150–151, 150*f*
    cystic, 150–151
    mucinous, 150–151
  peripancreatic fluid collections, 151, 151*f*
Pancreatic adenocarcinoma, 150, 150*f*
  hepatic metastases, 150
Pancreatic duct, dilatation, 151, 151*f*
Pancreatitis, 151, 151*f*
  chronic, 150, 151, 151*f*
  focal chronic, 150
  grading, Cambridge criteria, 151
  hemorrhagic, 151
Paraganglioma, carotid body, 118
Paranasal sinus(es)
  fungal infection, 121
  incidental findings in, 113
  inspissated secretions, 113–114, 114*f*
  mucosal thickening, 113, 114*f*
  mucous retention cysts, 113, 113*f*
  neoplasia, 116, 116*f*
  polyps, 113, 116
Parapharyngeal space
  infections spreading to, 121
  lesions in, 114–115, 115*f*
  masses, 117, 118
  neoplasia, 118
Parathyroid gland(s), tumors, 132
Parotid glands
  accessory, 117
  tumors, 118
PCA. *See* Posterior cerebral artery
PCL. *See* Posterior cruciate ligament
Pediatric abdomen
  disease, 152–153, 152*f*, 153*f*
  imaging
    sedation for, 152
    technique for, 152
  masses, 152, 152*f*
Pediatric retroperitoneal mass, 152, 152*f*
Pellegrini-Stieda disease, 171
Pelvis
  female, benign lesions, 157–159, 157*f*–159*f*
  imaging, technique for, 157
  male, 154–156, 154*f*–156*f*
Pericardium, imaging, 122
Peripheral vasculature, magnetic resonance angiography, 212–215, 213*f*–215*f*
Peritonsillar abscess, 120*f*, 121
Periventricular leukomalacia, 32, 32*f*
Pernicious anemia, cervical spine in, 71, 71*f*
Peroneal tendons, tears, 194
Perthes lesion (shoulder), 178, 178*f*
Pharyngeal space, lesions in, 114–115, 115*f*
Phenytoin, cerebellar atrophy caused by, 34, 35*f*

Pheochromocytoma, 147, 147*f*
in von Hippel-Lindau disease, 55
PICA. *See* Posterior inferior cerebellar artery
Pigmented villonodular synovitis, 199, 200
Pituitary adenoma(s), 12–13, 12*f*
Pituitary tumor. *See also* Sellar neoplasia
skull base involvement in, 117
Plantar calcaneonavicular ligament, 196–197
Plantar fasciitis, 199
Plasmacytoma, 104, 202–203
in parapharyngeal space, 117
Platybasia, 58
Pleural fluid, 132–133
exudative, 132–133
PLL. *See* Posterior longitudinal ligament
PML. *See* Progressive multifocal leukoencephalopathy
Pneumobilia, 144
POLPSA. *See* Posterior labral ligamentous periosteal sleeve avulsion injury
Polyarteritis nodosa, 219
Polycystic kidney disease, 148, 148*f*
and arachnoid cysts, 48
Polycythemia rubra vera, bone marrow in, 104–105
Polycythemia vera, bone marrow in, 202
Polymethylmethacrylate cement, MRI appearance, 90
Polymicrogyria, 47, 50, 51*f*
with Dandy-Walker malformation, 47
Pons, vascular supply to, 29–30
Popliteal aneurysm, 218
Popliteus muscle, 171
Popliteus tendon, 171
tears, 171, 171*f*
Pork tapeworm. *See* Neurocysticercosis
Portal hypertension, 143, 143*f*
Portal vein thrombosis, 143
Posterior cerebral artery, 31
infarction, 27*f*, 28, 29
Posterior communicating artery, 29
aneurysm, 24, 25*f*
Posterior cruciate ligament, 168, 169*f*
tears, 169, 169*f*
Posterior fossa
Chiari malformations, 46–47, 47*f*
congenital malformations, 46–47, 46*f*–47*f*, 58
Dandy-Walker malformation, 47
hemangioblastomas, 55
tumors, 4–5
vascular supply to, 29
Posterior inferior cerebellar artery, 30, 30*f*, 31
infarction, 30, 30*f*
Posterior labral ligamentous periosteal sleeve avulsion injury, 178
Posterior longitudinal ligament
injury, 61
MRI appearance, 61, 62, 62*f*
ossification, 65–66, 66*f*
Posterior talofibular ligament, 196
Primary biliary cirrhosis, 145
Primary sclerosing cholangitis, 145, 145*f*
Primovist/Eovist, 205
hepatic imaging, 138
in magnetic resonance cholangiopancreatography, 144
Progressive multifocal leukoencephalopathy, in immunocompromised patient, 44, 45*f*
ProHance, safety, 207, 207*f*
PROPELLER technique, 152
Prostate gland. *See also* Benign prostatic hypertrophy
cancer
detection, 155–156
metastases, 155–156
postoperative recurrence, 155
staging, 154–155, 155*f*
normal, 155
Pubic insufficiency fracture, 182, 182*f*
Pulmonary embolism, 130, 131*f*, 219, 219*f*
Pulmonary hypertension, 130, 131*f*
Pulmonary hypoxic vasoconstriction, 130
Pulmonary perfusion studies, 130
Pulmonic valve
insufficiency, 127, 127*f*
stenosis, 127
PVL. *See* Periventricular leukomalacia

R

Radial collateral ligament, 192, 192*f*
Radiation therapy, effects on bone marrow, 80, 80*f*
Ranula, 117
Rathke cleft cyst(s), 13
Recurrent artery of Heubner, 29
Reidel thyroiditis, 121
Renal artery
aortic dissection and, 218, 218*f*, 219*f*
magnetic resonance angiography, 216–217, 216*f*, 217*f*
stenosis
causes, 216
in fibromuscular dysplasia, 216, 217*f*
measurement, 216

Renal cell carcinoma, 148–149, 149*f*
  adrenal metastases, 147
  clear cell, 149
  hepatic metastases, 141
  metastases, to brain, 7
  papillary cell, 149
  staging, 148–149, 149*f*
  venous thrombus caused by, 219
Renal failure, and nephrogenic systemic fibrosis, 206–207, 207*f*, 213, 217
Renal masses, 148–149, 148*f*, 149*f*
Restrictive cardiomyopathy, 122
Retinal detachment, 119, 119*f*
Retinoblastoma, 118–119, 119*f*
Rhabdomyosarcoma, 201
  cardiac, 132
  in parapharyngeal space, 117
Rheumatoid arthritis
  cervical spine involvement in, 67, 67*f*
  wrist involvement in, 189
Right ventricular outflow tract, stenosis, 127, 127*f*
Rokitansky plug, 162, 163*f*
Rotator cuff
  tears, 174–175, 175*f*
    complete, 174, 175*f*
    full-thickness, 174, 175*f*
    partial, 174
    small full-thickness, 174
  tendinosus, 174, 175*f*

S

Sacral insufficiency fracture, 182, 183*f*
Sacral insufficiency fractures, 90–91, 91*f*
Sacral plexus, plexiform neuroma, 106
Salivary gland(s)
  abscess, 121
  tumors, 118
Salivary rest carcinoma, 117
Sanfilippo syndrome, 52
Sarcoidosis, 7
  mediastinal involvement in, 133, 133*f*
Sarcoma
  synovial, 200
  wrist, 189
SCA. *See* Superior cerebellar artery
Scaphoid fractures, 188–189
Scaphoid nonunion advanced collapse, 189
Scapholunate advanced collapse, 185
Scapholunate angle, 185
Scapholunate gap, widened, 184
Scapholunate ligament, 184
  tears, 184–185
    and dorsal intercalated segment instability, 184–185
Schizencephaly, 50, 51*f*
Schmorl nodes, 88, 89*f*, 90
Schwannoma(s)
  acoustic, in neurofibromatosis, 55, 55*f*
  cerebellopontine angle, 10–11, 11*f*
  facial, in neurofibromatosis, 55, 55*f*
  lumbar spine, 106, 106*f*
  malignant, 82
  recurrent, 10
  of thoracic spine, 82, 83*f*
  vestibular, 10, 11*f*
    bilateral, 10
Scrotal abnormalities, 156
SDH. *See* Subdural hematoma(s)
Segond fractures, 168, 171
  medial (reversed), 169
Sellar neoplasia, skull base involvement in, 117
Seminal vesicle(s)
  bladder cancer metastases to, 154
  congenital abnormalities, 154
  cysts, 154
Seminoma, testicular, 156
Septooptic dysplasia, 50
Shading sign, 162, 163*f*
Shoulder
  bursitis, 174, 175*f*
  imaging technique for, 174, 175*f*
  osteophytes, 175
Shoulder impingement syndrome, 174–175
Sialadenitis, 121
Sickle cell anemia, 35
  bone marrow in, 105, 202, 202*f*
  vertebral morphology in, 72
Sinonasal carcinoma, of skull base, 117
Sinus(es), paranasal. *See* Paranasal sinus(es)
Sinus disease, in brain, 40–41, 41*f*
Sinusitis
  in brain, 40–41, 41*f*
  paranasal, 113, 120, 120*f*
    acute, 113
    chronic, 113
    subacute, 113
    with Wegener's granulomatosis, 120–121
Skip lesions, 201, 201*f*
Skull, lesions, 14–15, 15*f*
Skull base, neoplasia, 117
SLAC. *See* Scapholunate advanced collapse

SLAP. *See* Superior labrum anterior posterior lesions
Slipped capital femoral epiphysis, 181, 181*f*
SNAC. *See* Scaphoid nonunion advanced collapse
Soft tissue tumor(s)
  benign, 200
  malignant, 200–201
Sphenoid dysplasia, in neurofibromatosis, 55
Spina bifida, with Chiari malformation, 46
Spina bifida occulta, with Chiari malformation, 46
Spinal artery(ies), 85
Spinal cord. *See also* Tethered cord
  arteriovenous fistula, 84–85
  cervical
    atrophy, 60
    compression, 60, 60*f*, 64, 64*f*, 65, 65*f*
      rheumatoid-related, 67, 67*f*
    compromise, by metastatic disease, 72, 73*f*
    disk herniation and, 62–63, 62*f*, 63*f*
    edema, 60, 61*f*
    hemorrhagic lesion, 60
  cystic lesions, differential diagnosis, 74
  hemangioblastomas, 55
  infarction, 85
  ischemia, 85, 85*f*
  in multiple sclerosis, 36, 69–70, 69*f*, 70*f*
  thoracic
    compression, 80–81, 80*f*
    impingement, 77–78, 78*f*
  wall thinning, 58, 58*f*
Spine
  abnormalities, with Chiari malformation, 46, 58
  cervical. *See* Cervical spine
  C1-occiput fusion, with Chiari malformation, 46
  cystic lesions, 88–89, 89*f*
  focal fatty deposits, 88, 88*f*
  incidental findings in, 88–89, 88*f*, 89*f*
  intervertebral disk, MRI appearance, age-related changes in, 96
  localizing scan, 77, 77*f*
  lumbar. *See* Lumbar spine
  thoracic. *See* Thoracic spine
Spinocerebellar ataxia, 34
Splenomegaly, 143, 143*f*
Spondylodiskitis, lumbar spine, 100, 100*f*
  contiguous spread, 101, 101*f*
Spondylolisthesis, 97, 98
Spring ligament (tibiospring; ankle), 196–197
Squamous cell carcinoma (SCC), of head and neck, 116–117, 116*f*
SSFP. *See* Steady-state free precession
Steady-state free precession, 122, 217
Stenogyria, 50
  with Chiari malformation, 47
Steroids, and bone infarction, 202, 202*f*
Stress testing, 124
String of beads appearance, 211
Stroke
  acute, 26, 27*f*
  arterial thrombotic, 30*f*, 31
  chronic, 26, 27*f*
  embolic, 31
  hemodynamic, 31
  hemorrhagic, 31
  hyperacute, 26, 27*f*
  lacunar, 29, 30*f*
  pontine, 29, 30*f*
  subacute, 26
Stroke volume, 126
Sturge-Weber syndrome, 20, 23, 57, 57*f*
Subarachnoid cyst(s), arachnoiditis and, 101
Subarachnoid hemorrhage, 18–19, 19*f*, 24, 42
  with dural AVMs, 21
Subarachnoid space, widened, secondary to atrophy, differential diagnosis, 48
Subdural effusion, in meningitis, 42–43, 43*f*
Subdural empyema, in meningitis, 42–43, 43*f*
Subdural hematoma(s), 18, 18*f*
  in children, 18, 19*f*
Subdural hygroma, 18, 48
Sunburst sign, 201, 201*f*
Superficial tibiotalar ligament, 196–197
Superior cerebellar artery, 29–30
  infarction, 30, 30*f*, 31
Superior labrum anterior posterior lesions, 178–179, 179*f*
Supraspinatus tendon
  tear, 174, 175*f*
  tendinosus, 174, 175*f*
Susceptibility artifact, 95, 96
Sustentaculum tali, 196–197
Syringobulbia, 58
Syringohydromyelia, 46, 46*f*
Syringomyelia, arachnoiditis and, 101
Syrinx, 77, 77*f*
  cervical, 60
  differential diagnosis, 74
Systemic lupus erythematosus, brain in, 34–35, 35*f*

T

Taenia solium. See Neurocysticercosis
Takayasu arteritis, 218–219
Talus
  aneurysmal bone cyst, 200, 200*f*
  avascular necrosis, 198, 199*f*
  osteochondral lesions, 198, 199*f*
Tarlov cysts, 88–89, 89*f*
Tay-Sachs disease, 52, 53*f*
Tectum, abnormalities, with Chiari malformation, 47
Temporomandibular joint
  disease, 190–191, 191*f*
    sequelae, 191
  dysfunction, 190–191
  imaging technique for, 190
  locked condyle, 190
  meniscal cartilage, myxomatous degeneration, 190
  meniscus
    anterior reducible dislocation, 190, 191*f*
    fixed-type dislocation, 190, 191*f*
    medial or lateral displacement, 190
  motion, evaluation, 190, 191*f*
  osteoarthritis, 191
Tentorium, abnormalities
  with Chiari malformation, 47, 47*f*
  with Dandy-Walker malformation, 47
Teratoma(s)
  mediastinal, 132
  ovarian, 162
Testes
  acute infarction, 156
  cysts, 156
  hydrocele, 156, 156*f*
  neoplastic masses, 156
  nonseminomatous tumors, 156
  seminoma, 156
  torsion, 156
Tethered cord, 86–87, 86*f*, 87*f*, 109, 109*f*
  retethering, 86, 86*f*, 87
Tetralogy of Fallot, 127, 128–129
TFC. *See* Triangular fibrocartilage complex (wrist)
Thalamoperforating artery(ies), 29, 30*f*
Thalassemia
  bone marrow in, 105, 202
  extramedullary hematopoiesis in, 105
Thecoma(s), ovarian, 162
Thoracic neoplasia, 132–133, 133*f*
Thoracic outlet tumor(s), 132
Thoracic spine
  arachnoid cyst, 80*f*, 81
  astrocytomas, 74
  canal compromise, 80–81, 80*f*, 81*f*
  compression (burst) fractures, 61, 61*f*, 80, 80*f*
    with malignancy, 80
    osteoporotic, 80
  disk herniations, 77–79, 77*f*–79*f*
  epidural lipomatosis, 98
  hemangioblastoma, 74
  metastatic disease in, 80, 80*f*
    blastic, 81, 81*f*
    lytic, 81
  multiple myeloma and, 81, 81*f*
  in multiple sclerosis, 70
  neoplasms, 82–83, 83*f*
  osteophytes, 77, 78*f*
  paraspinal mass, 105
  vascular abnormalities, 84–85, 84*f*, 85*f*
Thrombus, intracardiac, 132
Thymoma(s), 132, 133*f*
Thymus gland, tumors, 132
Thyroglossal duct, 117
Thyroid gland, tumors, 132
Thyroiditis, 121
Tibialis anterior tears, 195, 195*f*
Tibialis posterior tears, 194
Tibiocalcaneal ligament, 196–197
Tibionavicular ligament, 196–197
Tibiotalar ligaments, 197
TMJ. *See* Temporomandibular joint
Torcular herophili, abnormalities, with Dandy-Walker malformation, 47
Tornwaldt cysts, 114–115, 115*f*
Toxoplasmosis
  CNS manifestations, 44–45, 45*f*
  neonatal, 45
Tracheobronchial cyst, 133
Transposition of the great arteries, 128–129
  dextro, 128–129
  levo, 129, 129*f*
Transverse myelitis, 71
Trauma, cervical spine, 60–61, 60*f*–61*f*
Triangular fibrocartilage complex (wrist), 186
  defects, Palmer classification, 186–187, 186*f*
  degenerative tears, 187, 187*f*
  injury, 186–187, 186*f*, 187*f*
    associated lesions, 187
Tricuspid valve
  area, 126
  regurgitation, 123, 123*f*
Tuberculosis, adrenal involvement, 147
Tuberous sclerosis, 56–57, 56*f*
Turf toe, 195

U

Ulnar collateral ligament(s), 192, 192*f*
  tears, 193, 193*f*
Uncovertebral joint, 64
Urinary bladder. *See* Bladder
Urticaria, contrast agent–induced, 206
Uterine cancer, 160–161, 160*f*
  cerebral metastases, 6
Uterus
  adenomyoma, 159, 159*f*
  arcuate, 157–158, 158*f*
  bicornuate, 157, 158*f*
  didelphys, 157, 158*f*
  focal adenomyosis, 159
  leiomyoma, 158–159, 159*f*
  septate, 157
  T-shaped, in utero DES exposure and, 158
  unicornuate, 157

V

Vagal reaction, contrast agent–induced, 206
Valvular heart disease, 126–127, 127*f*
Vascular malformations. *See also* Arteriovenous malformation(s)
  in brain, 22–23, 22*f*, 23*f*
  spinal, 84–85, 84*f*, 85*f*
Vasculitis, 211
  brain in, 34–35, 36
Vein of Galen aneurysm, 21
Venous angioma(s), in brain, 23, 23*f*
Venous sinus, meningioma in, 9, 9*f*
Venous thrombosis, 219
  in brain, 40–41, 41*f*
Ventricle(s), cerebral, fourth, enlargement, with Dandy-Walker malformation, 47
Ventricular noncompaction, 123
Ventricular septal defect, 128, 129*f*
Vertebrae, wedge-shaped, in cervical spine, 59, 59*f*
Vertebral artery
  dissection, 210–211
  evaluation, in trauma patient, 61
Vertebral body fractures, benign *versus* malignant, 91
Vertebral fusion, 59
  with Chiari malformation, 46
Vertebrobasilar arterial system, 29
VHL. *See* von Hippel-Lindau disease
VIBE. *See* Volume-interpolated breath-hold examination; Volumetric interpolated breath-hold examination
VISI. *See* Volar intercalated segment instability (wrist)
Vitamin B_{12}, deficiency, cervical spine in, 71, 71*f*
Volar intercalated segment instability (wrist), 185
Volume averaging, 69
Volume-interpolated breath-hold examination, 79
Volumetric interpolated breath-hold examination, 138
von Hippel-Lindau disease, 5, 55, 108
von Recklinghausen disease. *See* Neurofibromatosis
VSD. *See* Ventricular septal defect

W

Wallenberg syndrome, 29–30
Wallerian (anterograde) degeneration, 27, 27*f*
  in multiple sclerosis, 36
Warthin tumor, 118
Watershed areas, 31
  parieto-occipital, injury, 31
Wegener's granulomatosis, sinusitis with, 120–121
Wernicke encephalopathy, 34, 35*f*
Wilson disease, 142
Wrist
  dorsal intercalated segment instability, 184–185, 189
  fractures, 184–185, 185*f*, 187, 188–189, 188*f*
    nonunion, 188–189, 188*f*
  ganglion cyst in, 189, 189*f*
  giant cell tumor of tendon sheath in, 189
  imaging technique for, 184
  osteoarthritis, 189
  pain, causes, 187, 188–189, 188*f*, 189*f*
  rheumatoid arthritis in, 189
  sarcoma, 189
  triangular fibrocartilage complex, 186
    defects, Palmer classification, 186–187, 186*f*
    degenerative tears, 187, 187*f*
    injury, 186–187, 186*f*, 187*f*
      associated lesions, 187
  volar intercalated segment instability, 185
Wyburn-Mason syndrome, 20